Aural Rehabilitation

DEREK A. SANDERS

State University of New York at Buffalo
Buffalo, New York

PRENTICE-HALL, INC.   Englewood Cliffs, New Jersey

13-053223-1
Library of Congress Catalogue Card No.: 70-134920
Printed in the United States of America
Current printing (last digit):

15

PRENTICE-HALL INTERNATIONAL, INC., *London*
PRENTICE-HALL OF AUSTRALIA, PTY., LTD., *Sydney*
PRENTICE-HALL OF CANADA, LTD., *Toronto*
PRENTICE-HALL OF JAPAN, INC., *Tokyo*
PRENTICE-HALL OF INDIA PRIVATE LIMITED, *New Delhi*

Introduction

The purpose of this book is to examine aural rehabilitation as a process rather than as a procedure. Its concern is to provide you with a knowledge of the basic factors involved in interpersonal communication, and with insight into the impact which a hearing impairment may have upon the individual.

The text develops, step by step, a theoretical framework within which to examine the nature of the communication problems arising from impaired hearing, and to help the reader to understand the principles underlying several approaches to rehabilitation.

This book is not intended to settle conclusively the major controversies relating to aural rehabilitation. On the contrary I hope that, through examination of theoretical concepts and research from other disciplines, it will help to present a new approach to these various issues.

The success of the text should be measured in terms of the degree to which it stimulates you to seek a better understanding of the task which confronts you. It is hoped that the ideas contained in this book will prove to be sufficiently challenging as to foster the growth of new approaches to aural rehabilitation, and that it will contribute to the effectiveness of our efforts to enrich the lives of the child or adult with impaired hearing.

Although the ideas presented in this book represent my personal bias at the time it was written, its completion leaves me indebted to many people. I first wish to acknowledge the influence of Dr. Louis M. DiCarlo and Sir Alexander Ewing, who were responsible for my graduate training. To Stuart Horton of Prentice-Hall, Inc. I owe my appreciation for nurturing the original idea and for his encouragement during its development. I wish to express my thanks to my students who read and criticized the early drafts of each chapter, and to Mary Moore who in addition to doing all the typing, kept track of all the figures and references which seemed predestined to get lost. To my colleague Robert McGlone I owe most of the credit for Chapter 3 and my thanks for his never-failing confidence that I could complete the manuscript. Among the other people influential in the writing of the book, I wish to thank Ruth Holden and Bob Briskey for their advice in the chapter on amplification and hearing aids, and the various manufacturers who contributed photographic material.

To my wife Cynthia, and to my daughters Jennifer and Hilary I am grateful for the patience, understanding and moral support that contributed so much to my achievement of the goals I set.

Buffalo, New York   Derek A. Sanders

Contents

vii

CHAPTER ONE

A General Consideration of Aural Rehabilitation

The problems encountered by individuals suffering from impaired hearing are many and varied. A hearing loss may result in difficulties in emotional and social behavior, in educational progress, or in vocational placement. However, at the core of these problems rests a breakdown in the process of communication. Human communication involves a process by which we evoke in others the thoughts and ideas that we ourselves have. We achieve this by use of a system of symbols that permits us to put a message into a common code that may be transmitted from one person to another. A system of signs or symbols, including the rules that govern the way in which they may be used, is known as a language. The process of using a language to cause another individual to be aware of your own thoughts is known as communication. Language is commonly thought of as being synonymous with speech—that is to say, only oral in nature. However, though speech constitutes the predominate method by which thoughts are made known to others, ideas can be, and are, evoked in other ways.

The development and use of speech as the major component of human communication is primarily dependent upon the possession of normal hearing by the individual. Normal hearing is necessary because speech signals are transmitted in the form of sound waves that can only be received by the listener via the auditory pathway. The nerve impulses that the acoustic signals trigger in the organ of hearing travel by way of the sensory nerves to the appropriate part of the nervous system. Simultaneously, additional information may be received by the listener through other sense receptors, such as those of vision, taste, touch, and smell. The complex signals used in communication then require analysis and interpretation at higher levels of the nervous system, a process involving the integration of the various sensory data into a meaningful whole. In doing this, the listener depends upon his perception of the immediate situation, his memory of previous related situations, and a familiarity with the various aspects of the code or language used. Therefore, in considering the problems arising from auditory impairment, it is essential to direct attention to this total process of communication. An understanding of the nature of the communication breakdown that may result from a hearing loss is made easier if conceived in reference to the components and function of a normal system. The techniques by which the teacher or therapist may attempt to circumvent or compensate for the deficiencies within the system may then be developed within this framework.

THE NORMAL COMMUNICATION SYSTEM

When we consider the process by which we are able to make our thoughts known to others, it is apparent that there are a number of distinct stages. After careful observation of normal communication behavior, it is possible for us to develop a theory concerning how the system functions. Several theories have been suggested, each of which may be illustrated by the use of models.* A communication model constitutes a schematic representation of the stages and functions that a particular theory suggests are involved in human communication. It is theoretically constructed since we have virtually no concrete evidence of what actually occurs within the individual. The theory can be developed only on the basis of a careful comparison of observed changes in behavior associated with a specific stimulus presented to the listener. It generally results from a consolidation of experimental and empirical data supported by philosophical reasoning. Although the model may prove to be an imperfect representation of what actually happens, it provides us with a valuable basis for our approach to rehabilitation. A model of communication will be developed together with an explanation of its relevance to the philosophy of aural rehabilitation proposed in this book.

*For more specific discussion of the term "model" the reader is referred to Irwin D. J. Bross, "Models," *Dimensions in Communication,* ed. J. H. Campbell and H. W. Hepler (Belmont, Calif.: Wadsworth Publishing Co., Inc., 1965), Sec. 1, pp. 10–26.

THE ACOUSTIC AND VISUAL COMPONENTS OF SPEECH

The utilization of a model in our attempt to understand the communication breakdown occurring as a result of a hearing loss necessitates familiarity with the components of the speech stimulus, since these will be embodied in the model. The hard-of-hearing individual experiences communication difficulty because the speech of others appears to him to be distorted. This occurs because the perception of speech or other sound stimuli is dependent upon the ability of the auditory mechanism to receive and analyze accurately the various physical characteristics of the acoustic stimulus.

Speech is comprised of complex sound waves that are constantly changing. Each of these wave forms can be reduced to a number of fundamental components, the most important of which are frequency, intensity, and duration. The relationship between these components gives the sound wave the particular quality that permits a listener to differentiate it from other sound waves. Any factor, such as hearing impairment, that results in the unintentional distortion of the wave form imposes a limitation upon its effectiveness as a vehicle for the transmission of the message. We shall attempt to assess the distortion that might be expected to occur as a result of different patterns of hearing loss by comparing the frequency components of particular speech sounds with the audiogram. It is hoped that this will result in a better understanding of the reason for the auditory-discrimination errors that may occur with different patterns of loss. This information may then be integrated with the results obtained from clinical tests of speech discrimination, and a program of auditory training planned accordingly.

It has already been pointed out that, in addition to the information transmitted in the form of sound waves received by the auditory mechanism, relevant information may be received through the other senses. Vision plays the major role as a supporting pathway. Many cues are derived from observation of the setting in which a speaker is talking and from the speaker's manner of dress, posture, bodily movements, gestures, and facial expressions. These observations help us to predict and evaluate the spoken message. More specific information about the spoken message is obtained from observations of the speaker's lips. The production of the speech sounds involves the movement of the organs of articulation, which are, to varying degrees, visible to the listener. Since they are directly related to the production of the auditory signal, they provide additional information concerning the nature of the message. However, the total information value is reduced by a number of factors. The articulation of speech involves movements that occur too rapidly for them all to be perceived. Furthermore, many of the movements associated with the production of speech sounds are partially or completely concealed within the mouth, while others are either identical or so similar in appearance as to make visual discrimination impossible. These limitations lie both in the nature of the signal transmitted and in the sensitivity of the receiver. If the visual pathway is to be utilized in a compensatory manner in a program of visual communication, then the therapist must be familiar with its function and limitations.

EVALUATION OF THE PROBLEM

Once the student has a fundamental understanding of the essential elements of normal oral communication, it is possible to discuss the evaluation of the communication difficulties of the hard-of-hearing person.

The first factor that it will be necessary to consider is the nature and effect of the distortion of the acoustic signal. In view of what has been said about the acoustic structure of speech sounds, it will be realized that an initial appreciation of frequency distortion can be obtained by the examination of pure-tone audiometric thresholds. From these we gain some insight into which sounds will probably be inaudible to the subject and those that may be expected to suffer distortion due to the inability of the listener to hear some of their components. The audiogram also provides us with information regarding how well the subject will be able to hear speech at various intensity levels. From this we can make some predictions concerning the type of speech situations that one may expect to present difficulty. In addition to the pure-tone data, we shall also discuss the significance of speech audiometric results obtained for different types of speech samples administered under various listening conditions.

It has been suggested [9, p. 5; 10, p. 165] and to some extent demonstrated [11] that, as the information obtained through one channel decreases, the dependence upon alternative channels as sources of information becomes more important. We may observe this in the greater awareness of auditory stimuli shown by a blind person and the greater dependency upon visual cues seen in the deaf person. We shall therefore wish to consider how well the subject is able to compensate for the auditory defect by the utilization of the visual pathway as an additional source of information. For this reason, it will be necessary to make an independent assessment of the contribution to the comprehension of a message made by these two major pathways. We shall, further, need to consider the effect upon communication of such psychological influences as attention, emotional tension, self-confidence, and motivation. While these may not directly affect the signal received, they play a vital role in determining whether the listener will be able to analyze and synthesize the raw data. The ability of the subject to follow rapid shifts in the nature of the message, to avoid perseverative thinking, and to make logical inferences may determine the ultimate success achieved by the subject operating on reduced cues.

Having completed the assessment of the communication problem, the therapist is faced with the task of integrating the information obtained from the case-history report, the audiological evaluation, and the results of specific tests generally alluded to above. The case report should present the therapist's assessment of the relative importance and significance of the information available. From this assessment, an outline of a program of rehabilitation may be developed that takes into account as many of the variables as possible.

AN APPROACH TO REHABILITATION

Throughout our discussion, the problem of the hearing-impaired individual will be approached from the standpoint of communicative ability. The advantage of this approach is that it provides a theoretical framework for a program of rehabilitation that is as valid for subjects with mild-to-moderate hearing losses as it is for subjects with severe impairment. The aim of the evaluation of the person's communicative abilities is to establish a model for the system being used and to assess the areas of relative strengths and weaknesses within the system. The rehabilitation program will be designed to strengthen areas of weakness through specialized training whenever possible or to circumvent the weakness through the development of the use of conpensatory channels.

A person with a mild-to-moderate impairment of hearing will still depend primarily upon the auditory signal as the major source of information. It is possible that this person's problem may be almost eliminated by the use of a hearing aid. This may increase the amount of information that he can deduce from the acoustic signal to the point where the residual distortion of signal amplitude and frequency pattern is insufficient to impair the adequate comprehension of the message. If, however, the auditory pathway is more seriously impaired, amplification may fail to reduce signal distortion enough to permit understanding. In cases of profound deafness, the improvement of auditory function that results from amplification is often so slight that very little additional information is received through this pathway. However, the nature of our approach to the rehabilitation of the hearing-impaired subject emphasizes that the degree of auditory impairment does not change the structure of the remedial program. Our concern with each case is the development of the maximum possible communication ability. It is only the *relative emphasis* that will be placed on the auditory and visual aspects of training that will vary.

In considering these two aspects of the training program, it is customary to discuss them separately. This serves the purpose of facilitating the instruction of student teachers and therapists in the underlying principles and techniques of each procedure. To some extent it is necessary and valuable to separate the two in a program of rehabilitation. We must, however, constantly bear in mind that maximum communication for the hard-of-hearing individual occurs when the auditory and visual pathways act in an integrative manner. Consequently, after separate discussions of auditory training and visual communication training, we shall attempt to draw the two together.

Auditory Training and Hearing Aids

Since oral communication utilizes the auditory pathway, it is reasonable to direct our initial efforts in rehabilitation toward the maximum use of residual hearing through auditory training. Before it was possible to make sound louder by electrical means, the value of auditory training as a remedial technique was severely limited. The remarkable advancements that have been made in the design and efficiency of amplifying units have resulted in a far greater potential for the use of residual hearing. The availability of a variety of amplifying units, commonly referred to as hearing aids or auditory training units, makes it possible to compensate to varying degrees for the loss of signal intensity and to a lesser extent for the frequency distortion. In consequence, a basic change is called for in the rehabilitation approach, shifting the emphasis from a visual to a combined auditory-visual training program. Courses entitled "Lipreading and Auditory Training" frequently fail to include an adequate consideration of the use of amplification in the rehabilitation program for the hard-of-hearing. Evaluating the current status of auditory training from an even broader viewpoint, J. J. O'Neil and H. J. Oyer [8, p. 70] express the opinion that this whole area is neglected by the therapist. They suggest that even in audiology clinics it is given only moderate attention. It is believed that the cause of this neglect lies primarily in the therapist's unfamiliarity with the principles and procedures of auditory training and appropriate equipment. No therapist or teacher can hope to develop optimum use of residual hearing in a subject without a thorough understanding of various types of amplifying units and the advantages and limitations of such units. Although the more technical aspects of amplifying units constitute a topic more applicable in an advanced course on hearing aids, a familiarity with the manner in which the audiologist evaluates the benefit provided is considered to be appropriate to the teacher of the hearing-impaired.

It is not uncommon for a child or adult to acquire and use a hearing aid without any form of counseling. This, together with inadequate evaluation procedures, probably constitutes the major reason why many subjects who acquire an aid fail to adjust to it favorably [4, p. 61]. Counseling may well be the responsibility of the therapist or teacher who must be able to offer intelligent and informed advice.

The provision of amplification generally makes audible sounds that were previously below the subject's threshold of hearing or that were so soft that they were not useful to him in the communication process. For very young children with congenital deafness, the sounds that become audible will be heard for the first time. The child will not only need to listen to and become familiar with environmental sounds, including those of speech, but he will also have to acquire an auditory memory for these sounds and learn to associate them with their sources. This is essential if the child is to associate meaning with the sounds he hears. The therapist is concerned with teaching these children to listen to sounds and to realize that the auditory stimulus serves as a reference to objects or events. In addition, the child with a significant impairment of hearing will frequently show retardation in the development of linguistic skills. Any program designed to develop visual and auditory communication in young children with a moderate or severe hearing loss must, therefore, be part of a more comprehensive program of language development. Thus, in considering the methods used in working with young children, we shall include the role language training must play in an integrated program of speech reading, auditory training, and language development.

When the onset of the hearing impairment occurs after the acquisition of speech, the nature of the communication problem is noticeably different. In this event, the child or adult is already aware of the referential nature of the auditory stimulus and has built up an extensive auditory memory, which makes sound differentiation of most stimuli automatic. Furthermore, the person with acquired deafness has become familiar with the rules of his language and can, as a result, deduce more information from limited cues than the person who lacks this familiarity. The result of the hearing loss is to distort the auditory pattern of sounds with which he has already become familiar. Because of this distortion, he will experience various degrees of difficulty in identifying the referent by its acoustic symbol. The auditory training program in this situation is, therefore, primarily concerned with a relearning process designed to help the pupil to match the now-distorted auditory signals he receives with the auditory memory patterns that he established before the onset of deafness. The subject has already acquired listening habits. He is motivated in the relearning situation by the fact that, prior to the onset of deafness, his system of communication had been structured around the analysis of auditory signals. The success of an auditory training program with such an individual will depend on the extent to which we are able to train him to differentiate among the distorted patterns that he is now receiving.

The problem may be further complicated by the psychological change that may be expected in an individual who is suddenly cut off from the world of sound or for whom the sounds being received have to a great extent lost their value as carriers of information. As in the case of the congenitally deaf child, the training program should be organized in progressive steps involving the reidentification of gross sounds in the environment, the identification of simple speech materials, and finally the identification and differentiation of isolated speech sounds and sound combinations with which the student has particular difficulty.

Training in Visual Communication

As previously mentioned, it is possible that some cases will require only a program of counseling in the use of the hearing aid, together with a relatively short program of listening training. In cases involving a moderate-to-severe degree of hearing loss it is unlikely that amplification, even with a program of auditory training, can completely compensate for the reduction in information received. A reevaluation of the amount of information that may be received through the auditory channel after a period of training will indicate the extent to which the subject will need to develop use of the visual pathway as a supplementary source. It is true, as we shall see later, that speech can be coded in such a way that it may be received through the sense of touch. This sensory pathway is, in fact, a valuable one in the training of the deaf-blind child. However, with the child who has normal vision, far more meaning can be derived from the observation of the articulatory movements of the speech organs, of facial expressions, of posture and gestural movements of the speaker, and from the observation of other events occurring in the environment at the time of transmission of the message by the speaker. It is for this reason that we turn to vision as the supporting sensory pathway when hearing proves inadequate.

It has been traditional in the past to use the terms "lipreading" or "speech reading" to refer to the training program designed to develop in the hard-of-hearing individual the ability to utilize the visual channel as a means of obtaining information. These terms have been criticized by many authors because of the fact that they tend to concentrate our attention only upon those visual cues that are directly associated with the articulatory movements involved in the production of speech sounds. In doing this, we tend to ignore the amount of information that may be deduced from a careful observation of other events that may be connected with the message being transmitted. A number of writers have suggested other terms in attempts to overcome this limitation. For example, M. K. Mason [6] uses the term "visual hearing" to encompass both the recognition of articulatory movements and the role of the mind in correlating the other relevant data received through the eyes. Oyer and O'Neil [8, p. 70] suggest that the term "visual listening" might provide a helpful orientation to this particular process of obtaining information. They suggest that, as in listening, the ability to attend and interpret the visual stimulus is a learned form of behavior. In both cases the subject has a mental set that directs his attention toward the comprehension of the message rather than the simple recognition of its components. In spite of this suggestion, the term that O'Neil and Oyer select to use in the title of their book is "visual communication."

The author believes that the term "visual communication" is the most useful of the terms that have yet been suggested, because the word "visual" specifies quite distinctly the channel involved, while the word "communication" implies the reception and comprehension of any symbolic representation of the idea that is being transmitted. For this reason, the term "visual communication" will be adhered to throughout the text when referring to any form of information pertinent to the encoded message that reaches the receiver by way of the visual pathway.

History of Visual Communication Training

It is customary in courses concerned with the teaching of visual communication to spend part of the course reviewing the historical development of the various methods of training the hard-of-hearing subject to utilize visual clues. It is the author's impression that the student is generally left rather puzzled as to why this section of the course is necessary, since it frequently bears little relation to the remainder of the material covered. It will, perhaps, be helpful to the student to realize that the early work in this area was oriented toward the needs of the deaf subject. Since amplification was not at that time available as a rehabilitative tool, most of those individuals whom we consider to be partially deaf were almost entirely dependent upon vision as the major channel for receiving information concerning the spoken message. The emphasis that began to be placed upon the oral method of communication as a substitute for manual communication systems gave added impetus to the development of programs of training in visual communication. Although as far back as the sixteenth and seventeenth century some writers were beginning to voice the opinon that it was possible for some deaf subjects to learn to be able to interpret spoken language [3], it was not until the early 1900s that widespread use of specific methods of teaching visual communication occurred.

The early pioneers of programs of training in visual communication were almost entirely connected with private schools for the education of deaf children. Many of them, in fact, founded their own schools to permit them to develop their particular techniques. In the thirteenth century, many of the teachers were anxious to confine the use of their techniques to their own school. As a result, very few of the specific methods that had been developed were published, thus limiting the general application of these principles. During the early part of the twentieth century, the methods established by such people as Martha Bruhn [1], Karl Braukmann (Jena method) [2], Cora Kinzie [5], and Edward B. Nitchie [7] began to be widely known. These specific methods, with subsequent development and modification, still constitute the major schools of visual communication training as taught today. The various schools may be generally classified as primarily analytical or synthetic in their approach to the problem. They are important to our present discussion of the problem of rehabilitation of the hard-of-hearing subject in that they provide us with examples and justifications for several approaches to the teaching of visual communication. Each of the various schools advocates a somewhat different approach and permits us to examine the advantages and disadvantages of the components of each of the particular methods. Our ultimate goal is to develop an eclectic approach to visual communication that will incorporate the advantages of each of the schools that we shall discuss. If, after careful consideration of a particular school of lipreading, the student feels that the methods advocated by this school can be successfully utilized in their entirety, then there is no reason why the student should not adopt these particular methods. Since the processes of which we are speaking are constantly being submitted to experimental research, it is believed that the student will find it necessary to modify the established schools in order to permit him to incorporate some of the more recent knowledge concerning the processes under discussion. Furthermore, it will be observed that most of the lesson programs advocated by the schools that have been mentioned are geared toward the older subject who has already acquired normal language before the advent of the hearing problem. We shall be equally concerned with meeting the needs of the hard-of-hearing child, who in many instances may be expected to have associated retarded language development. We shall attempt, therefore, to develop certain general principles to be considered when planning rehabilitation for a child or adult in need of training in the area of visual communication. We shall also provide examples of the particular ways in which these principles may be utilized in the development of lesson plans. Illustrative lessons, appropriate to various age groups and designed to develop specific abilities, will be presented.

The student is finally concerned with the problem of integrating the techniques advocated in the development of both visual and auditory communication. With the exception of the chapter "Lip Reading, Auditory Training, and Hearing Aids" in O'Neil and Oyer's book, little specific attention has been given to the correlation of the two remedial techniques. We shall therefore be concerned with bringing these two techniques together in such a way that the teacher or therapist concerned with aural rehabilitation will find it easy to move naturally from the utilization of one channel to the other within the same lesson plan. At the same time, we should be well versed in the techniques that may be used in developing the use of each specific channel separately in individual lessons devised for this purpose. Examples of such lessons will be presented.

Other Aspects of the Rehabilitation Program

To suggest that the rehabilitation of the hearing-impaired child is concerned only with the development of the use of residual hearing and the use of compensatory visual information is to underestimate the problem gravely. The therapist or teacher must concern himself with the suitability of the school placement of the child, a subject that should constantly come up for review, and the need for counseling of parents and the classroom teacher in how the child's needs may best be met at home and at school. The need for speech and language therapy for a child who may be indicating problems in both of these areas may arise, and one must not neglect the consideration of the emotional problems that may present themselves as patterns of behavior that have become integrated into the child's personality, or that may arise from time to time as a result of a change in some aspect of the child's environment, such as progression to a higher grade level. Often the therapist or teacher is the only person who is in frequent contact with the child and who is able to pull together the various reports that have been obtained on the child. Speech and hearing specialists, psychologists, and educational counselors in universities and clinics are frequently not in a position to accept the responsibility for providing an ongoing supervisory service to the child with a hearing problem. The teacher or therapist should therefore check to see who has assumed such a role. If it proves that no person is responsible for integrating the available information and for arranging a periodic reappraisal of the child's total needs, then the therapist may feel morally responsible to undertake this task. A discussion of the role of the therapist and teacher in this respect will conclude our consideration of the basic features of a sound rehabilitation program for the hearing-impaired.

REFERENCES

1. Bruhn, Martha E. *The Mueller-Waller Method of Lipreading for the Hard of Hearing*. Washington, D.C.: The Volta Bureau, 1949.

2. Bunger, A. *Speech Reading Jena Method*. Danville, Ill.: The Interstate Press, 1961.

3. DeLand, F. *The Story of Lipreading*. Washington, D.C.: The Volta Bureau, 1931.

4. Johnson, J. C. *Educating Hearing-Impaired Children in Ordinary Schools.* Washington, D.C.: The Volta Bureau, 1962.

5. Kinzie, Cora E., and Rose Kinzie. *Lip-Reading for the Deafened Adult.* Chicago: The John Winston Co., 1931.

6. Mason, M. K. "A Cinematic Technique for Testing Visual Speech Comprehension." *Journal of Speech Disorders* 8 (1943): 271–78.

7. Nitchie, Edward B. *Lip Reading: Principles and Practice.* New York: Frederick A. Stokes Company, 1912.

8. O'Neil, J. J., and H. J. Oyer. *Visual Communication for the Hard of Hearing.* Englewood Cliffs, N.J.: Prentice-Hall, Inc., 1961.

9. Ruesch, J., and W. Kees. *Nonverbal Communication.* Berkeley and Los Angeles, Calif.: University of California Press, 1956.

10. Streng, A., et al. *Hearing Therapy for Children.* New York: Grune & Stratton, Inc., 1958.

11. Sumby, W. H., and I. Pollack. "Visual Contribution to Speech Intelligibility in Noise." *Journal of the Acoustical Society of America* 26 (1954): 212–15.

CHAPTER TWO

The Human Communication System

In the opening paragraph of Chap. 1 it was suggested that human communication involves the exchange of information about our thoughts and ideas. Since thoughts and ideas do not exist in physical form, they cannot be directly exchanged. It is therefore necessary to embody the information about these thoughts in some physical form that can be passed between individuals. The embodiment of the idea or message is the message signal. We may therefore consider communication to be the process of reproducing at point B a message signal that originates at point A.

A network must exist to carry the message signal. The units that comprise the network may be considered its components; the particular arrangement and interaction between the components within the network constitutes a system. A system is, then, any group of components organized in a particular manner to serve a specific function. This chapter suggests a model of the human communication system, together with a possible explanation of how it may function.

A COMMUNICATION MODEL

Figure 2.1 illustrates what are considered the essential components of a communication system.

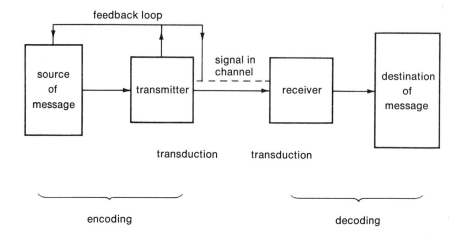

Fig. 2.1. Simplified version of the basic components of communication
through speech.

1. *Source:* The source is the originator of the information or message that
   is to be fed into the system. In speech this is the cortex.
2. *Message:* The message constitutes any form of information that may be
   conveyed by meaningful behavior. Passage through the system is made
   possible by encoding the message into some form of conventional symbols, at which point we may consider the message to exist in the form
   of a message signal.
3. *Message signal:* The message signal constitutes the encoded message put
   into a form appropriate to the particular channel through which it is to
   travel. In speech communication the message signal travels from the
   source (cortex) to the transmitter (speech organs) in the form of electrical
   nerve impulses; the energy is then converted into sound waves. On
   reaching the ear of the listener, the energy is converted into mechanical
   movement of the middle ear and finally back into nerve impulses by the
   inner-ear mechanism.
4. *Transmitter:* A transmitter is a device that projects the message signal
   from its source into another medium. In speech, the vocal folds serve to
   change the message signal existing as nerve impulses into the molecular
   movement of air particles that constitutes sound waves.
5. *Channel:* The channel is the pathway or medium through which the
   message signal travels, both within the individual (neurological) and in
   the external environment (physical). In human communication, the auditory, visual, and tactile channels are most frequently used.

6. *Receiver:* A receiver is a device capable of picking up the message signal. In man the sensory end organs serve as receivers.
7. *Destination:* The destination is the message signal terminal. In man this is the appropriate areas of the cortex where the message signal, which has been partially analyzed at various subcortical nerve centers, is finally interpreted.
8. *Feedback loop:* A feedback loop is a monitoring system that permits the maintenance of a desired quality of production by making possible the constant comparison of the output with a predetermined internal standard.

Figure 2.2 illustrates the application of the communication model to the essential components of a human communication system, utilizing only the spoken word as a means of conveying information. Subject A has a thought or idea that he wishes to communicate to a friend, subject B. This thought, which constitutes the message, must be encoded into some symbolic form before it can be communicated. In fact, for most of us it is probably only when we put the idea into words, either aloud or in silent thinking, that we are able to formulate the thought clearly. This process takes place in the brain, where the message is converted into a message signal in the form

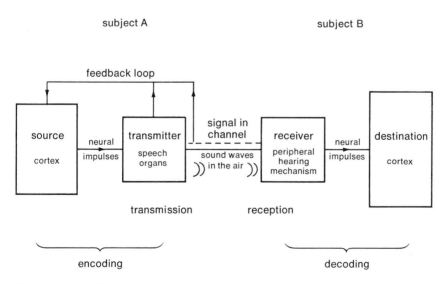

Fig. 2.2.   Simplified version of the basic components of communiction through speech.

of language symbols represented by nerve impulses. These impulses activate the vocal mechanism and the articulators of speech, which change the neural message signal into complex sound waves.

Subject B, who at this stage in the conversation is playing the role of the listener, receives the message signal through his hearing mechanism, which converts the sound waves back into nerve impulses. These travel by way of a series of subcortical nerve centers to the auditory cortex, where they are analyzed and interpreted, providing subject B with the meaning content.

Quality Control

If we wish to be certain that a production unit maintains a particular standard of operation, then it is necessary to devise a means of assessing and controlling the quality of the product. This is necessary in the production of speech as it is in the production of automobiles. To make this quality control possible, we must feed back into the system information concerning its output. The system must have incorporated within it a means of detecting any errors that occur in the message signal that it is transmitting, and it must also have the ability to make the appropriate corrections. An error is said to occur whenever a discrepancy exists between the generated message signal and an internal standard against which the output signal may be compared. This comparison will reveal any discrepancy that may exist between the intended and actual message signal, permitting immediate corrective action to be taken to eliminate the error. Such self-regulating mechanisms are commonly referred to as *servo-mechanisms* or *servo-systems*.

A much used, but simple illustration of such a system is that which automatically regulates the heat in a house (Fig. 2.3). The "message signal" being conveyed is heat, generated by the boiler (source), transmitted into the air by a radiator or warm-air ducts. Feedback of information concerning the air temperature in the room is made possible by a thermostat, which we set at a desired temperature. This temperature represents the internal standard of the system. Whenever the output of heat from the boiler causes the heat in the room to rise above the prescribed temperature, the sensing mechanism of the thermostat, detecting the discrepancy (error) between the actual and the desired temperature, operates to turn down the boiler. When the temperature falls below the required level, the thermostat will cause the heat to be turned on again.

Feedback must be considered an integral part of the communication system itself; without it effective communication is impossible. It is of particular importance to an understanding of the communication problems resulting from impairment of hearing, since these problems result primarily from an impairment of the feedback process. We shall, for this reason,

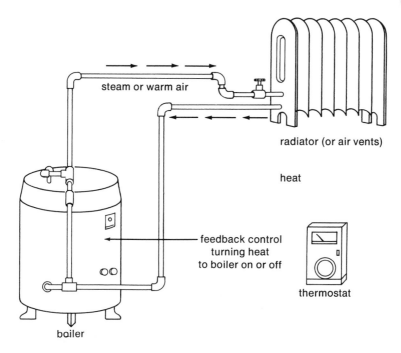

Fig. 2.3. A common servo-mechanism (boiler and radiator).

consider it in rather more detail than is usual in an introductory chapter on communication.

The continual monitoring of the message signal (speech sound, written symbols, gestures, etc.) is necessary to insure the greatest possible accuracy of the message. G. Fairbanks [3] has proposed a model (Fig. 2.4) that is helpful in understanding the internal feedback mechanism by which we control the quality of our speech production. The system is divided into two linked units, one concerned with converting the neural message signal into speech sounds (effector unit), the other (sensor unit) concerned with feeding a copy of the output back to a control unit which modifies future signals.

A message signal originates within the language system in the cortex. It first passes through a storage component (1)* that is capable of storing for a short period of time a copy of a few units of the message.† The message-signal then passes through a mixer (2) that provides the impulse needed to drive the effector unit (effective driving signal). The effector unit

---

*Numbers in parentheses refer to Fig. 2.4.

†Message units are the individual components from which the message is constructed. The smallest unit in speech is the phoneme; the largest unit, for the purpose of this discussion, will be considered to be the construction, as explained on page 26.

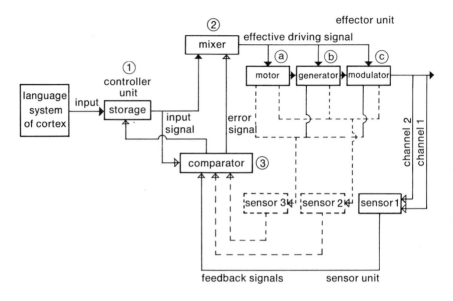

Fig. 2.4. Model of a closed-cycle control system for speaking proposed by Fairbanks [3].

consists of three divisions: (a) the motor, which corresponds to the breathing mechanism; (b) the generator, representing the vocal folds; (c) the modulator, which represents the articulators and resonators of the speech system.

The effector unit is responsible for transmitting the message signal into the external environment. Information concerning the behavior of the various components of the effector unit is carried by feedback pathways to associated sensor units. The first unit (sensor 1) represents the ear. Information concerning the output reaches it via two channels: channel 1 is the airborne route through the middle-ear structures, while channel 2 is the tissue and bone conduction route resulting from vibration of the skull and its tissues. The message signal received by sensor 1 travels directly to the comparator (3).

Information concerning the tactile and proprioceptive aspects of the message signal reaches the comparator by individual channels from sensors 2 and 3. Thus, the information arriving at the comparator consists of the total of all the available sensory data concerning the message signal being transmitted. A copy of the original message signal that was fed into the mixer unit also reaches the comparator from storage. In this way, the intended message signal and that which is actually being transmitted are brought together for comparison. Any difference between the two constitutes an error. An error-correction signal is immediately fed into the mixer, where it is combined with the driving signal in such a way as to modify the impulses to the effector unit. This is done so that future output more closely approximates the input signal. It will be seen from the diagram that the error signal travels from the comparator to the storage unit, where a modified input is established before the previous unit has been utilized by the effector unit. This is necessary, since the storage unit provides the input signals to both the mixer and the comparator.

Fairbanks stresses the importance of this final aspect of the system as a means of providing for the role of prediction of the system's output. He states:

> The essence of a speaking system, however, is control of the output, or prediction of the output's future. In this kind of system the significance of the data about the past is that they are used for prediction of the future.

Fairbanks' model is only concerned with an explanation of the manner in which the output of the spoken word is monitored by the speaker. This internal monitoring is referred to by J. V. Irwin and C. Van Riper [10, p. 113] as an intrapersonal communicative circuit. An understanding of the total communicative process necessitates that we expand this model to include the monitoring of other forms of symbolic output, such as those transmitted by the hands, face, and other body parts.

Figure 2.5 illustrates a model that includes the monitoring of communication through such means as writing, gesturing, facial expressions, and bodily movement. The message is encoded into a particular symbolic form and travels as neural impulses to an error-detection and control unit. At this point, a copy of the encoded message is stored while impulses travel to one or more of four transmitters. These transmitters represent the organs of speech production (T1), the hands and arms (T2), the face (T3), and other body parts (T4). At the transmitter, the encoded message is transduced into a signal. The nature of the signal will differ depending upon which transmitter is being used. Speech production involves the movement of the organs of speech, the laryngeal mechanism and the articulators. The hands and arms are used for such forms of communication as writing, signaling, or gesturing, while the facial muscles transmit the message through facial expressions and grimaces. Impulses to other body parts will be transmitted in a variety of body movements and postures, as is seen in the communication that takes place through the medium of dance or pantomime. Internal sensory feedback of tactile and proprioceptive information travels from each of the transmitters to the error-detection and control unit for comparison with the stored copy of the intended signal. External feedback of the acoustic signal travels by way of the hearing mechanism.

The signal leaving each of the transmitters will travel in one or more

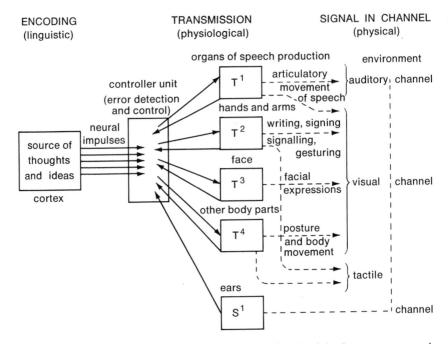

Fig. 2.5. Model of the transmission processes involved in human communication.

of three major channels. The speech signal travels as complex sound waves
through an acoustic channel. Simultaneously, the visible aspects of the
articulatory movements involved in speech production travel through a
visual channel in the form of light energy. Signals transmitted by hands and
arms, face, and other body parts also travel in the visual channel. The third
channel utilized in human communication is the tactile channel, through
which information may be transmitted as in a handshake or embrace, the
aggressive pounding on a rostrum, or by the tap of a foot on another foot
beneath a table.

So far, we have concerned ourselves only with intrapersonal feedback.
We must also take into consideration the influence exerted upon the speaker
by the reception of information concerning the effect of his message upon
the person to whom it is directed. This constitutes the interpersonal communicative circuit.

The information transmitted by subject A in the form of a message
signal has passed through the appropriate channels and has been received
and analyzed by subject B, for whom the message was intended. If the
message is satisfactorily decoded, subject B will give evidence of having
received the message by some form of change in his behavior. The nature

of this change will, in itself, be informative to subject A. Cues to the success with which the message is being received and decoded are, in fact, transmitted by the receiver even as the message is being received. The dichotomy of the communication situation into speaker and receiver is an artificial one. We really assume both roles simultaneously, though one may dominate at a given time. As I am speaking to a person I am also receiving information from him about his response to my message. This necessarily means that in his role of listener or receiver he is also sending information. Oral communication involves the constant and simultaneous interaction of people. The behavior elicited by the message may involve the use of a verbal reply, spoken or written, or it may take the form of a nonverbal vocalization, such as a gasp, sigh, or laugh. It may evoke a gesture, a facial grimace, or the adoption of a particular posture, or it may cause the subject to perform a particular task. The effectiveness of the signal carrying the encoded message is therefore evaluated on the basis of how well it brings about a desired response. The response made by subject B may reach subject A through his sensory end organs of hearing, vision, touch, and pressure. From the peripheral sensory receptors, the encoded message travels to the brain by way of a number of nerve centers situated enroute to the cortex. Thus, a variety of stimuli are reaching subject A concerning his own speech production and its effect upon his listener, subject B. In addition, subject A will receive other stimuli from the environment; these may be both related and unrelated to the message. All of this data must be sorted and that which is relevant must be integrated into a meaningful whole, a function that also involves the incorporation of information based on associations drawn from a memory of relevant past experiences. The final result of this process is total perception.

It has been generally held that the process of synthesizing sensory data in order to provide a total perception of a situation takes place only at the association level of the cortex. Research evidence is, however, available which suggests that the specialized sensory pathways are, in fact, neurologically related at levels below the cortex. The concept of the nervous system as comprised of a number of separate circuits, each responsible for a particular function, has been increasingly challenged by research evidence [7]. It may, however, reasonably be presumed that there exists a complex system involving reception, integration, analysis, association, and interpretation of data from all sensory end organs. Thus, Fig. 2.6 indicates by dotted lines the existence of interconnecting fibers traveling between the various subcortical nerve centers.

The information that is derived from this process of total perception of the effect upon B of the signal that was originally transmitted by A is then utilized by Subject A to modify his future output. The model suggested in Fig. 2.7 depicts the total process involved in the act of communication

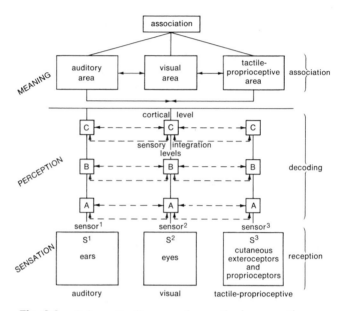

Fig. 2.6. Schematic diagram of synesthesic perception.

between two individuals. Although at first glance this diagram may appear overwhelming, closed examination will reveal that, in fact, it contains nothing that has not been previously discussed. The diagram simply puts together the information contained in Figs. 2.5 and 2.6. It represents two people in a communication situation, each with a transmitting and a receiving system serving the language system.

INFORMATION*

The purpose of the human communication system is to provide us with a means of informing others about our thoughts and ideas and to make it possible for us to be aware of their thoughts. We recognize that we are unable actually to pass the thought from one person to another. What we

*The term "information" was first applied to this concept by two mathematicians, C. E. Shannon and W. Weaver who, in a series of publications commencing in 1948, developed a theory of communication orientated to such communication systems as the telephone, television, and radar.

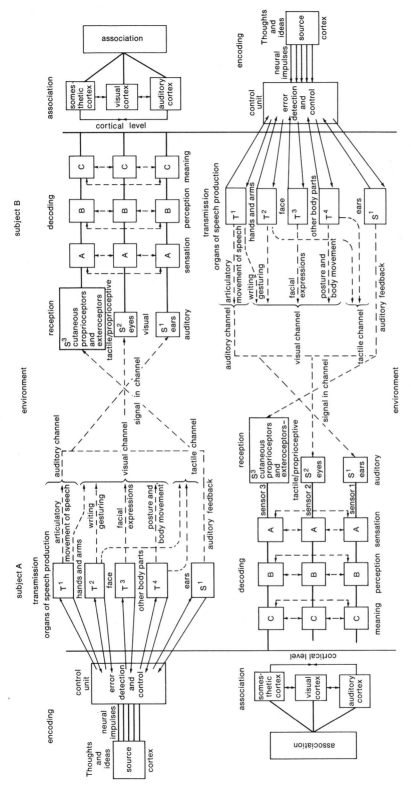

Fig. 2.7. The communication cycle.

attempt to do is to make it possible for the other person to reconstruct for himself as exact a replica of our thoughts as possible. In order to bring this about, we transmit to our listener a series of coded physical stimuli by various channels. These stimuli do not, in fact, represent an embodiment of the message itself, but rather, they are a set of coded instructions that direct the listener in his attempt to reconstruct the message.

Imagine, for example, that I wish to convey a secret message to you. We may agree to do this by means of the words contained in this book. Since we both have a copy before us, I can send you a set of directions concerning the page, line, and word number that will make it possible for you to select the words I have chosen to express my thought.

The directions I send you do not themselves convey the message meaning, but they guide you in your selection of words from the page: they limit the number of alternate word choices and permit you to reconstruct my idea.

Shannon [8] describes "information" as "the informativeness of the symbols in a message relative to one's expectation of those symbols." That is to say that, in reconstructing my secret message, the amount of information you derive from each of my directions to select words will depend upon how well you can predict these words without my instructions. It might be helpful to consider such directions to be analogous to the symbols involved in speech communication. The result of information is, as M. Valentine [9] points out, to eliminate confusion.

Shannon has shown that the amount of information in a symbol is directly related to the total number of symbols from which one has to choose. The value of each symbol as a vehicle for carrying information is decreased if the symbols are not random but are to some extent dependent upon, and therefore predictable from, each other.

Linguistic Constraints

In most communication systems the selection of a message-signal unit is not completely random. Certain constraints are placed upon the manner in which the units may be linked together in sequences. That is to say that immediately a particular message-signal unit has been selected, the choice of a second unit is limited by virtue of certain rules governing its relationship to the first. The selection of a third unit is further restricted, since it is influenced, not by one, but by two previous units. The number of constraints placed upon the selection of each new unit increases as the number of units increases. Different sets of constraints exist for the written and spoken language systems. Since we are interested in communication through speech, we shall consider only the constraints of spoken English, though it will be necessary to resort to the written form for purposes of illustration. These constraints may be classified under three major headings: (1) structural, (2) contextual, and (3) situational.

Structural Constraints

The three types of structural constraints to be considered are those at the level of the phoneme, the form, and the construct.

PHONEMES. In the conventional form of any language, the basic unit from which words are built is the phoneme.* Any speech sound that, in at least one instance in the spoken vocabulary of the language, can be shown to differentiate one word from another is designated a phoneme. For example, in the spoken form of the words sit [sɪt], sat [sæt] set [sɛt], soot [sʊt], the initial and final sounds remain constant; only the middle sound permits a difference in meaning to be recognized. These words demonstrate that the vowel sound in each example constitutes a phoneme.

The general American dialect, spoken in the midwestern and western areas of the United States, contains a total of 38 phonemes (16 vowels, 22 consonants) [6, pp. 66–170]. This number represents the first structural constraint. The speaker of general American dialect must construct his words from sounds within this phonemic inventory. Whenever he begins to utter a particular phoneme, he limits the number of phonemes from which his second phoneme may be selected. C. F. Hockett [4] illustrates this by pointing out that if the initial utterance of a speaker is the phoneme /p/, he may be said to be in a "post-/p/" state. He is now limited in his choice of the next phoneme to any of the vowel sounds or /r/,/l/,/y/,/w/. He may not in English select, for example, /t/,/k/,/ʃ/ among others. The probability with which he may select a particular sound will vary for each phoneme. If he selects an /r/, then he is in a "post-/pr/" state, with a new set of limitations and probabilities, e.g., any vowel but not, for example, /r/ or /p/ or /l/. The effect of phonemic constraint will be apparent to the reader if he attempts to make up a nonsense language. He will find himself using the phonemic patterns of the English language, and he will experience difficulty in avoiding sound combinations that constitute meaningful English words.

FORMS. The second level of structural constraint therefore concerns itself with the manner in which phonemes may be strung together in sequences acceptable to the linguistic culture. These sequences are known as forms, and they constitute the basic elements of the grammatical structure of a language. C. F. Hockett [5, p. 133] states that a form may be recognized by asking whether a sequence of phonemes reoccurs in various utter-

---

*Phonemes will be designated by slash marks // throughout the text.

ances with approximately the same meaning. If it does, the particular sequence may be considered to be a grammatical form. It may be noted that a form may be as small as a single morpheme* or it may be made up of several morphemes. The following examples illustrate some of the forms that exist in the English language.

spare	un	good
ing	inhibit	ness
ly	ed	me
sparingly	uninhibited	goodness me
in	ambi	re
differ	valent	form
ent	ambivalent	ation
ly		reformation
indifferently		

CONSTRUCTIONS. Just as the phonemes of English must conform to certain acceptable sequences, the forms themselves may be strung together in certain sequential patterns referred to as *constructions*. J. B. Carroll [1, p. 19] suggests that it is helpful to consider constructions as a series of "slots" into which particular types of material may be fitted. In the phrase "the boy fell," the word "the" may, for example, be replaced by "a," "this," or "that." The word "boy" may be replaced by a variety of different nouns, while "fell" may be substituted by, for example, "ate his dinner," said he had a good time." Carroll points out that if the slot contains a different kind of material, it either belongs to a different construction or is meaningless: e.g., "the boy green." The speaker is therefore limited in the ways in which he may combine constructs in order to convey a message. The sentence "Go you with him today?" is not an acceptable interrogative construction in formal English. This is, however, the accepted construction in Norwegian.

The Role of Structural Constraints

Each of these structural constraints influence the degree to which a person who understands a language well is able to predict a given unit of a message signal. Lack of familiarity with structural rules lies at the roots of the language retardation of deaf children. The structural constraints affect the relative statistical probability of occurrence of a given phoneme immediately following or preceding another phoneme, of a form occurring in a particular position in a word, or a word or construct occurring in a particular

---

*Morphemes are the smallest individually meaningful elements in the utterances of a language [7].

position in a phrase or sentence. It has already been pointed out that the amount of information a message signal or a unit of a message signal contains is closely related to the ability of the listener to predict accurately its content. If one is in a position to know in advance the exact message-signal content, then the message signal itself imparts very little information. For example, if a person receives by phone a dictation of a telegram, providing the dictation is accurate and correctly received, the written confirmation of the telegram arriving later will provide almost no further information. If, on the other hand, a faulty telephone connection results in the poor reception of a number of dictated words, the written confirmation will convey a certain amount of information. The amount of information will increase as the ability to correctly predict the message units decreases.

Carroll [1, p. 55] illustrates this with three strings of ten-letter messages with the tenth letter missing:

$$P \quad R \quad R \quad N \quad W \quad B \quad I \quad T \quad K \_\_$$

$$A \quad A \quad A \quad A \quad A \quad A \quad A \quad A \quad A \_\_$$

$$G \quad E \quad N \quad E \quad R \quad A \quad T \quad I \quad O \_\_$$

He points out that the informativeness of the missing symbol is great in the first example, since the symbols are in a random sequence. The probability of a given letter occurring in the tenth position is uninfluenced by those preceding it and is, therefore, low. The ability of the reader correctly to predict the letter is very poor. In the second example, if the selection of the letter *A* for the missing symbol proves correct, it will convey little information since one would have had little difficulty in predicting it. If, on the other hand, it proves not to be *A*, then the missing letter would be very informative. The missing *N* in the third string of letters may be predicted with a high degree of success, since the choice of letters is severely limited by the preceding letters and, therefore, may be said to convey little information.

The role of structural constraints was demonstrated in an experiment conducted by the author. Thirty college students were divided into three groups of ten. Each subject was presented a series of dashes which, he was told, represented groups of letters. The students were further advised that the letters might or might not constitute meaningful words, and that the units might or might not be related to each other. All of the letters were drawn from the sentence "The cat sat on the mat."

In the first test item (A), administered to student group I, the letters were arranged at random. That is to say, they were not subject to any structural constraint. In the second test item (B), student group II, the letter order constituted words, but the word order was randomized; the subjects were therefore subject to phonemic constraint but not to constructional rules. The test item (C), student group III, constituted the complete sentence which obeyed the rules of formal English construction.

Test item A. OTT / TAS / CHA / NE / MTT / EHA.

Test item B. MAT / THE / THE / ON / SAT / CAT.

Test item C. THE / CAT / SAT / ON / THE / MAT.

Each subject was given the following instructions:

The dashes on the sheet (Table 2.1) represent letters of the alphabet. With one exception these are grouped in threes. You are asked to guess the letters in each group, letter by letter. The letters may or may not constitute meaningful words or sentences. The alphabet lists below permit you to record each letter you use for each blank. Beginning with the first dash (examiner indicates this on subject's sheet), which corresponds to Alphabet List No. 1 below, try to guess the missing letter. I will tell you if your guess is right or wrong. If you name the correct letter, fill in the dash. If your answer is incorrect, cross that letter off in Alphabet List No. 1 and try again. Continue guessing until you choose the correct letter. We shall repeat this for each dash.

TABLE 2.1

1	2	3		4	5	6		7	8	9		10	11		12	13	14		15	16	17
__	__	__	/	__	__	__	/	__	__	__	/	__	__	/	__	__	__	/	__	__	__

ALPHABET LISTS

1. A B C D E F G H I J K L M N O P Q R S T U V W X Y Z
2. A B C D E F G H I J K L M N O P Q R S T U V W X Y Z
3. A B C D E F G H I J K L M N O P Q R S T U V W X Y Z
4. A B C D E F G H I J K L M N O P Q R S T U V W X Y Z
5. A B C D E F G H I J K L M N O P Q R S T U V W X Y Z
6. A B C D E F G H I J K L M N O P Q R S T U V W X Y Z
7. A B C D E F G H I J K L M N O P Q R S T U V W X Y Z
8. A B C D E F G H I J K L M N O P Q R S T U V W X Y Z
9. A B C D E F G H I J K L M N O P Q R S T U V W X Y Z
10. A B C D E F G H I J K L M N O P Q R S T U V W X Y Z
11. A B C D E F G H I J K L M N O P Q R S T U V W X Y Z
12. A B C D E F G H I J K L M N O P Q R S T U V W X Y Z
13. A B C D E F G H I J K L M N O P Q R S T U V W X Y Z
14. A B C D E F G H I J K L M N O P Q R S T U V W X Y Z
15. A B C D E F G H I J K L M N O P Q R S T U V W X Y Z
16. A B C D E F G H I J K L M N O P Q R S T U V W X Y Z
17. A B C D E F G H I J K L M N O P Q R S T U V W X Y Z

The examiner also checked, on a duplicate sheet, the letters the subject chose. The mean number of guesses required to correctly identify each letter was calculated for each student group. Also computed were the mean number of guesses made by each group per unit and for the complete test item.

The results shown in Table 2.2 indicate that, as the number of structural constraints increase, the ability of a subject to predict missing symbols also increases.

Group I subjects were constrained only by the 26 letters of the alphabet. They tended at first to guess according to the rules of English, e.g., most subjects first guessed the initial letter to be "t," predicting that the word was "the." Once they realized that the letters did not constitute meaningful words, they resorted to random guessing. It will be noticed that in each instance, with the exception of the first letters, the vowels required fewer guesses in this item than any of the consonants. This results from the fact that a large number of subjects, when guessing, first ran through the vowels. Therefore, when the missing letter was a vowel, it was quickly guessed. It will be seen that the number of guesses per letter does not improve as the number of known letters increases, since each letter is independent of the preceding or succeeding letter.

The results for Group II indicate that the effect of phonemic constraint is progressively to reduce the number of alternative letters from which the subject may choose. Within each unit (word), knowing the first letter obviously reduces the number of guesses needed to identify the second. Note, however, that correct identification of the first unit does not reduce the number of guesses necessary to identify the succeeding units, since each unit is independent of adjacent units.

In Group III, the effect of phonemic and constructional constraints is clearly seen to reduce the mean number of guesses per letter and per unit.

Contextual Constraints

Even familiarity with the structural rules of a language frequently proves insufficient to permit a message to be understood under conditions of distortion. If, however, the topic of conversation is made known, the distorted signal may be interpreted because it is in context. The effect of contextual and/or semantic constraints is to limit the choice of words and phrases that may be used to convey a particular meaning. A conversation on the topic of baseball eliminates the use of most vocabulary that might be appropriate to a discussion of, for example, music. It is in this way that we often reject a particular interpretation of a distorted message because it appears to be unrelated to its context. Certainly a relationship exists between the semantic and syntactical constraints. We are aided in our interpretation of the signal by the knowledge that nouns are naming words, that

TABLE 2.2. The Effect of Different Degrees of Structural Constraint

TEST ITEM

A

STUDENT GROUP	Mean number of guesses corrected to nearest whole number	O	T	T	A	S	C	H	A	N	E	M	T	T	E	H	A
I	Letter mean	13	14	13	9	5	12	10	13	3	12	7	10	16	14	8	12
	Unit mean	13			9				9					14			8

B

STUDENT GROUP		M	A	T	T	H	E	T	H	E	O	N	S	A	T	C	A	T
II	Letter mean	8	3	7	12	9	1	11	5	2	7	4	10	3	2	11	3	4
	Unit mean	6			7			6			6			5			6		

C

STUDENT GROUP		T	H	E	C	A	T	S	A	T	O	N	T	H	E	M	A	T
III	Letter mean	11	4	1	4	1	1	4	1	1	1	1	2	3	1	4	1	1
	Unit mean	6			2			2			2			1			2		

	Group	Item	Mean number of guesses per item
	I	A	10
	II	B	6
	III	C	2

verbs designate activities, and adjectives, properties or characteristics. Yet, as C. Cherry [2, p. 119] points out, meaning may be conveyed by a chain of nouns, e.g., woman, street, crowd, traffic, noise, haste, thief, bag, lost, scream, police.

The reader, by virtue of his knowledge of syntax, can predict the missing elements, but he has also experience of the types of contexts in which these words may occur, particularly when they occur in this order.

Situational Constraints

In addition to the effect that context has on the choice of vocabulary, the speaker is further limited in his mode of expression by the actual situation in which he is to communicate his message. The same message may be expressed in a variety of different ways, different words and phrases being used according to the speaker's evaluation of the nature of his audience. A message may be communicated to a roommate in a form that may be totally inappropriate for use in conveying the same information to one's parents. Situational constraints may be considered to be a function of the people present, the relationship of the speaker to these people, and the social structure of the particular environment. The form of expression of a message that passes between a professor and his student may reasonably be predicted as being different from the same message passing from the student to the professor. This will be influenced by the relationship that exists between these two people. Between individuals who have had little or no previous contact, the message will be influenced primarily by the speaker's evaluation of the role and social standing of the listeners.

The influence of environmental factors upon a topic of discussion and upon the manner in which the information is conveyed will be appreciated by the listener if he envisages himself in each of the following situations: in the main aisle of a large cathedral just before morning service, at an informal student party, in a seminar group, at the question period in a large lecture meeting, or on a first date in a small cocktail bar.

Redundancy

The result of these various constraints is to produce what is known as redundancy. This may be defined as that part of a message that can be eliminated without a significant loss of information. Carroll [1, p. 56] explains it as "the property of texts (language contexts) that allows us to predict missing symbols from the context." It must not be confused with simple repetition of all or part of the message signal, though repetition may affect redundancy. The idea of redundancy is perhaps more easily understood if it is considered as the result of the interaction of certain factors within the speaker (and therefore the message signal), the environment, and the listener. It is not possible to state a redundancy figure for a given message signal without considering these three variables. What may prove to be redundant for one listener may not be so for another. A message signal in one set of environmental conditions may have high redundancy, while in a different environment the redundancy of the same message signal may be severely reduced. Similarly, a message spoken by a person whose native tongue is English, may become extremely difficult to understand when spoken by a foreigner whose English is characterized by a heavy dialect. The most important factors influencing redundancy are shown in Table 2.3. Shannon has shown that for the average adult reader the redundancy of written English over any series of not greater than eight letters is approximately 50 per cent. Thus, when we are operating under the constraints of written English, half of what we write is freely chosen, while the other half is deter-

TABLE 2.3.   Factors Influencing Redundancy

FACTORS WITHIN THE SPEAKER

   a. Compliance of the speaker to the rules of the language
   b. Compliance to the patterns of articulation, stress, intonation
   c. Size of vocabulary from which the message is composed
   d. Appropriate choice of words to convey the message

FACTORS WITHIN THE MESSAGE SIGNAL

   a. Number of syllables within the word
   b. Number of words within a sentence
   c. Number of different words (i.e., type-token ratio*)
   d. Amount of context
   e. Amount of repetition
   f. Frequency bandwidth of acoustic signal
   g. Intensity of acoustic signal

FACTORS WITHIN THE ENVIRONMENT

   a. Amount of acoustic noise
   b. Amount of reverberation
   c. Amount and intensity of other environmental stimuli
   d. Number of potential clues related to the message

FACTORS WITHIN THE LISTENER

   a. Familiarity with the language rules
   b. Familiarity with the speech patterns of the speaker
   c. Familiarity with the vocabulary used by the speaker
   d. Familiarity with the topic of conversation
   e. Fidelity of reception of the acoustic message signal
   f. Awareness of and ability to interpret related stimuli

*Type-token ratio: $\dfrac{\text{number of different words}}{\text{total number of words}}$.

mined by the structure of the language. In normal conversational speech, under favorable conditions, the level of redundancy is higher. Most of us can recall instances in which we have been able to maintain a conversation with one person while listening to the conversation of two people standing close to us.

Noise and Redundancy

Closely related to the concept of information is the concept of noise. In communication terminology this term is far more inclusive than the concept of audible noise. Noise may be considered the effect of any factor that adds confusion and so reduces the amount of information conveyed. In any communication situation the listener is faced with varying amounts of noise in the system. This may be inherent within the message signal itself,

TABLE 2.4. Sources of Noise

WITHIN THE SPEAKER

    a. Inadequate vocabulary
    b. Poor syntax
    c. Semantic ambiguity
    d. Imprecise or deviant articulation of speech
    e. Poor vocal production
    f. Improper stress and inflection

WITHIN THE ENVIRONMENT

Acoustic signal

    a. Acoustic noise resulting in masking of the message signal
    b. Distortion of the frequency pattern of the message signal
    c. Reverberation

Visual signal

    d. Poor lighting
    e. Visual field limited
    f. Competing visual stimuli

WITHIN THE LISTENER

    a. Unfamiliarity with the vocabulary and rules of the language
    b. Failure to identify correctly the topic of the message
    c. Incorrect recognition of auditory and/or visual signals because of similarity between sounds or between the visible characteristics of some articulation patterns
    d. Distracting stimuli
    e. Psychological factors, such as poor intellectual ability, poor motivation, poor attention span, high distractibility, preoccupation with something else, prejudice against the speaker or topic of conversation, etc.

may be a function of limitations in the listener's ability to receive and decode the message signal accurately, or may exist in the channel through which the message signal travels.* Table 2.4 indicates the major sources of noise in oral communication.

The importance of redundancy lies in the role it plays in helping to combat these noise factors. If the redundancy of a particular message is relatively high, then its resistance to noise or distortion is also great, permitting the receiver to obtain enough information to enable him to predict the missing elements of the message. The amount of redundancy in any given speech sample is therefore a function of the interaction between the speaker, the listener, and the message signal. It must be stressed that the value of redundancy is limited by the extent to which the receiver is able to utilize it. Unfamiliarity with the linguistic structure or ignorance concerning the context of the message will seriously affect the benefit that the listener can derive from redundancy of speech material.

An understanding of the role of noise and redundancy in communication helps us to appreciate how it is that a person, with what appears to be quite a severe auditory handicap, can often function adequately in a communication situation. At the same time, it emphasizes the need for developing in the individual an awareness of an ability to capitalize on other factors that contribute to redundancy.

The concept of human communication being a process based upon the ability to predict the next "bit" of information has been very succinctly summarized by Peter Laurie in an article entitled "The Explorers" in the British *Sunday Times Supplement.* He writes:

> The idea of the mind computing the probabilities of what's coming next has proved an essential key in the fast-growing new branch of psycholinguistics. One of the problems here is to elucidate the processes of hearing speech and decoding it into ideas. A good deal of experimenting has been done on this now, starting with the work of Professor Colin Cherry at Imperial College, London, at the beginning of the 1950s. It appears that hearing and understanding a spoken message involves several layers of computation. At the first level we can pick out from the noise around us—a cocktail party, say—one voice. We can tell the rate it's speaking and the direction it's coming from. Even something as apparently simple as this is in fact very sophisticated. It involves, to keep track of the tone of voice, making a statistical analysis of the characteristic sounds of that voice, storing this and comparing all the incoming sounds with this to pick out the ones we want. Then to find its direction we have to store the last second or so of *this* voice's input into each ear and shuffle the two records until they match to find the time delay between the two ears.

---

*The term "channel" refers to the pathway through which the message signal travels. This includes both the neurological and the environmental pathways; e.g., auditory channel: hearing and sound waves; visual channel: vision and light waves; tactile channel: touch and low-frequency vibrations.

The sounds from the selected voice are stored for less than a second and passed on to the next level where they are translated into the equivalent sounds one could make oneself, and stored again—this is how one can make a stab at the last few syllables of something in a foreign language. This transfers again into a store where the sounds are identified with meaningful words—the short term memory we use to hold a telephone number between directory and dial. Unless the number is consciously repeated and reinserted, it fades after six seconds or so. Then the words are recoded again as ideas and transferred into long term memory. Interest focuses at the moment on this transfer from short term into long term store and back again. It is suggested that as one listens to a speaker, one runs ahead, using the statistical structure of the language to throw up the probable next words out of the long term store and matching them in one's head against those in the short term store. What we remember, or understand, is not the *sound* of the word we hear, but the *idea* stored in our heads that would generate the sound nearest to it. It's as if we were using a dictionary, flipping through it until we find a word that seems to match the word we hear and reading off the meaning. The fact that there's only one central dictionary is shown by the impossibility of speaking effectively while reading, writing, or listening.

This dictionary is not, however, arranged alphabetically, but by a continuously shifting scale of probabilities, and these are influenced by who is speaking, the situation we are both in, and particularly by what has just been said. So when one goes to answer the phone, one's dictionary already has some likely phrases ready to hear, like "Hold on, I have a call," and when you've got that far you hear "for you" automatically. But if the operator said, "Hold on, I have a call for umbilical hippopotamus," the last two words—having a low assigned probability—would not be found until it was too late, and so wouldn't be heard. That the brain works somehow like this was shown by an English psychologist, David Bruce, who made a record of a voice speaking against a background so noisy that nothing could be understood. He played this to a group of listeners who were told it was a talk about football. Then he played them one about hire purchase, and another about politics. Each time, given a cue, they could follow the sense; they were astonished to be told afterwards he'd played the same record each time.

We must, however, bear in mind the fact that our understanding of the process of human communication is still very much theoretical and that the development of any theory is subject to certain qualifications.

QUALIFICATIONS CONCERNING THE DEVELOPMENT OF THE THEORY

Any explanation of the process of human communication must be based upon a theory or philosophy. In all areas of human behavior, emphasis is increasingly placed upon experimental study. This sometimes leads the beginning student to conclude that the techniques used in philosophical reasoning are rather suspect as a research tool. It is important to recognize that even when it is possible to examine physically each component of a network, a particular orientation or approach is necessary. What is selected for examination, why it is selected, and how the results are integrated are all determined by the approach of the investigator. The particular orientation of an investigator must be founded upon a carefully constructed hypothesis arrived at after systematic evaluation of the factors known to be involved. Ideally it should then be possible to prove or disprove the hypothesis by experimental studies. However, many problems prove to be so complex that they defy experimental study within the limits of current knowledge and equipment.

Certain aspects of the communication process present this problem. Parts of the process are easily observable. We can study the mechanics of respiration, the nature of the laryngeal mechanism, the physical characteristics of sound waves, the operation of the middle ear. This still leaves inaccessible to us most of the complex processes concerned with the exchange of information. We are not able to examine the exact process involved in the formulation of ideas, the coding into language, the analysis of the acoustic signal by the ear and auditory nerve centers, and the final deciphering of the message signal by the listener.

For these reasons, the student must recognize that the greater part of what has been presented in this chapter is in fact theoretical. In his outside reading, he will encounter a number of other models of the communication process based upon different theoretical approaches. For the therapist or teacher, the advantage of any model rests in the fact that it provides us with a basis for understanding the communication problems associated with impairment of hearing, and it affords a rationale for the rehabilitation program.

REFERENCES

1. Carroll, J. B. *Language and Thought.* Englewood Cliffs, N.J.: Prentice-Hall, Inc., 1964.

2. Cherry, C. *On Human Communication.* New York: John Wiley & Sons, Inc., 1957.

3. Fairbanks, G. "Systematic Research in Experimental Phonetics: Speech as a Servo-mechanism." *Journal of Speech and Hearing Disorders* 19 (1954): 133–139.

4. Hockett, C. F. Review of *The Mathematical Theory of Communication,* by Claude Shannon and Warren Weaver, in *Psycholinguistics,* ed. Sol Saporta. New York: Holt, Rinehart & Winston, Inc., 1961; reprinted from *Language* 29 (1953): 69–93.

5. _____. *A Course in Modern Linguistics.* New York: The Macmillan Company, Publishers, 1958.

6. Kantner, C. E., and R. West. *Phonetics.* 1st ed. New York: Harper & Row, Publishers, 1941. pp. 66–170.

7. Pangborn, R. M. "Influence of Color on the Discrimination of Sweetness." *American Journal of Psychology* 73 (1960): 229–38.

8. Shannon, C. E., and W. Weaver. *The Mathematical Theory of Communication.* Urbana: University of Illinois Press, 1962.

9. Valentine, M. "Information Theory and the Psychology of Speech." in *The Psychology of Communication.* Edited by J. Eisenson, J. Auer, and J. Irwin. New York: Appleton-Century-Crofts, 1963.

10. Van Riper, C., and J. V. Irwin. *Voice and Articulation.* Englewood Cliffs, N.J.: Prentice-Hall, Inc., 1958.

CHAPTER THREE

The Acoustic Aspect
of Speech*

This chapter will attempt to familiarize the reader with those aspects of acoustics that are considered essential to a basic understanding of the nature of speech communication. Although the acoustic structure of speech is highly complex, it is best approached by first examining sound in its most fundamental form.

SIMPLE HARMONIC MOTION

Sound energy results from the movement of air particles, a movement that may be induced by any vibrating body. Vibration occurs when a force causes an object to move from its position of rest. Since all objects possess some degree of elasticity, the maximum possible displacement, the *amplitude*, is limited; once the initial energy has been exhausted by resistance, the natural elasticity of the object will cause it to reverse its direction of movement. It travels back toward its rest position, but is carried beyond it by momentum to a position of maximum displacement in the opposite direc-

*Associate Professor Robert E. McGlone, State University of New York at Buffalo, is co-author of Chap. 3.

tion, and finally returns to its position of rest. This simple form of vibration is called *simple harmonic motion.*

The movement thus described by the vibrator is induced in the air molecules surrounding it, causing them to vibrate in an identical pattern. Each molecule sets adjacent molecules in a simple harmonic motion, creating a pressure wave, referred to as a *sinusoidal wave,* which moves away from the source. The backward and forward movement of the particles occurs in a straight line; however, it is possible to depict this repetitive event as circular motion. This is done by dividing the particle movement into parts of a circle by degrees: 360 degrees represents a full cycle; 180 degrees represents a half cycle; 90 degrees, a quarter cycle. The portion of a cycle that has been completed at a particular instant of time is called the *phase of the motion* and may be referred to by degrees. Although the phase of a sound does not affect its normal perception, it will be seen later that the phase does play an important role in the perception of speech under adverse listening conditions.

When the rate of the simple harmonic vibration of air particles falls within the sensitivity range of the ear, the sound that is perceived is called a *pure tone.* The complete simple vibration of either the vibrator or the air particles is called *one cycle*; while the number of cycles through which these vibrating bodies move in a given unit of time is referred to as the *frequency* of the motion. For example, if one cycle of vibration is completed in one second, the unit of time that is most commonly used in acoustics, the frequency of the activity is said to be one cycle per second. Frequency is designated by the term *Hertz* (Hz), after Heinrich Hertz, who confirmed the existence of electromagnetic waves. The frequency, phase, and amplitude of a sinusoidal wave are illustrated in Fig. 3.1.

To displace a particle from rest, set it in motion, and maintain that motion requires energy. The rate at which energy is given off by a sound source, or the energy in a pressure wave when it strikes an object, is called *intensity,* which is dependent upon the frequency and the amplitude, both of which can affect the energy in the sound wave.

For the student who does not understand the concept of simple harmonic motion and its components as described here, there are several texts which deal with this topic in detail. Two that may be helpful are *Elements of Acoustic Phonetics,* by P. Ladefoged [7], and *Bases of Speech,* by G. Gray and C. Wise [4].

COMPLEX SOUNDS

Unfortunately, the study of speech is complicated by the fact that the human speech mechanism does not produce a pure tone but a variety of

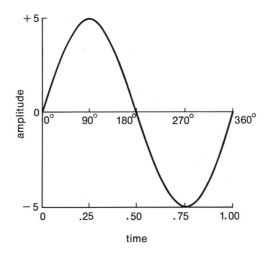

Fig. 3.1.   A graphic representation of a sinusoidal wave illustrating its frequency, amplitude, and phase.

complex sounds, not all of which are used for communication. The speech organs move the particles of air in such a manner that they produce patterns of vibration that contain more than a single frequency. If these frequencies are related to each other so that each is an exact multiple of the lowest frequency, all are called *harmonics*. If they are not arranged in any organized pattern, the resultant sound is called an *inharmonic sound*, or *acoustic noise*. Figures 3.2(a) and 3.2(b) illustrate an inharmonic and a harmonic complex sound. It can be seen from Fig. 3.2(a) that the graphic display of the harmonic complex sound is no longer the smooth upward and downward movement that is found in simple harmonic motion as shown in Fig. 3.1. The wave form depicted results from related vibrations occurring at each of the harmonic frequencies. On the other hand the complex inharmonic tone, as shown in Fig. 3.2(b), is made up of particle movements at frequencies that are unrelated to each other.

HARMONIC COMPLEX SOUNDS

All sounds that are produced by the normal vibration of the vocal folds are harmonic complex sounds. These consist of a *fundamental*, which is the lowest frequency at which energy is present and which reflects the number of times the vocal folds open and close in a given unit of time, and a series of *harmonics*, which occur because the vocal folds do not vibrate in a simple manner. In Fig. 3.2(a) the fundamental frequency is 100 Hz, the second harmonic is 200 Hz, and subsequent harmonics occur at 300 Hz, 400 Hz, 500 Hz, etc. We refer to the division of a harmonic complex sound into its frequency and amplitude components as *harmonic analysis.*

The wave shape of a complex tone is often difficult to describe; however, a complex, but repetitive, wave form can be divided into a number of sinusoidal waves of different frequencies, amplitudes, and phases. Figure 3.3 shows how a complex wave may be built from three sinusoidal components of different frequencies and of different amplitudes. The simple summation of the amplitudes of each of these waves provides the complex harmonic sound illustrated in this figure.

The most usual way of specifying the amplitudes of the components of complex harmonic sounds is by the use of the line spectrum, which illus-

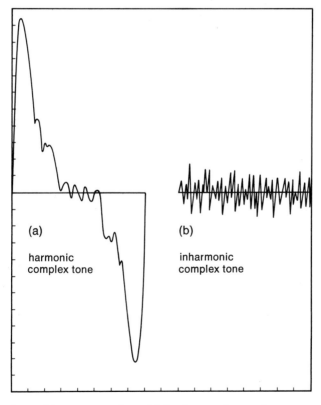

(a)

harmonic complex tone

(b)

inharmonic complex tone

Fig. 3.2. A graphic representation of (a) a harmonic complex wave, and (b) an inharmonic complex wave.

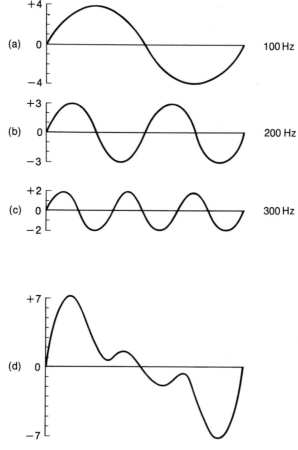

Fig. 3.3. A harmonic complex wave and its sinusoidal components.

trates the amplitude of each of the frequency components. Such a spectrum for the complex wave shown in Fig. 3.3 is presented in Fig. 3.4, which depicts the frequencies at which energy is present and the relative intensity of each component. The total energy of the sound is equal to the sum of the amplitudes at each harmonic frequency.

INHARMONIC COMPLEX SOUNDS

Many speech sounds exist that have component frequencies that are not harmonically related to each other; the particle vibrations occur randomly. Just as occurs in harmonic complex sounds, the amount of energy present at each frequency may vary or may be equal.

RESONANCE

We have said that air molecules are set in motion by the action of a vibrator. It is equally possible for the vibrator to set in motion a second potential vibrator, a resonator, in close proximity to it. If this occurs, the frequency of vibration of the second vibrator will be the same as, or close to, the frequency of the first.

One of the characteristics of all vibrators is that as a result of their particular construction and composition they exhibit greater sensitivity to vibrations at some frequencies than at others. The band of sensitivity varies from vibrator to vibrator and represents the frequency vibrations at which it will most easily be set in motion. The center of this frequency sensitivity band is called the *natural frequency* of the resonator. If the vibrating frequency of the sound source and the natural frequency of the second source are close, the resultant sound will be of greater amplitude than that produced by the original vibrator. On the other hand, if the natural frequency of the second source is *not* close to the vibrating frequency of the first, the energy from the vibrator will be absorbed and the sound weakened or *damped*. In such cases, when frequencies are *not* matched and the sound source does *not* continue to maintain a driving force to the second vibrator, the energy gen-

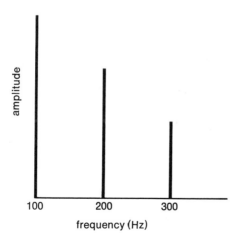

Fig. 3.4. A line spectrum of the harmonic complex wave shown in Fig. 3.3.

erated by the vibrator will be quickly absorbed and the sound will last for only a short period of time. If, however, the sound-source vibration is maintained, it will continue to drive the second vibrator, though little energy will be transmitted. This loss of energy results from the mismatching of the frequency of the driving source and the natural frequency of the second vibrator. This is termed *impedance mismatch*, since the transmission of energy is impeded by the incompatibility of the vibrators. The modifying effect that the second vibrator will have on the sound emitted from the source is called *resonance;* the second vibrator itself is called a *resonator.* The pattern of sensitivity of the resonator at frequencies on either side of the natural frequency will vary; it may be depicted by joining the peaks of the spectral components. This joining line results in a pattern which we refer to as the *envelope.*

For complex sounds with energy present at many frequencies, it is possible that some of the frequencies higher than the fundamental will correspond to the natural band of the resonator. When this occurs, the amplitude of those components of this complex wave will be greatly increased as a result of resonance. Figure 3.5(a) illustrates a spectrum of a complex sound, and Fig. 3.5(b), the envelope of a resonance chamber. When the complex sound, represented in Fig. 3.5(a), is introduced or *coupled* with the resonant chamber, the resultant sound resembles the spectrum illustrated in Fig. 3.5(c).

FREQUENCY AND PITCH OF THE VOICE

As indicated earlier, the term *frequency* is used to describe one of the physical parameters of a sound. The perception of this parameter is referred to by the term *pitch.* When a sound of 100 Hz strikes the ear and is transmitted on to the higher neural centers involved in hearing, we perceive not 100 pulses striking the eardrum each second, but a tone that has a particular pitch characteristic. If a second tone of 1000 Hz is heard immediately following the 100 Hz tone, we recognize it not as a vibration ten times greater than the first, but as a tone of a higher pitch than the first. The frequency of the vibration is thus a purely physical measure, though it does have a definite effect on the perceived pitch. Generally speaking, the higher the frequency, the higher the perceived pitch.

As a person grows from infancy to adulthood, his mean vocal pitch level changes; both the cries of newborn infants and the speech of children are of a higher pitch level than the speech of adults. The mean vocal pitch levels of persons of different ages have been studied by many investigators, and a composite of the results of these studies is shown in Fig. 3.6. You will

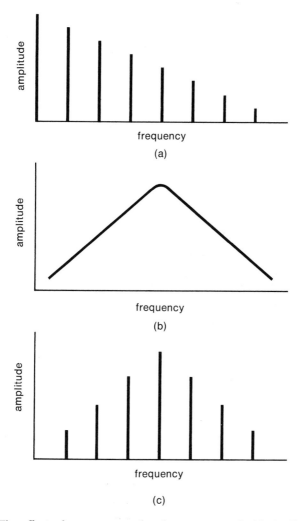

frequency

(a)

frequency

(b)

frequency

(c)

Fig. 3.5. The effect of a resonance chamber on a sound: (a) the line spectrum of a sound at its source, (b) the envelope of the resonance characteristics of a resonant cavity, (c) the result of passing sound (a) through the resonant chamber (b).

see from this figure that the fundamental frequency of newborn children and of children within the first two years of life is extremely high [9, 12]. As the child grows older, the pitch level becomes lower, with a marked drop occurring during adolescence for both boys and girls [1, 2, 5]. After people reach young adulthood, the fundamental frequency of the voice tends to

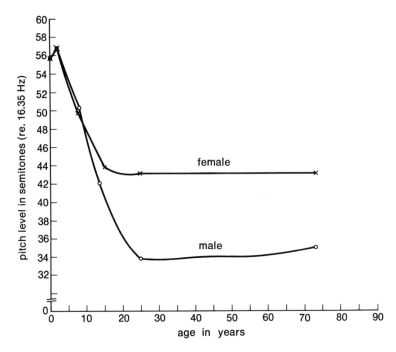

Fig. 3.6.   Pitch-level trend for males and females, from data collected at various ages (after R. Ringel et al.; R. McGlone; J. Michel et al.; G. Fairbanks et al.; E. Linke; H. Hollien et al.; E. Mysak).

level off and remain constant [8]. However, there is an indication, especially in the voice of male speakers of older ages, that mean pitch level appears to rise again [10, 11].

The range of frequencies that the vocal mechanism is capable of producing covers approximately two and one-half octaves when the speaker is asked to progress from the lowest tone he can sustain to the highest. However, for conversational speech, the speaker uses nowhere near his total range. He tends to use a more restricted range centering around the 25 per cent point of the total frequency span from the lowest sustained vocalization. Table 3.1 presents the general pitch range used by males, females, and children, along with their mean vocal pitch level. The average habitual pitch for male speakers will be seen to be around 120 Hz, for females 200 Hz, and for children 400 Hz. From what has already been said about the relationship between the fundamental frequency and the harmonics, it will be apparent that when the fundamental tone is raised each of the harmonics will also be moved to a higher frequency. For this reason, some people with high-frequency hearing loss experience considerably more difficulty in understanding the speech of small children and sometimes that of women than

TABLE 3.1. **Mean Speaking Fundamental Frequency Level and Speaking Frequency Range Used by Males, Females, and Children**

SPEAKERS	AGE	MEAN FREQUENCY (HZ)	RANGE (S.D. IN TONES)
Children (9)	16.5 mos.	443.3	1.70
Pre-adolescent girls (1)	8 yrs	288.0	1.40
Pre-adolescent boys (2)	8 yrs	297.0	1.00
Post-adolescent girls (6)	17.5 yrs	211.5	1.67
Post-adolescent boys (5)	18 yrs	115.9	2.21
Females (8)	adult	199.8	1.52
Males (11)	adult	113.2	1.45

they do in comprehending male speakers. This occurs because the higher fundamental frequency of the child's or woman's voice raises some of the identifying higher overtones beyond the range of their residual hearing.

INTENSITY AND LOUDNESS OF THE VOICE

The same relationship exists between intensity and loudness as between frequency and pitch. The listener does not perceive a sound as having an intensity (actual energy) but hears the sound varying in *loudness*. The perceived loudness of a sound usually depends upon the intensity of the physical stimulus; generally, if we hear two sounds, the one with the greatest amount of energy present will seem the loudest, providing the pitches of the two tones are not far apart. Table 3.2 presents measurements of the energy present in various vowel and consonant sounds [3]. The vowel values were obtained when each was surrounded by the same consonants; however when the consonants surrounding a particular vowel are changed, the loudness or energy present in the vowel also changes. It is apparent, therefore, that the phonetic environment of a vowel sound significantly affects its perceived loudness. For this reason, specific statements about one vowel being louder than another cannot be made unless the environment of the sounds is held constant. In speech, the phonetic environment must change in order to communicate; therefore, the intensity or loudness of vowels usually differs within sentences and even within words. Table 3.2 shows the amounts of energy present in the consonants used in American speech. Note that the intensity of consonant sounds is considerably less than the intensity of vowels. Because of this difference, vowels carry most of the energy in connected speech. The purpose of consonants will be discussed later in this chapter.

Since many of the sounds of speech are vocalized, the intensity of these sounds may be varied by the manner of vocal-fold vibration. Figure 3.7

TABLE 3.2. Relative Phonetic Powers of Speech Sounds as Produced by an Average Speaker

ɔ	680	l	100	t	15
ɑ	600	ʃ	80	g	15
ʌ	510	ŋ	73	k	13
æ	490	m	52	v	12
ʊ	460	tʃ	42	ð	11
ɛ	350	n	36	b	7
u	310	dʒ	23	d	7
ɪ	260	ʒ	20	p	6
i	220	z	16	f	5
r	210	s	16	θ	1

illustrates the spectrum of a sound recorded just above the larynx and produced at a soft level, compared to the spectrum of a sound produced more
loudly with the pitch of both held at essentially the same level. The difference
between these two spectra is seen in the higher harmonics. More energy is
present at higher frequencies and the number of higher harmonics also
increases. Therefore, one manner of making sounds louder occurs in the
addition of energy in higher frequencies where no energy was present for
softer sounds.

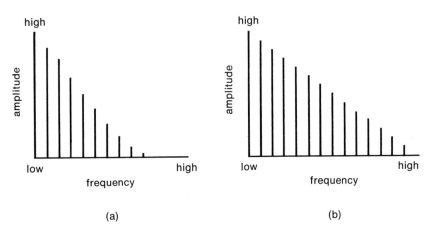

(a)   (b)

Fig. 3.7. A line spectrum of the sounds produced by the vocal folds recorded
just above the larynx: (a) a soft tone, and (b) a loud tone.

THE PRODUCTION OF SPEECH SOUNDS

The vocal folds, when activated, produce a sound wave that is transmitted into the pharyngeal, oral, and nasal cavities. The air contained within these cavities has the potential of vibrating when excited, constituting a resonance system. However, from what is known of the resonance cavities, there appears to be no chamber tuned to a frequency low enough to match the fundamental. When we compare the spectrum of a sound produced above the larynx with the spectrum of the same sound after it has passed through the speech resonance system, the fundamental is always found to have been attenuated and higher harmonics amplified. This comparison may be seen in Fig. 3.8. Yet the listener does not perceive the pitch of a sound to be as high as the frequency that contains the most energy. Usually the speaker's pitch level is perceived as near the fundamental. This occurs even when all, or nearly all, of the energy at the fundamental has been damped. The explanation may rest in the ability of the hearing mechanism to make an analysis of the differences between the harmonics.

Complex harmonic sounds of various pitches differ in structure because the fundamental frequencies are not the same. When these sounds pass through the same oral resonance chamber, they do not produce the same spectral distribution and, therefore, will differ in their perceived quality. The vibration of any segment of the resonance system is dependent upon the presence of energy in the vibrating tone at or near the natural resonant frequency. A sound with a fundamental frequency of 400 Hz and harmonics at multiples of this frequency may not have overtones to activate certain resonators that would be activated by a sound with a fundamental of 100 Hz and a difference of 100 Hz between harmonics. The resulting spectrum of each of these sounds is shown in Fig. 3.9. The wave compositions of these sounds are different because the overall spectrum of sounds, including speech phonemes, results from an interaction of the fundamental frequency and the cavity shape. Practically all the information necessary for speech discrimination can therefore be derived from the sound spectrum.

Vowels

When we define vowel-sound production, it is necessary to designate both the amount of jaw opening and the tongue position. The vowel /i/ and the vowel /u/ are considered as closed vowels with the maxilla and the mandible in close approximation, while the vowel /ɑ/ is essentially an open vowel. As a speaker assumes a particular cavity posture for each of the vowels progressing from /i/ and /u/ toward /ɑ/, the mandible becomes progressively more separated from the maxillary arch. Still another articulator that can affect the shape of the resonance tube is the lips. The most common position used for the production of the /i/ sound is the retraction or spread of the lips; the production of the /u/ sound generally involves lip rounding, while for the /ɑ/ sound the lips are unrounded. The lip positions for each of eight vowels are shown in Fig. 3.10.

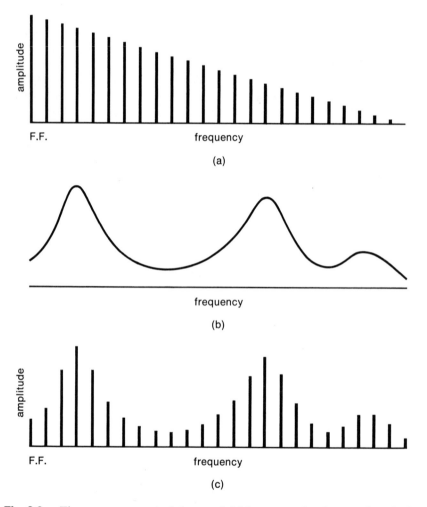

Fig. 3.8. The rearrangement of the vocal-fold spectrum by the speech articulatory cavities. The vocal-fold spectrum before it passes through the resonant cavities is shown in (a). The fundamental frequency is designated f.f. The resonant-cavity characteristic is illustrated by the envelope in (b). The spectrum of the sound after it passes through the cavities is shown in (c).

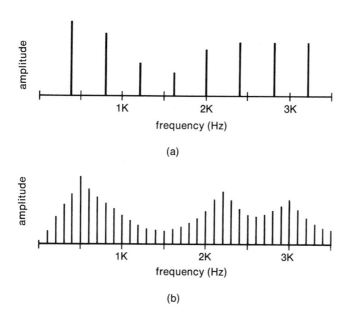

Fig. 3.9. Spectra of harmonic complex tones with different fundamental frequencies passed through the same oral cavity: (a) a tone with a fundamental frequency of 400 Hz, and (b) a tone of 100 Hz.

Usually vowels are produced with vocalization. The complex harmonic sound produced by the larynx is rearranged depending upon the shape of the cavities above the larynx. The rearrangement of the total energy that occurs when the cavities are in the general shape that they assume for the vowel /i/ is shown in Fig. 3.11. When the cavity shape is changed to the configuration for the vowel /ɑ/ and the pitch level is held constant, the spectrum of the sound changes (Fig. 3.11).

Actual line spectra of eight different vowels are shown in Fig. 3.12. Note that the amplitude of the various frequency components is different for each vowel sound. Two or three major amplitude peaks occur for each vowel and reflect the natural resonant frequencies of the cavities when articulating these vowels. This concentration of energy around each peak is called a *formant*.

The reception of the first and second formants is essential for vowel identification. Figure 3.13 presents the first and second formant values for each of the vowels shown in Fig. 3.12. For example, it will be seen that the vowel /ɑ/ has an F_1 value of 500 Hz (ordinate), and a value of 2100 Hz for F_2 (abscissa). It must be noted that seldom, if ever, does an individual or a group of individuals produce the same vowel in the same way. Since vowel-sound production varies, the formants' structure also varies; therefore, a

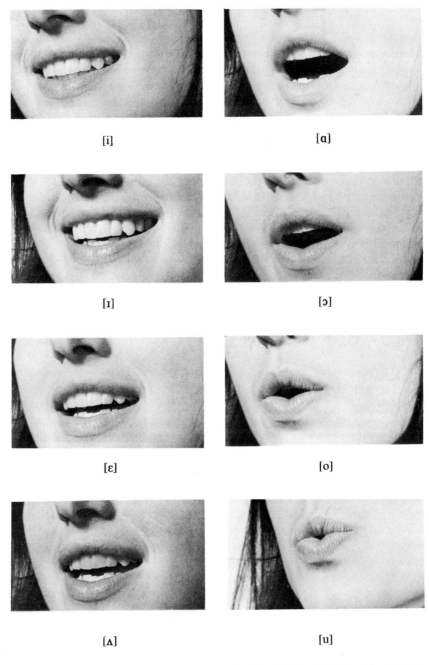

Fig. 3.10. A speaker producing the vowels: [i], [ɪ], [ɛ], [ʌ], [ɑ], [ɔ], [o], [u].

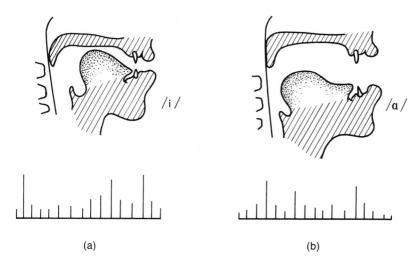

(a)   (b)

Fig. 3.11.   A diagrammatic representation of the position of the speech articulators of a person producing /i/ and /ɑ/ and the resulting spectra of
these vowels.

precise statement of the formant frequencies associated with vowel production is not possible. However, formants do tend to fall within a range that
can be specified. Cavity configurations that produce this range of acoustic-
signal modifications result in phonemes that have been assigned a specific
identification value and, within a language, are invariant. That is, if the
oral-cavity shape is changed to a configuration outside this range, the resulting acoustic signal is no longer identified as the original vowel. When this
occurs, the sound may be confused with another vowel, or it may be considered only as a sound without linguistic value.

Of the two vowel formants, a wider span of frequencies are found for
the second formant. Although changes in formant frequency occur from
vowel to vowel for F_1, these are relatively slight when compared to the variations which occur for the frequency range of F_2. The second formant of
vowels coincides with the most sensitive frequency range of the ear.

Consonants

Vowels alone comprise just a small part of the sounds used in speech;
in fact, few words consist only of vowel sounds. As previously mentioned,
vowel sounds do apparently carry most of the energy of speech. However,

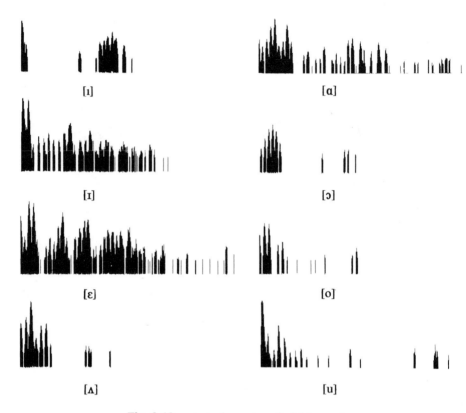

Fig. 3.12. Actual spectra of eight vowels.

it is consonants that contribute most to the identification of words and phrases. Consonants may, or may not, contain vocalization and therefore may, or may not, have wave forms which have a harmonic complex structure. A few consonants, notably /m/, /n/, /l/, and /r/, present harmonic complex wave forms very much like a vowel. Some of these sounds, depending upon their use in a syllable combination, have a semivowel characteristic. Generally, what discriminates a vowel from a consonant is that a consonant, unlike a vowel, contains an articulatory movement that obstructs or greatly restricts a flow of air from the laryngeal mechanism through the articulatory mechanism. The most common method of describing consonants is by specifying the place and manner of articulation. The place of articulation refers to the major anatomical-structure position for the production of each consonant, while the manner of articulation is based upon a subjective description of the acoustic nature of the sound. For example, the consonants /p/, /b/, and /m/ are called *bilabials* because both lips must come together for adequate production of these sounds. The /t/, /d/, and /n/ sounds are made by the contact of the tongue to the alveolar maxillary ridge and hence are called *lingual alveolar* sounds. Definition by acoustic nature describes the phonemes /p/, /b/, /t/, /d/, /k/, and /g/ as *stops* because the air stream associated with their production is completely blocked. Similarly, *fricatives* are made by constricting the air flow, somewhere in the mouth, enough to make the air turbulent, resulting in a sound that has a characteristic hissing quality as /ʃ/. The consonants /m/, /n/, and /ŋ/ are made by directing the air stream through the nasal passages, hence adding the effect of nasal resonance to the production. Many articulatory positions may be used either with or without voicing, thus further delineating phonemic categories.

The rapidity of speech precludes the precise production of speech sounds. The ability of our system of speech communication to tolerate slight changes in articulatory placement for both vowels and consonants without affecting their value is therefore vital to speech comprehension. Since speech is not made up of sounds used individually, but of sounds put together in a series, this tolerance permits us to maintain values at high rates of transmission. In connected speech, the movement from one articulatory position to another is often as important as the position itself. This movement is called the *transition*. The spectrum of connected speech shows that much of speech is transitional. Figure 3.14 shows a spectrum of a word. This type of spectrum differs from a line spectrum in that the ordinate now represents

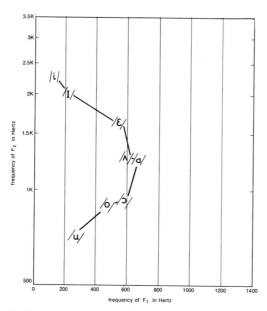

Fig. 3.13. A plot of the frequencies of formants 1 and 2.

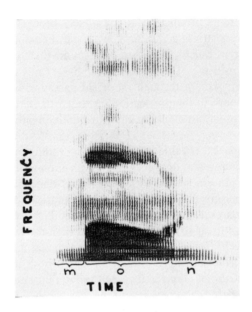

Fig. 3.14. An actual bar spectrum illustrating transition.

frequency while the abscissa depicts time. The amplitude of these formants is shown by the darkness of the frequency bars. The transitions indicated by arrows above this spectrum show that the articulators, primarily the tongue, are moving toward the place of articulation for each consonant sound, but do not necessarily have to reach a specific frequency. The articulators are moving toward a target—the target being the place of articulation for each consonant sound. However, because of the rapidity of speech, it is often necessary to move the articulators into another position before the target is reached. This movement toward the target is sufficient to give the consonant its proper identification value.

RECEPTION OF SPEECH

The chief mechanism for the normal reception of speech is the auditory system. However, the entire auditory range, 20 to 20,000 Hz, is not necessary for the identification of speech sounds, since as will be seen in Fig. 3.15, which also shows the relative sensation levels of each formant, the major frequency components fall within the range 250 to 8000 Hz, sometimes

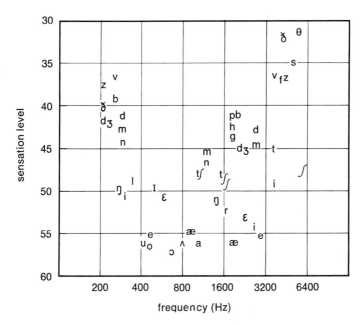

Fig. 3.15. Sensation level and frequency characteristics of speech sounds (modified from H. Fletcher [3]).

referred to as the speech range of hearing. This range includes the first and second formants of vowels as well as those of voiced consonants. The major energy concentrations of voiceless consonants also fall within these frequency limits.

You will recall that we explained that the first two formants are essential for the discrimination of vowel sounds; however, consonant-sound identification is more dependent upon the ability to receive the higher frequency components. If these are inaudible, the place of consonant articulation cannot be determined, thus precluding identification. Such a situation can arise when a listener suffers from high-frequency deafness and may be aggravated by the presence of environmental acoustic noise. Under such circumstances, the listener will become dependent upon other sources of information, usually the visual channel, as a means of obtaining the necessary cues to the identity of the consonants.

Consonant discrimination may also be significantly affected by a decrease in signal intensity. As is shown in Fig. 3.14, consonant components contain less energy than vowel sounds; thus, they are affected by loss of intensity far more rapidly than vowels. If a speech signal is made softer, it is often difficult to distinguish the consonant sounds. However, in syllables and words, vowels provide many cues to the recognition of consonants.

Actually, it is probably the transitional part of the syllable rather than the vowel itself that assists in this identification. Since vowels contain the greatest energy of all speech sounds, and transitions are similar to vowels, the information transmitted in these sounds requires considerable attenuation before it is lost.

If the reception of speech sounds is in any way interfered with, the intensity of the sound will be diminished, and thus it will sound softer. For the sound to have full intensity, all of the harmonics must be received. The removal of any harmonic by filtering or by attenuation, including that imposed by an impairment of auditory sensitivity, will reduce the overall intensity or loudness, even though intelligibility may not be affected. The effect that this will have upon the identification of the pitch characteristics of the voice will be minimal, providing the listener possesses enough hearing to permit him to receive several harmonics. Failure to receive either high or low frequencies will not destroy pitch identification. Pitch perception is possible even without understanding of what is said.

This chapter has dealt with the production and reception of sounds used in speech. It is these sounds that constitute the basic units of a spoken language. When the sounds are "strung together" in a predescribed manner, communication through speech may occur. Perception of the message communicated requires a more complex process than the simple reception of sounds. However, if the basic units cannot be accurately produced or received, this language cannot be used.

REFERENCES

1. Fairbanks, G., E. Herbert, and J. Hammond. "An Acoustical Study of the Vocal Pitch of Seven- and Eight-Year-Old Girls." *Child Development* 20 (1949) 71–78.

2. Fairbanks, G., J. Wiley, and F. Lassman. "An Acoustical Study of the Vocal Pitch of Seven- and Eight-Year-Old Boys." *Child Development* 20 (1949): 63–69.

3. Fletcher, H. *Speech and Hearing in Communication.* Princeton: D. Van Nostrand Company, Inc., 1953.

4. Gray, G., and C. Wise. *The Bases of Speech.* New York: Harper & Row, Publishers, 1959.

5. Hollien, H., E. Malcik, and B. Hollien. "Adolescent Voice Change in Southern White Males." *Speech Monographs* 32 (1965): 87–90.

6. Hollien, H., and P. Paul. "A Second Evaluation of the Speaking Fundamental Frequency Characteristics of Postadolescent Girls." *Language and Speech* 12 (1969): 119–24.

7. Ladefoged, P. *Elements of Acoustic Phonetics.* Chicago: University of Chicago Press, 1962.

8. Linke, E. "A Study of the Pitch Characteristics of Female Voices and Their Relationship to Vocal Effectiveness." Ph.D dissertation, University of Iowa, 1953.

9. McGlone, R. "Vocal Pitch Characteristics of Children Aged One and Two Years." *Speech Monographs* 33 (1966): 178–81.

10. McGlone, R., and H. Hollien. "Vocal Pitch Characteristics of Aged Women." *Journal of Speech and Hearing Research* 6 (1963): 164–170.

11. Mysak, E. "Pitch and Duration Characteristics of Older Males." *Journal of Speech and Hearing Research* 2 (1959): 46–54.

12. Ringel, R., and D. Kluppel. "Neonatal Crying: A Normative Study." *Folia Phoniatrica* 16 (1964): 1–9.

CHAPTER FOUR

The Visual Aspects
of Communication

Our concern with the visual aspects of communication arises from recognition of the increased role that vision plays for the hard-of-hearing person as a result of the reduction of the amount of information received through the auditory channel. Since vision is to play such an important part in communication, it is essential to check to be sure that the hearing-impaired child or adult is not doubly handicapped by a visual pathway that is not functioning at the best possible level.

In order to understand the contribution that may be made by vision in the communication process, we need a basic familiarity with the eye, the way in which it functions, and the types of visual disorders that may impair the person's ability to derive information from visual cues to speech. The next few pages constitute a brief review of the salient aspects of this material.

THE HUMAN EYE

An examination of the structure of a human eye reveals a marked similarity to the structure of a camera (Fig. 4.1). The reason for this is that the two instruments are designed to perform essentially the same functions.

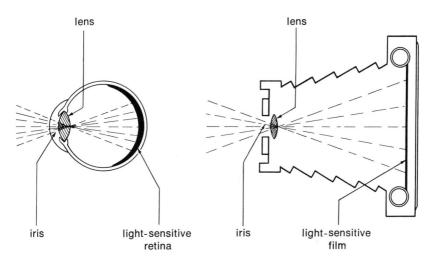

lens　　　　　　　　　　　　　lens

iris　　　light-sensitive　　　iris　　　light-sensitive
　　　　　retina　　　　　　　　　　　　film

Fig. 4.1. The structure of the human eye is fairly analogous to that of a camera.

This similarity makes it helpful to use the analogy of the camera in explaining the various components of the eye and their associated function. Figure 4.2 represents a cross-sectional diagram of the human eye. Close to the front of the eye, where the light enters, is the colored *iris*. In the center of the iris is a small hole to which we refer as the *pupil*. Embedded within the iris are a number of small muscle fibers that, by contraction and relaxation, control the size of the pupil, and thus the amount of light that is permitted to enter. When the light source is weak, the muscles of the iris contract, widening the pupil to permit more light to enter. Conversely, in a bright light, the pupil is narrowed to prevent an excess of light from entering the eye. The function of the iris is therefore identical to the opening and closing of the diaphragm of a camera.

In front of the pupil, at the front of the eye, is the curved, transparent *cornea,* which acts as a powerful lens. Just behind the pupil is a second lens. The purpose of the lenses in the camera and in the eye is to concentrate and focus light on photosensitive materials. In the camera, the focusing is achieved by varying the distance between the lens and the film. In the eye, focusing is accomplished by adjusting the curvature and thickness of the lens by the action of the *ciliary muscle.* This results in the bending of light rays passing through the various parts of the eye in order to focus them on the retina, a process known as *refraction.* In this way, the eye is able to be focused on near or far objects.

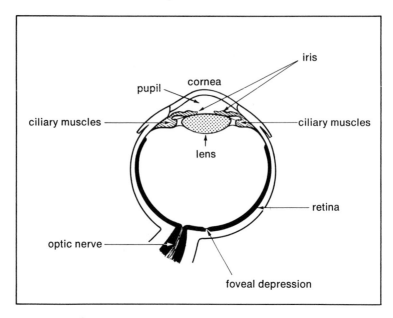

Fig. 4.2.　Horizontal section of the human eye.

The light passing through the lens of the camera is focused on a photo-sensitive film. In the eye, the light is focused on a thin membrane that lines the rear of the eyeball. This membrane, called the *retina,* contains the photo-sensitive nerve cells from which nerve fibers run to the brain. The function of the retina of the eye, with respect to light energy, is similar to that of the cochlea, with respect to sound energy. The role of the retina is to transduce the light stimulus into an electrical code that can be transmitted to the brain in the form of nerve impulses.

At a position on the retina directly opposite the pupil is a small depression known as the *fovea,* which constitutes the center of clear vision. When we concentrate our attention on a small object in order to see it clearly, we turn our eyes so that the light reflected from the object is focused upon the fovea. As one moves away from the foveal depression, both form and color are less clearly perceived.

The movement of the eyes within their sockets is achieved by the action of the optic muscles. Two distinct patterns of movement may be observed. In the first, the eyes perform an identical movement, working together in unison. This type of movement is used for distance vision, as occurs when viewing scenery. The second type of movement involves the independent movement of each eye, resulting in the convergence of the eyes upon a given point. This movement is obvious when a person is asked to fixate his gaze on a pencil point that is then moved closer and closer to his face.

Factors Influencing Visibility

The efficiency of the human eye is markedly reduced when the light intensity is either strongly increased or reduced. The reader will be familiar with the effect of extinguishing the lights in a bright room. The initial reaction is that one is in total darkness. However, one gradually becomes able to distinguish the shapes of objects that were previously not visible. This phenomenon is known as *dark adaptation*. Similarly, sudden exposure to bright light after a period in a relatively darkened room results in a sensation of glare until one's eyes adapt to the new light conditions. To the hard-of-hearing subject, adaptation is very important in communication, since he is dependent upon the visible aspects of speech as an aid to comprehension. If he moves from brightness to a dimly lighted environment, he will experience a temporary decrease in visual sensitivity because of the low light. He will experience similar difficulty in bright light.

Visual acuity can be defined as the ability of the eye to distinguish fine details. Perhaps the most important factor affecting visual acuity is the light intensity. The amount of light that needs to be present in the environment to permit the clearest vision will vary depending upon the nature of the visual task. Generally speaking, the finer the nature of the work the eyes are required to do, the more illumination is required. For example, one may be able to peal an apple, count coins, or arrange flowers in a relatively poor light. However, the threading of a needle, removal of a splinter from a finger, or the reading of small print on a label, all necessitate a much greater amount of illumination. Up to a point, one's performance on even larger tasks may be improved by the provision of extra light; however, too much intensity will produce glare, which reduces acuity. It must be remembered that the light must be directed on the activity or object being observed; if the light is directed towards the viewer, it will tend to decrease his ability to perform the task accurately.

Another important factor in determining the fineness of details observed by the eye concerns the angle at which the light strikes the retina. When one focuses upon an object, the light reflected from that object is directed upon the fovea of the retina. One's ability to see an object 20° to one side of the center of focus is reduced to a visual-acuity level approximately one-tenth of the foveal vision, since the light rays at this position will not be as sharply focused [5]. This is why, in teaching deaf children the names of objects or in talking about a picture, we try to bring the object or the book close to the speaker's face so that both may be seen in clear focus.

Visual acuity is also affected by the distance between the eye and the object being observed. The greater the separation, the poorer visual acuity becomes. The background against which the object is placed will also affect the clarity with which it may be seen. The use of the defensive technique of camouflage illustrates this. An object is most easily seen when it stands out clearly against the background. For example, lip movements may be more noticeable when a woman wears bright red lipstick; they are also more clearly seen from the front of the room than from the rear. In teaching hearing-impaired persons and when giving advice concerning the seating position of a child in class or an adult at a committee or group meeting, we should remember that adequate lighting on a speaker's face and protection of the viewer from glare will facilitate the use of vision as an aid to communication. Seating that permits the hearing-impaired person to hold the speaker's face in clear focus from a short distance will considerably aid speech communication.

A major part of all information reaching a normal hearing individual comes to him through his eyes. For the hard-of-hearing subject, the amount is increased. Even mildly defective vision may prove to affect significantly the understanding of speech.

It will be recalled from our discussion of the function of the human eye that the process of focusing light energy upon the retina is achieved through bending or refracting the light waves. When the light is reflected from objects close to the individual, it tends to spread outwards. This requires a much greater amount of refraction in order to obtain the necessary focus than is essential for distance vision.

The relatively few people who possess perfect vision do so because the eyeball is so shaped that it provides focus for distance vision without adjustments to the shape of the lenses. The amount of adjustment necessary for close vision is very small; neither near nor far vision places the eyes under strain. An abnormality in shape or size of the eyeball is liable to result in a distortion of the normal refractive process, to the extent that it may cause a decrease in visual acuity, discomfort, or interference with the coordinated action of the two eyes. These defects in vision are known as refractive errors, and they fall under three headings: *myopia* (nearsightedness), *hyperopia* (farsightedness), and *astigmatism*.

Myopia

Myopia results from an abnormal elongation of the shape of the eyeball (Fig. 4.3). As a result, the light rays emanating from distant objects come into focus at a point before they reach the retina. Thus, the image of distant objects is blurred. Near vision remains unimpaired, since the light rays from near objects come into focus farther back and fall on the retina. A child with such a defect would not have difficulty in observing facial expressions and lip movements of a speaker close to him, but would be unable to make use of these visual clues to speech on a person at twenty feet from him. He might be unable to recognize faces at this distance.

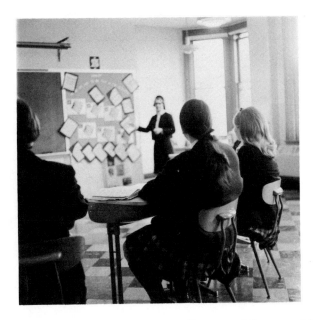

Fig. 4.3. Myopic vision blurs objects at a distance, while near vision remains unimpaired. (Courtesy of St. Mary's School for the Deaf, Buffalo, New York.)

In the classroom or therapy session, the child with a hearing impairment depends heavily on visual aids and information presented on the blackboard. He derives great help from seeing new or difficult vocabulary written up, from seeing the written outline of subject material and key words associated with it, and from written instructions or assignments. A myopic child without glasses will encounter difficulty in seeing the blackboard. He may be unable to read or may misinterpret what has been written. More serious is the general overall reduction in the amount of information that he is receiving. A hard-of-hearing person with normal vision may be able to manage adequately in communication situations when supported by a program of aural rehabilitation. The same person deprived of adequate visual information to augment the auditory signal may find it quite impossible to function in the same situations. This is particularly true for the child in school.

Hyperopia

Hyperopia results from a shorter-than-normal distance between the cornea and the retina (Fig. 4.4). As a result, the visual image is still not in focus by the time the light waves reach the retina. In an attempt to com-

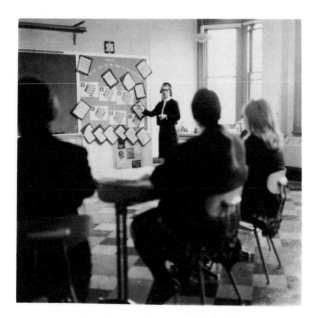

Fig. 4.4.   Hyperopia results in the blurring of objects close to the viewer, while those at a distance remain clear. (Courtesy of St. Mary's School for the Deaf, Buffalo, New York.)

pensate for this loss of focus, the ciliary muscles, which control the shape and thickness of the lens, must contract strongly. This process, called *accommodation*, is necessary even for distance vision, while a much greater amount of contraction is involved in producing a clear image of objects close to the viewer. If the ciliary muscles are strong, as is common in children, a person may be able to māke the necessary adjustment in order to be able to carry out close work without difficulty. This, however, involves placing a strain upon the optic muscles, and it may give rise to such symptoms as periodic blurring of the visual image, a short visual attention span, or headaches. These symptoms are most likely to occur in connection with tasks requiring fine visual acuity, one of which is the interpretation of the visual articulatory movements of speech. Hyperopia may therefore seriously impair a hard-of-hearing person's ability to capitalize on the visual cues of speech. A speaker may appear quite clear when seen at a distance, as will any visual aids that are used. In a more personal communication situation, however, in which the speaker is much closer, as in a tutoring relationship or in a small group, the face and lip movements will appear blurred, depriving the listener of the cues embodied in the visible articulatory movements of speech.

Astigmatism

An astigmatism arises from an irregularity in the curve of the cornea. This results in the uneven focusing of light rays originating from the same source. The fact that some of the rays are focused farther back than others produces a blurred distortion of the image on the retina. Objects may appear fuzzy, may be elongated or flattened. Astigmatism is a condition that may be found both in isolation and also associated with either hyperopia or myopia. With this type of visual problem, the observer may find part of the object viewed to be in focus while other parts are out of focus. This can be particularly disturbing to a person who is attempting to focus vision upon a speaker. As the speaker moves, different parts of the image of him will be in focus.

In addition, problems may arise that affect the fusion of the image from both eyes. These conditions are *impairment of binocular vision.*

Since the human being has his two eyes placed in a single plane in the front of his head, the visual images of the same object are focused simultaneously on the retina of each eye. A brain mechanism, unique to man, fuses these images so that the observer perceives only a single object. An even subtler feature of binocular vision is made possible by the separation of the two eyes by an average of sixty-five millimeters in the adult. Due to this separation, a slight disparity exists in the positions of the two corresponding images on the two retinae. This disparity is responsible for depth perception, known professionally as *stereopsis.* There are several visual clues available for the judgment of distance, such as parallax and differences in size and brightness, but true depth perception is possible only as a result of this image disparity associated with binocularity. Any disfunction in this fusional ability and stereopsis, especially in children, will interfere with the spatial orientation of the individual. In severe cases this may result in double vision (*diplopia*).

A loss of binocular vision may also occur in the condition in which the eyes are crossed, or in which a single eye turns outward or inward. This condition may result from a severe refractive error in one eye. If the amount of accommodation necessary to correct this refractive error is too great for the ciliary muscles to achieve, the poor eye will cease the attempt, leaving the task of maintaining visual acuity to the better eye. Since the distorted vision of the poor eye will no longer be of use, that eye will tend to converge. In time, this inactivity leads to a complete suppression of the visual image received from the poor eye, resulting in what may prove to be permanent changes in the function of the ciliary muscles. For all practical purposes, the eye becomes blind. To a hard-of-hearing person, either of these conditions would constitute an added handicap, since there would be serious impairment of his sense of distance as well as direction, both of which may already be affected by the hearing impairment, as will be explained in the next chapter.

These five types of visual problems are common to children and adults alike. Two additional visual hazards are encountered by adults, both of which may result in serious damage to vision. These are *glaucoma* and *cataract*.

Glaucoma

Usually an ailment found in adults, glaucoma affects 2 per cent of people over 40, though occasionally it may be present in children and young adults. An increase in the pressure of the fluid in the eye jeopardizes both the optic nerve and its blood supply. Glaucoma may develop so slowly that the subject is unaware of the gradual loss of vision until the condition is fairly advanced. Some early symptoms may be: mild headaches or aching eyes, both of which may occur after viewing television or movies; transitory blurring of vision; poor vision in dim light; halos around lights; or partial loss of side vision.

Cataract

Cataract involves "a cloudiness of the lens of the eye which blocks the normal passage of light rays through the pupil to the retina [12]." This may produce blurring of near and distance vision, black spots in the visual field, or a phenomenon by which parts of objects appear to be missing. The symptoms vary according to the part of the lens that is affected.

Any of the symptoms listed for either of these conditions necessitates prompt consultation with a medically qualified eye specialist (ophthalmologist). The effect these problems produce upon visual communication cues will be similar to those produced by the other visual defects discussed.

It is important to note that the two periods in life when visual problems are most likely to appear first are during the early school years and during middle age. These are the same periods when impairment of hearing is also most frequently detected. Furthermore, some of the conditions that cause deafness are also likely to result in defects in vision. The most noticeable of these are maternal rubella, which affects the infant, particularly when the mother contracted the disease during the first three months of pregnancy, and increasing age in the adult, which produces a deterioration of both the visual function (*presbyosis*), and the auditory function (*presbycusis*).

Although many adults become aware of the fact that they are experiencing difficulty with visual acuity, the amount of deterioration is often fairly marked before it draws attention to itself. Up to this time, the person has been unconsciously compensating for the problem he is experiencing.

It is also possible that he will, to a certain extent, psychologically reject the idea that he might need glasses. A person who wears them might not want to go to the expense of reexamination and possible replacement of his current pair. The visual difficulty may therefore only evidence itself for the hard-of-hearing person as part of the total deterioration in the ability to communicate. The person is unable to compensate to any marked degree for the loss of hearing by greater dependence upon vision. In a visual communication training class he may suggest all manner of reasons why he has been unable to develop this skill. It may not occur to him that he may be calling upon his eyes to perform a task that is too fine for his visual acuity to handle.

The problem of poor visual acuity in young children is even more likely to remain undetected unless the eyes are tested. The child with a visual defect may be quite unaware that the world should appear any differently from the way he sees it. Furthermore, in the early years most children tend to be farsighted. Thus, the gradual onset of myopia, most commonly occurring during the first few years of school, may escape detection. It is not until the visual deterioration evidences itself in the child's failure to make progress in school that visual acuity is questioned. The hard-of-hearing child stands in double jeopardy in this respect. We are only too likely to attribute his educational retardation entirely to his hearing impairment and in doing so completely overlook the role of vision.

In keeping with our concern for the total process of communication, it is essential that we make particularly certain that, in addition to providing the hard-of-hearing subject with every possible help in receiving and interpreting the auditory signal, we also insure that the visual pathway is operating at its optimum level. This requires that each subject with a hearing impairment receive a thorough examination of visual function by an ophthalmologist or optometrist,* and that reexamination of vision is made every two years.

VISIBILITY OF THE MESSAGE SIGNAL

Up to this point we have been concerned with those factors that directly affect the ability of the eye to detect visible cues related to the message signal.

---

*Ophthalmologist: A medical doctor who specializes in the medical diagnosis and treatment of defects of the eye. This includes the use of surgery and the prescription of glasses.

Optometrist: A nonmedical specialist qualified to test vision, provide glasses, and conduct visual training. He is not qualified to treat diseases of the eye or to recommend medical or surgical treatment.

Optician: A person trained to grind lenses and fit glasses according to the prescription provided by the ophthalmologist or optometrist.

We must now consider the nature of the visible stimuli in human communication. Our discussion will concentrate upon the properties of visible cues that determine the degree to which they will be visible to the observer. The factors that affect the manner in which this information is actually perceived —that is, the way in which meaning is ascribed to what is seen—will be discussed in the next chapter.

The visible stimuli with which we are concerned may be divided into three categories:

1. Stimuli arising from the environment in which the communication occurs.
2. Stimuli associated directly with the message, but not part of speech production.
3. Stimuli directly associated with the production of speech sounds.

Environmental Stimuli

Communication between individuals necessarily takes place in a physical environment. It is against this background that the message signal, received by the listener, will be interpreted. Nonspeech stimuli arising from people or objects may therefore prove useful in the interpretation of the message signal if they are received by the eye. For the most part, environmental cues suffer least from poor viewing conditions. It is nevertheless important to recognize that such factors as low light intensity, dark adaptation, position of the stimulus object within the viewer's visual field will all influence to some extent the ability of the observer to make use of this background information. In a communication situation, a person is able to encompass a large number of objects and people at a single glance. It is from this massive amount of stimuli that he will select those that he considers to have a probable relationship to the content of the message signal being received by him.

The role of environment is easily understood if we consider the effect that theatrical scenery and costumes have on the interpretation of the actual words of a play. We interpret what is said in the light of the scene in which it is said. We must therefore be able to see the scenery clearly. The lighting director often makes use of this by opening the scene in darkness and then gradually raising the light intensity level until a background is provided against which the dialogue may be interpreted. Similarly, he may focus the lighting on one particular section of the stage, thus eliminating the remainder of the scenery from the context, changing the relative emphasis on various actors and items of scenery. In this way, variations of period, time, and place may be conveyed within a stage set.

In a more everyday setting, imagine yourself joining a group of people at a table in a dimly lit restaurant. The phenomenon of dark adaptation, together with the low intensity, may deny you the benefit of interpreting a spoken message about someone or something in the environment against the background of visual clues. Again, it may be emphasized that the limitations that this places on the already handicapped communication system of the hard-of-hearing person, may sufficiently reduce the total amount of information to a level that denies comprehension.

Nonspeech Stimuli Directly Related to the Speaker

Under this category we include body posture; body movement, including gesture; and facial expressions. Each of these aspects of communication behavior are capable of conveying information concerning events that have preceded the sending of a message, and concerning factors that lie behind the message at the time it is being transmitted [3]. The actual way in which these may be interpreted will be considered in more detail in the next chapter. At this point it will suffice to say that when a person is denied the benefit of seeing these cues clearly he is denied an additional source of information. We recognize this when, at a lecture or a discussion, we attempt to seat ourselves in a position that permits us to see the speaker clearly. We do this even when we know we will have no difficulty in hearing what is said. When the acoustic conditions are poor, as is frequently true for churches and some meeting halls, we are particularly anxious to insure that we are not denied the additional help that we, as normal hearing subjects, derive from watching the visible aspects of the speaker's delivery.

Poor visual acuity, resulting from defective vision or environmental conditions, is likely to have a marked effect upon the ability of a person to see the speaker's face clearly. If you wear glasses you will know how troublesome it is to attend a lecture without them, and as a result to have to listen to a speaker whose face appears blurred. The same annoyance is experienced when a theatre stage is poorly lit or a movie is slightly out of focus. In choosing a seat at a play or lecture, we like to sit near the front, since being seated at a distance deprives us of a clear view of facial expressions. This indicates that even persons with normal hearing utilize to some extent the additional information conveyed by the visual channel.

We may therefore conclude that the ability to receive both environmental stimuli and nonspeech stimuli originating from the speaker is important in determining whether we will be able to understand a spoken message, particularly when the acoustic signal is distorted.

Visible Aspects of Speech Production

The production of various speech sounds is made possible by the modification of air flow from the lungs brought about by the changes in the shape and size of the supralaryngeal resonators. These changes involve the movement and positioning of the jaw, lips, tongue, and soft palate. Each speech sound involves a distinctive articulatory movement. Under favorable viewing conditions, part, but seldom all, of this movement will be visible to an observer. A movement may be considered as having a *formative aspect* and a *revealing aspect*. The formative aspect includes the movement of all articulators essential to the production of a particular sound; the revealing aspect involves only those articulators that may be seen to be involved in or associated with its production. For example, the formative aspect of the speech sound *sh* /ʃ/ involves elevation of the soft palate, the grooving of the tongue, and the elevation of the sides of the tongue to make contact with the upper teeth. None of these movements are easily visible. The revealing movement associated with /ʃ/ is the puckering and protrusion of the lips, a movement associated with, but not essential to, the acoustic production of the sound.

In a number of phonemes some of the formative movements may also be revealing, as are the lip movements in the production of the bilabial plosives /p/ and /b/, or as is the tongue movement in the production of the voiced and unvoiced lingual dental fricatives /θ/ and /ð/.

Since these visible stimuli arise directly from the production of a specific phoneme, they provide a valuable source of additional information concerning the spoken word. If it were possible for the eyes to receive and identify each phoneme or word spoken purely on the basis of its visible characteristics, and if the conditions for viewing the speaker were always optimal, then the hard-of-hearing subject would not be handicapped by his inability to receive the auditory signal correctly. Rehabilitation of the hearing-impaired person would simply involve training the person to replace the use of his ears by his eyes in the reception of the message signal. Unfortunately this is not the case. The visible aspects of speech are subject to a number of important limitations that exist within the visual message signal itself, within the environment through which it travels, and within the person who is acting as the receiver. At this time, we shall concern ourselves only with the factors that pertain to the message signal and the environment. Factors within the receiver will be discussed later as an aspect of visual perception.

Four major factors influence the usefulness of the visual signal as a conveyor of information. These are as follows:

1. The degree of visibility of the movement.
2. The rapidity of articulatory movements.
3. The similarity of the visual characteristics of the articulatory movements involved in the production of different speech sounds.

4. Intersubject variations in the visible aspects of articulatory movements involved in the production of any given sound.

The Degree of Visibility

The visual recognition of the speech sound is dependent upon the revealing aspects involved in its production. These vary considerably for each phoneme. The only phoneme that can truly be said to possess no revealing visible characteristic in its production is the aspirate /h/; however for a considerable number of phonemes the revealing characteristics are relatively obscure, and accuracy of recognition can not be absolutely guaranteed even for a trained observer.

A study undertaken by the American Society for the Hard of Hearing [15], investigated the relative visibility of different phonemes. Using a value system that classified sounds into four categories ranging from complete visibility to zero visibility, they devised a system for calculating the measure of visibility for any speech sample. A modified table of the relative visibility of speech sounds, using this scale, is presented in Table 4.1. The percentage visibility of a word or sentence can be calculated by assigning each phoneme the maximum visibility value for its category; that is,

Category	Value
I	1.00
II	0.75
III	0.50
IV	0.25

The individual values are then added and divided by the total number of phonemes. Multiplication of the quotient by 100 provides a percentage-visibility figure. The formula for calculating percentage visibility is therefore:

$$\frac{\text{Percentage}}{\text{visibility}} = \frac{\Sigma \text{ individual phoneme values}}{\text{the total number of phonemes}} \times \frac{100}{1}$$

For example,

most speech sounds are fairly visible.

mou s p i tʃ sɑunz ə fɛəlɪ vɪzɪbl

TABLE 4.1. Degree of Visibility

CATEGORY

IV	III	II	I
0–0.25	0.26–0.50	0.51–0.75	0.76–1.00

CONSONANTS

[k] as in *k*ite	[s] as in *s*it		[l] as in let	[p] as in pay	
[g]	good	[z]	zebra		[b]	boy
[ŋ]	sing	[t]	toy		[ʃ]	ship
[h]	hat	[d]	dog		[ʒ]	pleasure
		[n]	no		[tʃ]	church
		[r]	red		[dʒ]	jump
					[f]	fish
					[v]	very
					[θ]	think
					[ð]	the
					[m]	mouse
					[j]	yacht
					[w]	weep

VOWELS AND
DIPHTHONGS*

[ɛ] as in pen	[eɪ] as in make		[ɑ] as in father	
[ɪ]	bid	[i]	he	[ɔ]	fall
[ɝ]	bird	[ɛɝ]	fair	[æ]	cat
[ʊ]	put	[ɑɪ]	my	[ou]	no
[ʌ]	hut	[ɪə]	here	[u]	move
[ə]	about			[ɔi]	boy
				[ɑu]	house

*Double consonants, such as [bl], [fr], involve one movement.

Value:

$$1 + 1 + .5 + 1 + .75 + 1 \quad .5 + 1 + .5 + .5 \quad + .5 \quad 1 + .75 + .75 + .5$$
$$1 + .5 + .5 + .5 + 1 + .75$$

Total phoneme value   = 15.5

Total number of phonemes = 21

Percentage visibility   = 73.8 per cent

$$\frac{15.5}{21} \times \frac{100}{1} = 73.8 \text{ per cent}$$

or: Her hat isn't in here Katy.

                            hə hæt ɪznt ɪn hɪə keɪtɪ

Value: .25 + .5 + .25 + .25 +.5   + .5 + .5 + .5 +.5   .5 + .5   .25 +
                            .75 + .5 + .5

        Total phoneme value   = 7.75
        Total number of phonemes = 17
        Percentage visibility   = 45.6 per cent

From these two examples it may be seen that the visibility of sentences can vary quite considerably. The range of visibility of normal conversational sentences was found to vary from a minimum of 47 per cent to a maximum of 83 per cent, with the average falling between 65 and 70 per cent.

Rapidity of Articulatory Movements

Edward B. Nitchie [9] has pointed out that in ordinary conversational speech a speaker averages approximately 13 articulatory movements per second. The eye, on the other hand, is capable of consciously recording eight or nine movements per second. According to these figures, the eye therefore misses approximately a quarter of all sounds produced, though it must be remembered that not all of the sounds are clearly visible to the observer in the first place. Nitchie draws our attention to the fact that although the average duration of the articulatory movement is one-thirteenth of a second, speech sounds are produced that are both shorter and longer in duration. Using a motion picture camera, filming at 16 frames per second, he found that many of the speech sounds were too rapid to be recorded by the camera, indicating a duration of less than one-sixteenth of a second. The consonants were found to be of shorter duration than the long vowels, which had a duration of two-sixteenths to three-sixteenths per second, although some short vowels were articulated as quickly as many of the consonants.

The importance of the rate of articulation is supported by the findings of Marigene Mulligan [7] in an investigation that included a study of the effect that speed of projection of a movie film had on the viewer's scores on a test of "lipreading." She showed the film at two speeds—slow, 16 frames per second, and normal, 24 frames per second—and found that the slowest speed resulted in higher scores on the test.

On the other hand, a later study conducted by V. W. Byers and L. Lieberman [1], produced contrary evidence. They subjected four groups of experienced lipreaders from a school for the deaf to a sentence lipreading test adapted from the Utley test [13]. By modifying the speed in filming and the speed of projection, they were able to produce controlled variations in the speaker's rate of utterance. Using four rates, normal (120 words per minute), and two-thirds, one-half, and one-third slower than normal rate, they studied the subject's performance on the test under each condition. The results indicated no significant differences between the four rates of presentation. The authors concluded that, within the range studied, variation in rate did not affect the degree of correct recognition of the visible aspects of the spoken word. This was found in spite of the fact that one of the rates was one-third of normal, and in spite of complaints from the viewers that the films were being shown at too slow a speed. They were of the impression that lipreading skill is adaptable to quite an extensive range of articulatory rates.

The reason for the discrepancy between the results in these two studies may rest within the subjects used. Mulligan's findings are based on the performance of college students with normal hearing, while those of Byers and Lieberman were obtained from a group of deaf subjects, all of whom had had at least two years of formal lipreading training. It may well be that we are not justified in generalizing data collected on subjects with normal hearing to the performance of subjects with hearing impairment. It has been demonstrated by W. H. Sumby and I. Pollack [11], Keith N. Neely [8], and S. J. Goodrich [2] that for subjects with normal hearing increased distortion of the auditory aspects of speech results in an increased dependence upon the use of visual cues. It may reasonably be presumed that a subject with a marked congenital auditory impairment will have come to depend heavily upon the contribution that vision is capable of making to speech intelligibility. This dependence will undoubtedly have resulted in a degree of skill in making use of this information, a skill that the subject with normal hearing has not been called upon to develop. When each of these two groups, the normal and the hard-of-hearing, are presented with a task involving the ability to obtain information through the recognition of visible speech characteristics, the hard-of-hearing subject is at an advantage. As a sophisticated user of visual information, his tolerance for changes in speech rate is much greater than that of the person with normal hearing who finds that he performs best when the material is presented at a slower speed.

If this is in fact so, then it has important implications for the training of beginning lipreaders. Factors that may not be important for the sophisticated lipreader may well be crucial in the early learning stages. The role of rapidity of articulatory movements in the learning and maintenance of visual communication requires more investigation before we can confidently say that rate is not important.

The Similarity of Visible Articulatory Movements

As was explained in our discussion of the acoustics of speech, each phoneme in the English language has a unique acoustic structure. The phonetic alphabet recognizes this in that, unlike the alphabet of written English, there exists a discrete symbol for each sound. The uniqueness in acoustic structure is due to the fact that no two sounds are articulated in exactly the same way. In other words, for a given sound the formative movements that constitute the total articulatory movements are different from the formative movements of all other sounds. This is not, however, true for the revealing movements, which are confined only to the articulatory movements that are visible. Many speech sounds are revealed by identical visible movements. Such sounds are known as homophenes.* The adjective *homophenous* may be applied both to individual phonemes such as /p/, /b/, /m/, which are identical in revealing movements; to groups of phonemes such as /nt/ and /nd/; or to words, such as *bad, mat, pan.* In normal conversational speech it is quite impossible to distinguish between homophenous items. A study of the vowels and consonants of English indicates that the vowels do not exhibit any strictly homophenous formation, though some of the vowel sounds do present difficulty and only appear different to a trained observer. A list of homophenous groupings of consonants is given in Table 4.2. The homophenous groupings of consonants indicated in this table were established by Mary F. Woodward [15]. She made a linguistic analysis of the phonological, grammatical, and lexical aspects of lipreading stimulus materials and hypothesized that the absolute visibility of a given speech item was dependent upon the area of articulatory placement involved. She presented a filmed series of paired syllables to a group of subjects with normal hearing who were asked to judge the two items as same or different. From an analysis of the results, she established the consonant classifications already indicated. Woodward concluded that, although in context it is possible to distinguish between many of the phonemes within a set, differentiation cannot be based upon visual comparison alone. It must be concluded, therefore, that the visual similarity of homophenes compels the observer to rely on the linguistic redundancy of the material to provide him with the information necessary to differentiate between them.

TABLE 4.2.   Homophenous Clusters of Initial English Consonants (after Woodward [15])

(a)	p	b	m						
		f	v						
	m	w	r						
(b)	ch	dȝ	ʃ	ȝ	j				
	t	d	n	l	s	z	θ	ð	
	k	g	h						

*The term *homophenes,* which refers to phonemes that are identical in the visible aspects of their articulation, should not be confused with the similar term *homophones,* which refers to letters or symbols that have the same sound as others.

On the basis of tests conducted with different passages representing colloquial English, Nitchie [9] estimated that almost every word contains one or more homophenous sounds, that more than 40 per cent of the total number of sounds in the test sample have one or more sounds homophenous to them, and furthermore, that approximately 50 per cent of the words in the sample constitute homophenes of one or more other words.

Intra- and Inter-subject Variation of Articulatory Movements

Careful analysis of the speech of a given individual reveals that the manner of articulation of a given speech sound varies at each production. It has been demonstrated experimentally that exact duplication of the manner of production is not possible, even when a subject makes a special effort to achieve this. The variation, which always exists to some degree, is frequently found to be quite considerable. While these deviations are observed in the production of all speech sounds, they are especially noticeable in the production of vowels. In spite of these variations, there exists for each phoneme a fundamental movement pattern, which remains essentially the same. C. E. Kantner and R. West [4, p. 29] use the analogy of movements involved in writing to illustrate this point. They explain that while letters of the alphabet may be produced in a variety of different ways, the movements tend to become stereotyped within an individual, making it possible to identify a person by his handwriting. The expert is able to recognize these stereotypes even when an attempt has been made to disguise them.

In the production of speech sounds within the individual, this stereotyping occurs as a result of the necessity to insure that the acoustic characteristics remain within the limits of a phoneme in order that the meaning of a group of phonemes (word) is not interfered with. A second factor is the influence of a physiological tendency to stereotype movements.

When we extend our interest in the variability in speech-sound production to the changes occurring in a way in which different people produce a given speech sound, we find that the differences are frequently quite marked. It has been suggested that these interpersonal variations can be attributed to three causes: (1) variations in anatomical structure of the speech mechanism; (2) interpersonal differences in auditory perception of speech sounds; (3) regional or social variations occurring where speech sounds have developed in a different manner from those of people in other areas or social milieux.

Obviously, the stereotyping of sound production between individuals is dependent upon the acoustic factor. Auditory feedback insures that the output, that is, the acoustic pattern of the speech sound, stays within the person's perceptual limits for that particular phoneme. It is these limits, rather than the specific articulatory movements, that different speakers have in common. Since within the phonemic limits it is possible to produce a sound in a variety of ways, it is understandable that the visible, or revealing, characteristics may vary somewhat from person to person.

As we have already noted, a careful comparison of the visible characteristics of English phonemes indicates that for some the movements essential to the normal production of the sound, that is, those upon which the phonemic value of the sound is dependent, are quite visible to an observer. In these instances, the sound may be considered to be formed and revealed by the same movement. For other sounds, the formative movement is concealed from the observer. However it has been demonstrated that the articulation of certain phonemes commonly involves movements of groups of facial muscles that are quite unnecessary for the normal production of the acoustic properties of the sound [6]. These movements constitute associated, but under normal conditions of oral communication, unessential, accompaniments to the formative movements.

It would seem rather odd that an organism should preserve such apparently useless movements. The answer rests, perhaps, in the underlying philosophy of this text, namely, the totality of the act of communication. Viewed in the light of this, we may presume that these seemingly unimportant movements do, in fact, have a role to play. Although they do not contribute to the recognition of the acoustic aspects of the sound, they are directly associated with it. They constitute, therefore, part of the total identity of the sound. Under normal listening conditions, we do not need to make use of these visible characteristics; however, under conditions of auditory distortion, recognition of the sound may be dependent upon the ability of the listener to utilize this built-in visual redundancy. For example, for many hearing-impaired subjects, the recognition of such sounds as /sh/ and /s/ is dependent upon the associated secondary lip rounding and lip spreading, since the formative movement, which is lingual alveolar, is practically invisible.

It is the secondary movements that are most subject to variation. The visible aspects of a sound that is revealed by its associated rather than by its formative movements may vary sufficiently from one speaker to another to present a problem of identification. As will be explained in the following chapter, the recognition of vowel phonemes is a function of auditory judgment rather than the exact nature or the extent of the movement. The pitch, resonant qualities, and duration are all important contributing factors. The actual articulatory movements of vowel production vary considerably, making it difficult to differentiate between them on the basis of their visible appearance. Consonants, on the other hand, require more exact positioning of the articulators and tend, therefore, to exhibit somewhat less variability of revealing characteristics. When we examine the visual nature of the articulatory movements in consonant production, we find that a number are revealed by their secondary characteristics alone. Those that are considered visible are /r/, /s/, /z/, /t/, /ʃ/, /ʒ/, /j/. It is these consonants which are particularly subject to interspeaker variability.

We have discussed the four major factors that influence the usefulness of speech as a form of visual communication. We have also considered some of the conditions that are known to affect the efficiency of the human eye. These included the phenomenon of dark adaptation, variations in light intensity, the position of the object in the visual field of the observer, the distance between the eye and the object viewed, and the background against which the object is seen. In addition to these, we also discussed the affect of certain defects of vision. Unfortunately, when we look to the literature to provide us with data concerning the relationship between these various conditions and the communicative value of the visual aspects of speech, we find virtually none available. This is an area that urgently requires systematic investigation. Our conclusions must therefore be based upon information concerning how environmental conditions affect visual performance on other tasks. In general, we know that environmental conditions become increasingly critical as the fineness of the visual task increases. Our previous discussion has familiarized us with the limiting factors inherent within the visual message signal. The difficulty of the visual task is apparent.

We may therefore conclude that the value of the visual message signal in communication will be significantly influenced by the environmental conditions mentioned above. Until we have definite evidence to indicate the contrary, we must take these factors into consideration when planning rehabilitational training in the area of visual communication.

REFERENCES

1. Byers, V. W. and L. Lieberman. "Lipreading Performance and the Rate of the Speaker," *Journal of Speech and Hearing Research* 2 (1959): 271–76.

2. Goodrich, S. J., and D. Sanders. "The Relative Contributions of the Visual and Auditory Components of Speech to Speech Intelligibility as a Function of Three Conditions of Frequency Distortion." To appear in a forthcoming issue of *Journal of Speech and Hearing Research*.

3. Hall, E. T. *The Silent Language*. Garden City, N.Y.: Doubleday & Co., Inc., 1959.

4. Kantner, C. E., and R. West. *Phonetics*. New York: Harper & Row, Publishers, 1941.

5. Kendler, Howard H. *Basic Psychology*. New York: Appleton-Century-Crofts, 1963.

6. Lightoller, C. H. "Facial Muscles: The *Modiolus* and Muscles Surrounding

the *Rima Oris* with Some Remarks about the *Panniculus Adiposus.*" *Journal of Anatomy* 60 (1925): 2–45.

7. Mulligan, Marigene. "Variables in the Reception of Visual Speech from Motion Pictures." Unpublished Master's thesis, Ohio State University, 1954.

8. Neely, Keith N. "Effect of Visual Factors on the Intelligibility of Speech." *Journal of the Acoustical Society of America* 28 (1956): 1275–77.

9. Nitchie, Edward B. "Principles and Methods of Lipreading." New York: Nitchie School of Lipreading, *n.d.* Mimeographed pamphlet.

10. Parmenter, S. N., and C. E. Trevino. "Vowel Positions as Shown by X-Ray." *The Quarterly Journal of Speech* 8 (June 1932): 351–69.

11. Sumby, W. H., and I. Pollack. "Visual Contribution to Speech Intelligibility in Noise." *Journal of the Acoustical Society of America* 26 (1956): 1275–77.

12. U.S. Department of Health, Education and Welfare. *Cataract and Glaucoma.* Public Health Service Publication No. 793, Health Information Series No. 99. Washington, D.C.: Government Printing Office, 1963.

13. Utley, Jean. "A Test of Lipreading Ability." *Journal of Speech and Hearing Disorders* 11 (1946): 109–16.

14. W.P.A. Lipreading Project of the Board of Education. *News Aids and Materials for Teaching Lipreading.* New York: U.S.W.P.A. for the City of New York, 1939.

15. Woodward, Mary F. "Linguistic Methodology in Lipreading Research." *John Tracy Clinic Research Papers* 4 (December 1957).

CHAPTER FIVE

Auditory and Visual Perception

SOME GENERAL PRINCIPLES OF PERCEPTION

We have discussed the physical aspects of the visual and auditory stimuli that are considered relevant to an understanding of the communicative processes. We have also considered the sensitivity of the peripheral receptors of vision and audition and the factors that may affect this sensitivity. It was suggested (Fig. 2.6) that this initial receptive level is concerned only with sensations, which arise as a direct result of the stimulation of the peripheral receptor by environmental stimuli. In theory this is a relatively passive procedure. The receptor is acted upon; no part of the organism contributes anything to the sensory experience, which is entirely dominated by the stimulus. In practice, however, the human organism is incapable of remaining passive in the presence of a complex stimulus. Active involvement is invariably evidenced in the form of discrimination, differentiation, and interpretation of the stimulus. The resultant awareness of ourselves and the world around us is known as perception. When you pick up the phone in response to its ringing, turn down the flame when the milk begins to boil, or develop an appetite when you smell and hear bacon sizzling in the pan, you have done more than receive a stimulus; you have responded in a dis-

82

criminative manner. You have perceived a difference between a particular group of stimuli reaching you and all other stimuli and can therefore attribute a particular meaning to it. The whole complex structure of human communication is utterly dependent upon this ability. The newborn child or a person suffering from some types of cortical damage lacks this ability to discriminate between stimuli. It is therefore not possible for them to make meaningful responses to groups of stimuli. In our own area of study we observe that a hearing loss frequently impairs auditory discrimination sufficiently to prevent the listener from differentiating between the various speech sounds or, in severe cases, between environmental sounds. As a result, the auditory stimulus alone loses its usefulness as a conveyor of information.

It is quite clear that sensory perception constitutes the basis of all forms of adaptive behavior. The adjustment that a hearing-impaired person has to make to his environment is an instance of this behavior. Ideally, we would like to raise the level of the handicapped person's perception of his environment to the point where it differs from the norm, not in its accuracy, but only in the nature of the information upon which the total perception is based. C. M. Solly and P. Murphy point out that "There is a redundancy of environmental information that an individual utilizes in anticipating environmental events" [37, p. 154]. We are aiming to train the hearing-impaired person to compensate for his auditory communication deficit by the maximum use of this redundant perceptual information.

THE ROLE OF THE SENSES

Though we are particularly concerned with the role of hearing in speech communication, we should not forget that hearing, together with the other senses, has a more fundamental purpose. The three major functions of sensory perception are to provide information, protection, and orientation.

Our knowledge of our external world is gained entirely through stimuli reaching us through our internal and peripheral sense organs. These provide us with a continual flow of data concerning changes that occur in our environment and within our bodies. In this way we are able to initiate appropriate behavioral responses. The information reaching the hearing-impaired person is severely limited by the reduction of the auditory input. His knowledge of the physical world in which he exists can never be complete since the auditory aspects of it cannot be incorporated into his perceptions. How limited our concept of a bird would be if we had never heard one sing, or of an orchestra if we had never heard a symphony. More seriously impaired is the intake of vicarious experience that we obtain primarily through the written or spoken word.

The most vital information we receive is that which provides warning of threats to our safety. The ability to perceive and react to these warnings is essential to the preservation of the individual. Warnings from our internal sense organs inform us of sickness or disease, while those received through our peripheral sensory receptors indicate potential external danger. The startle (Moro reflex) and eye blink response (auropalpebral reflex), occurring as a reaction to a loud sound, are examples of the most primitive of the auditory defense processes. We should expect that the person with a severe hearing loss will not be aware of the significance that intense or unusual sounds may have in alerting him to potentially threatening situations; for as long as these sounds are inaudible to him they can play no part in his perception of the situation. Once amplification has been provided and the sounds made more audible, we must attend to this most primitive aspect of hearing and incorporate it in the auditory training program.

Our orientation in space is also dependent upon the integration of information from external and internal sensory mechanisms. From these sources we obtain not only information relevant to posture and balance, but also information concerning the position of our body relative to objects around us. The role of hearing in spatial orientation is, perhaps, underestimated. You are probably unaware of the number of times you safely cross a road without looking, depending upon your ears to tell you that no cars are coming. Your ability to walk confidently down a familiar staircase in the dark without falling is partly due to the auditory feedback you receive from your footsteps, which tell where you are in relation to the bottom. In a strange house, you may literally need to feel your way down the stairs. We see this use of the auditory aspects of spatial perception most clearly illustrated in the blind subject. Several experiments [6, 8, 22, 34, 42], working under controlled laboratory conditions, have demonstrated that both blind subjects and sighted subjects temporarily deprived of vision are able to detect the presence or absence of target objects placed before them, purely on the basis of echo reflection from the objects. The sound made by a person's body movements and his footsteps as he approaches an object is sufficient for detection and avoidance [6, 22]. There is even evidence that it is possible to discriminate with a high degree of accuracy between various-shaped objects and to a lesser extent between materials of different qualities [32].

These studies emphasize the importance of recognizing that the sense modalities do not function as independent mechanisms. To consider hearing only in relation to its role in speech perception is to fail to understand the complexity of the problem of deafness. An impairment of hearing must be evaluated on the basis of the total adaptive or maladaptive behavior to which it gives rise, rather than upon the reduction in speech communication performance alone.

THE PERCEPTUAL PROCESS

Earlier in our discussion it was pointed out that, in responding to stimuli in a discriminative manner, we show that we have perceived a particular group of stimuli, a "stimulus complex," as different from all other stimulus complexes. This permits us to attribute a particular meaning to it. It may help you to understand this process of perception if you look up from this text for a moment and glance around you. Now ask yourself what you see and hear. Your answer will almost certainly include a list of people, things, and activities that you have observed, together with the sounds associated with them. Depending upon where you are, you may perceive your roommate sitting in a chair studying, a clock ticking on a bed table, a news program on television, or the siren of a fire engine or ambulance in the distance. The first thing to note is that the stimuli reaching you are all complex in nature and that you are aware not of the individual stimuli, but of the objects and activities that give rise to them. You see people, not rays of light, hear voices instead of the component sound vibrations. Your reaction is to *patterns* of stimuli; you are not usually aware of the component parts. Each of the pieces of this perceptual jigsaw may be looked at in isolation, but when you put them together they constitute a picture that you are only then able to recognize. As E. R. Hilgard says, "The total impression from organized stimuli has properties not predictable from the parts in isolation" [19, p. 363]. We will do well to bear this in mind when we discuss the analytic and synthetic approaches to the teaching of visual communication skills.

The second thing that you may note about your observation of your environment is that you are familiar with almost all of the things you see and hear in it. You have encountered them on previous occasions and in other settings. Nevertheless, your orientation toward them on this occasion may be somewhat different from what it was before. This is because your perception of the object or activity is determined not only by its immediate setting, but also by your past experience of the same or similar object, event, or idea. Note how, on separate occasions, you often respond differently to the same stimulus complex, and how different reports of the same event may be received from a number of observers.

We observe, then, that we react to groups of stimuli that are seen as an integrated whole, *a gestalt.* This gestalt is the result of the interaction of all the component stimuli; the identity of the individual components may not be consciously perceived. Indeed in the early stages of learning it may not be possible to consciously isolate and identify them. We respond to the "catness" of a cat, rather than to the individual attributes of a cat, a phenomenon referred to as physiognomic perception [3, p. 5–6]. We also notice that we are influenced in what we perceive by our previous experiences. How do we organize these multitudinous stimuli in order to make possible the designation of meaning? In communication two phenomena are particularly important in this process: figure-ground and closure.

FIGURE-GROUND PERCEPTION AND CLOSURE

The general constancy of most of our perceptions implies the existence of an underlying organizational pattern. The first of these is the phenomenon of *figure-ground*. This may be defined as the perceptual process by which a particular object or object quality is seen to stand out against a background constituted by the remaining objects or object qualities.

The world in which the newborn child finds himself consists essentially of a jumble of meaningless stimuli. In order to make a start toward perceiving the objects that give rise to this multitude of sensations, it is necessary to learn to organize the stimuli into complexes, to pattern them, to bring order and, therefore, predictability. This is only possible if some of them can be made to stand out more distinctly than the rest. A number of factors within the child and within the stimuli will determine which are most attention getting. The group of stimuli that at a given instance in time command the child's attention become the figure; the remainder constitute the background. This phenomenon of figure-ground perception appears to occur even when practice has been denied. The research findings of M. von Senden [34] on the experience of congenitally blind adults following surgical removal of cataracts showed that after an initial period of recovery his patients evidenced figure-ground perception ability. Without previous visual-perceptual experience, they were able to organize the stimuli into a figure-ground relationship. Chester A. Lawson has explained this function very clearly.

The code interpretation of how an infant learns to differentiate a primitive figure-ground unity to perceive an object as a whole is based on five related assumptions. The first of these is that every perception involves an etiology and a prognosis, i.e., any perception is based on past experience and contains a predictive element. In the code hypothesis both the S and T elements* are the results of past experience, while the operation of the T element produces the prediction. The initial code of the human infant is presumed to be the result of ancestral experience, i.e., heredity, rather than the infant's own perceptual experience. However, changes in this code that produce new S and T code elements are presumed to result from the infant's own experience.

The second assumption is that every visual perception includes a figure-ground unity. The third assumption is that every perception results in some behavior. The fourth assumption is that following perception of a

*S equals elements of the sensory code. T equals a connected code element.

unity there results an automatic shift of focus to some part or subfigure within the whole. The fifth assumption is that through eye movement (behavior) other parts or subfigures of the whole are sought and the perceived parts are then related and recorded in the memory code.

If we accept all these assumptions, we may say a human infant begins by perceiving a figure-ground unity. He then changes his focus from the figure as a whole to some part of the whole. If he can differentiate lines and angles and can follow the contours of the figure by eye movement, he can differentiate parts of the whole and relate them. If we assume that each movement of the eye is recorded and that the parts of the figure also are recorded, then after the record is complete, perception of any part of a figure would activate the record, firing the entire sequence and producing perception of the whole. [24, p. 17]

Figure-ground perception is not confined to vision; it also occurs in hearing. It makes it possible for you to attend to a particular sound source against a background of other environmental noises and to shift your attention from one sound source to another. It accounts for the fact that you are able to listen to what a person is saying at a cocktail party, in spite of the fact that everyone is talking, and that you can recognize the melody of a piece of music against the background of accompaniment. It is important to recognize that perception of figure-ground does not constitute the ability to attribute meaning to a stimulus. A person exposed to sound for the first time is able to hear something against a background but will not at first have any knowledge concerning what this something may be. Subjects studied by von Senden were unable to make even the simplest visual discrimination between shapes until they had been given extensive training. We recognize the need for such basic perceptual training in auditory discrimination as part of our program of aural rehabilitation. Lessons must be designed to progress from the discrimination of gross everyday environmental sounds to the difficult task of discrimination of conversational speech under adverse listening conditions.

The second factor of importance to us in our consideration of perceptual organization is *closure*. This term refers to the tendency we have to perceive an incomplete figure as being complete. It accounts, in part, for the ability of a person to recognize a spoken word or a sentence on the basis of limited visual cues, or for a person with a marked hearing loss correctly to perceive certain sounds that are inaudible to him. Closure is obviously dependent upon prior experience with the whole figure. It is impossible to complete correctly a figure with which one is unfamiliar. Given parts of a relatively unfamiliar sentence, you may be unable to complete closure:

_____ has a _____ suffered _____ _____ tragedy.*

*Never has a man suffered such great tragedy.

The task is relatively easy if you are familiar with the whole:

Don't _____ all _____ eggs _____ _____ basket.*

When you encounter an unfamiliar situation, you attempt to understand it by an analysis of its components. In doing so, you are able to establish the relationship that exists between the whole and its parts. On future occasions it may not be necessary actually to receive the total stimulus complex in order to recognize it. Perception of part of the stimulus will frequently be sufficient to call forth a memory of previous perceptions of the same or related experiences. Every stimulus complex has, for each of us, a minimal number of component stimuli necessary for its accurate perception (recognition). We may consider this minimum to constitute the *minimal perceptual invariant*. The minimal perceptual invariant need not constitute a consistent pattern of stimuli. It may be constituted differently on different occasions, but whichever combination of stimuli is utilized, it provides the essential elements for recognition.

In aural rehabilitation, we utilize this knowledge when we separate the visual and auditory aspects of the message signal. We break each of these down further into their individual parts (analytical approach) in order that the person may become familiar with the characteristics of individual speech sounds or groups of sounds. We then present the whole visual complex and the whole auditory complex. Finally, the integrated auditory-visual stimulus is presented (multisensory approach). If we can train the person to obtain through vision, audition, and the phenomenon of closure the minimal component stimuli necessary for recognition, it will be possible for a speech sound, word, sentence, or idea to be perceived even when only part of the stimulus has actually been received.

A PERCEPTUAL MODEL

Solley and Murphy have proposed a model to help clarify the perceptual process (Fig. 5.1). They state that perception is a process that "is extended in time, and which consists of a series of interdependent subprocesses, or stages, which can be partially ordered in their succession" [37, p. 18]. Their schematic model involves five stages: (a) perceptual expectancy, (b) attending, (c) reception, (d) trial and check, and (e) final perceptual organization.

The box on the extreme right constitutes the covert or overt behavior changes occurring as a result of the perception. Also incorporated in the

*Don't put all your eggs in one basket.

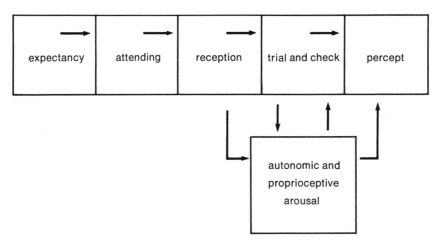

Fig. 5.1. A model of the perceptual process. After Solley and Murphy [36].

model is the autonomic and proprioceptive arousal system that, it is suggested, may exert control over some forms of perceptual behavior.

The external factors contained in the box on the extreme left represent those forms of readiness that give rise to "expectancy." Solley and Murphy point out that a perceptual act originates because an individual has certain needs and desires for which fulfillment is sought. It is this factor that serves as the primary motivation for communication between individuals. The perception of language stimuli serves to mediate between our personal needs and our environment. Motivation is therefore an important factor in communication since it serves to direct our attention toward the appropriate stimuli and heightens our awareness of them.

The first component of the perceptual model, *expectancy*, involves our ability to predict, with some measure of reliability, the probability of a given stimulus complex occurring in a given situation.

> We know from countless acts of commerce with our environment that we can expect such and such a stimulus to follow or occur with another set of stimuli. Often, before a given source can act as an input to our receptors, we are expecting it. The ebb and flow of experience is such that we are constantly being bombarded by stimuli, and it is only by developing expectancies and schemata that we are able to deal with this array of stimulation.
> [37, p. 156]

In human communication it is the effect of the situational and contextual constraints placed upon a speaker that permit the listener to develop expectancy. The importance of this ability increases considerably when the message signals are received under adverse listening conditions as are experienced by the hard-of-hearing person.

Our expectancy for given stimuli directs us to search for them and so increases our probability of becoming aware of them. *Attention* serves, therefore, to increase our chances of perceiving specific stimulus complexes. It determines the figure-ground relationship by increasing the degree to which we are conscious of certain stimuli. It is important to our consideration of communication to realize that this process of bringing a particular stimulus complex into focus does not exclude all other stimuli from consciousness; it serves, rather, to determine the relative importance of various stimulus groups. Elements of the background do not cease to contribute information, but they do contribute less than the figure.

> Successive acts of attending bring stimulations into close contiguity with one another, an important requirement for sensory integration. . . . The perceived environment becomes integrated into a meaningful whole. [37, p. 184]

We should also recognize the possibility of the existence of two types of attention. As Lawson points out:

> First, there is the awareness essential for carrying out a learned behavior pattern. A person who has driven an automobile for years performs the manipulations of driving automatically, without paying attention to the details of steering, accelerating, shifting, or braking, as long as the pattern unfolds as expected. However, should the accelerator get stuck, or the brakes fail, or any other event occur that is contrary to the normal behavior pattern, then the second kind of awareness or attention would go into operation. Specific attention is now directed to the cause of the disruption and the person is alert to new sensory input, unexpected in terms of normal driving behavior, but expected in view of the disturbance. [24, p. 98]

Reception, the third stage of the perceptual model, has been discussed in some detail in the two previous chapters. The nature of the stimulation itself is obviously of critical importance. The way in which we perceive stimuli will be dependent upon our previous experience in structuring them into complexes. If the receptive process is impaired, or if we lack previous experience, then we may be forced to develop our perceptions on the basis of inadequate information. We may fail to recognize the stimulus complex, or we may develop a misperception, resulting in an incorrect meaning being attributed to the stimulus.

Before the received stimulus is finally structured as a percept, it is suggested by the model that a process of *trial and check* takes place. This is the same process that we discussed when we considered the role of the comparator in Fairbank's model of a closed-cycle control system for speech. Solley and Murphy have borrowed their term, trial and check, from Woodworth [46], whom they quote:

> When a new percept is in the making—when an obscure stimulus complex is being deciphered, or when the meaning of a cue or sign is being discovered —an elementary two-phase process is observable. It is a trial and check, trial and check process. The trial phase is a tentative reading of the sign, a tentative decipherment of the puzzle, a tentative characterization of the object; and the check phase is an acceptance or rejection, a positive or negative reinforcement of the tentative perception. [37, p. 156]

The purpose of this stage, then, is to compare the expected perceptual pattern with what actually has been received. If the predicted event concurs with the perceived event, it is possible to attribute meaning to it. If a discrepancy is revealed, then the organism is directed both to obtain more information through re-observation and to recheck the files of associated memories in an attempt to identify the incoming stimulus complexes. Within-channel trial and check might occur, for example, when a friend introduces you to her fiancé. From her previous description of him you will have built up an expected perceptual pattern. When you meet him you may find that he is quite different from what you had envisaged; your predicted image does not concur with what you now perceive: "He's not a bit like I had imagined him." You then seek to eliminate the discrepancy between what you had previously anticipated and what you now observe in order to insure future recognition. Within-channel trial and check may cause you to fail to recognize a male friend who, unbeknown to you, has decided to grow a beard. Future recognition necessitates your restructuring your image. This process plays a role in verbal communication when, for example, a person expresses something about us that we had not expected. The discrepancy may cause us to ask him to repeat his statement, or we may seek through our files of memory to find something that would help us to understand what gave rise to the comment.

In attempting to understand this process, do not forget that it is not confined to one sensory channel. We recognize that a given object or event simultaneously emits stimuli of various types. We may see, hear, and touch a particular object. In doing so, we initiate a trial and check procedure for each channel. If you refer back to Fig. 2.6, you will see that it shows interconnecting fibers traveling between various subcortical nerve centers. These interconnecting fibers are indicated because we presumed the existence of a complex system involving reception, integration, analysis, association, and interpretation of data from all sensory end organs. The trial-and-check process occurs, therefore, not simply *within* a sensory channel, but also *between* sensory channels. When we perceive and attribute meaning to something, we do so because there is harmony between the perceptual structure in each channel. If, for example, you were to see what you thought to be a vase of freshly cut roses, but on touching them felt the texture of plastic and noted the absence of any scent, you would reject the visual percept that had already satisfied the trial-and-check process for that sensory channel.

An example of the effect of between-channel trial and check created considerable humor in one of the Candid Camera programs. In this situation, a young and unwitting participant was sent to a bakery to purchase a custard cream pie. The salesgirl was herself enjoying a slice of pie and offered a piece to the customer. His within-visual-channel trial and check was acceptable. He observed a custard filling with a thick cream topping; he also observed the girl obviously enjoying her portion. Not until between-channel trial and check had been carried out, when he bit heartily into his piece, did he reject his perception upon realization that his piece had, in fact, a thick layer of shaving cream for a topping. Between-channel trial and check would be important in a communication situation in which a speaker might perceive a person to say, "Did you hear that John Smith lost his life in a car accident?" This sentence would make sense in context and would pass an auditory trial-and-check stage. If, however, the observer noted that the word he heard as "life" showed lip rounding of the initial sound, he would not achieve auditory-visual, interchannel trial-and-check agreement. If the word has lip rounding for the initial sound, it cannot be "life"—it must be "wife." He will therefore reject his initial perception and replace it by, "Did you hear that John Smith lost his wife in a car accident?"

The amount of trial and check necessary is a function of the predictability of the event. When redundancy is high, as in favorable listening or viewing conditions, it is not necessary to carry out extensive trial and check. However, when high noise levels in one sensory channel reduce redundancy, then trial and check both within and between sensory channels becomes vital to comprehension. Our justification for training the hard-of-hearing person in visual communication skills is based upon this awareness of the part that intersensory-channel trial and check contributes to the correct decoding of the message signal.

Autonomic and Proprioceptive Arousal System

The evidence pertaining to the relationship that may exist between stimuli arising from the automatic and proprioceptive arousal system and our total perception of the external world is at best tenuous. In reviewing the existing literature, Solley and Murphy conclude that the research indicates the existence within the individual of specific and diffuse feedback systems. Through the process of conditioning, it becomes possible for these to be aroused by specific external stimuli. They explain that "in addition the occurrence of such feedback will also strengthen the perception (cortical integration) of that stimulus" [37, p. 242]. Referring to the work by R. L. Solomon [38, 39, 40], the authors suggest the perception may then become "linked or 'locked' to certain specific and general autonomic and proprio-ceptive feedback mechanisms so that perception and the feedback mechanism are mutually excited" [37, p. 243].

We should pay careful attention to the discussion by the authors of the manner in which this operates, for it has important significance in our attempt to understand the processes of communication and, in particular, the way in which figure-ground relationships and auditory and visual set may occur. They see at the heart of perception the organism's constant sensory scanning activities, occurring within the framework of readiness to perceive, resulting from homeostatic factors or from specific needs or sets. Initially random in character, this scanning for exteroceptive cues becomes progressively more patterned. The authors make the suggestion that we also scan for internal memory cues to attempt to identify a match between the incoming stimuli and memory traces left from previous stimuli. These central cues serve to direct the scanning and to influence the figure-ground relationship, momentarily stabilizing and then breaking up the relationship when what is sought has been found. "Scanning moves to that which is congruent with the established set, and excludes that which is noncongruent" [37, p. 253].

J. D. French is of the opinion that the internal scanning process prob-ably constitutes part of the function of the reticular formation, which, he suggests, develops differential sensitivity to stimuli [14]. He proposes that the attention pattern results from the action of both the arousal system and a cortical probability calculation. Perception is seen as being dependent upon a preliminary firing in the cortex followed by a firing pattern from sensory nerves. Such a hypothesis lends support to the concept of perceptual mobilization.

In addition to the exteroceptive feedback, which influences the motor and perceptual responses, further information is derived from the proprio-ceptive feedback of the perceptual act itself, such as the sensations arising from visual focusing.

We have talked repeatedly about total perception and the need to attempt to enrich this for the hearing-impaired person in all available ways. The question arises whether it is feasible to sensitize the student to such inter-nal cues. If this is possible, we may be able to evoke what Solley and Murphy refer to as a new "search set." The authors are reassuring; they refer to an experiment by J. P. Seward in which it was shown that on a repeated visual-perceptual task in which no results were given to the subject between trials the number of correct responses progressively increased [35]. This indicates that repeated exposure to the sensory data arising from a perceptual act, even in the absence of external feedback, may lead to the modification of the response to more closely approximate reality. Evidence that this may

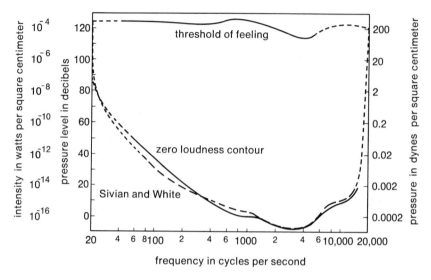

Fig. 5.2. The auditory area between the threshold of feeling and the threshold of hearing. (After Fletcher [11]).

be true for the perceptual act of interpreting visual speech cues can be derived from my work with S. J. Goodrich (Fig. 5.2).* If one examines the mean scores obtained by the subjects on four successive visual-discrimination tests of monosyllabic words with no feedback given, it is seen that the mean items correctly identified rose from 6.60 on the first presentation to 8.00 on the fourth. This tendency encourages us to persevere with many aspects of auditory and visual communication training for which as yet we lack experimental proof of value. In the words of Solley and Murphy:

> To the extent an individual can learn to discriminate and recognize these cues he can gain greater control over his perceptual system and, hence, become more viridical in his perceptions. [37, p. 260]

The ultimate result of these progressive stages is the *percept*. This final structuring of the perception permits meaning to be attributed to the stimulus

*Derek A. Sanders and S. J. Goodrich, "The Contribution of Vision to Speech Intelligibility under Three Conditions of Frequency Distortion," to appear in a forthcoming issue of the *Journal of Speech and Hearing Research.*

complex. The stimulus is interpreted in a particular way on the basis of previous experience. The phenomenon of figure-ground and closure play an important role in determining the final percept. We have seen that the determinants of the figure-ground relationship lie both within the stimulus and within the individual. It is a dangerous oversimplification to consider the environment and the individual as independent entities. They are, in fact, so interrelated as to constitute one system. It is rather like stirring chocolate cake batter into a white cake mixture to make a marble cake. In places, the two are clearly all white or all brown, yet in general, they run together so as to be inseparable.

The process by which we finally attribute meaning is highly complex but clearly involves the fusion of selected external stimuli with the memory of past experiences. This brings about an interpretation that most reasonably fits in with the information that has satisfactorily passed the within-channel and between-channel trial-and-check stage. This process is never completed; our perceptions can never be reality, since absolute reality is really non-existent. We are not attempting to specify a "something" out there, but rather to specify the significance of the result of our interaction with that "something." So the trial-and-check process constitutes a continuous servo-mechanism, causing us to constantly re-evaluate our perceptions in the light of the never-ceasing intake of additional sensory data. The amount of perceptual change must be a function of the ability of the individual to make use of the additional stimulus input, an ability determined by motivation, awareness, and a library of perceptual experiences. Through a systematic program of aural rehabilitation, we aim to provide the hard-of-hearing person with an enhanced ability to do this.

We have now set the stage for a consideration of the perception of the auditory and visual signal. From our earlier discussion of communication you will be familiar with the importance of the language system as a prerequisite for the understanding of speech. It has been explained that in order to communicate with another person we resort to the use of a code. We encode the thought or idea in such a way that it may be reconstructed by the person receiving the message signal. Our attention to the role of linguistic, contextual, and situational constraints and to the visual aspects of speech production leads us to the realization that a simple relationship does not exist between the sound and the meaning. We are dealing, then, not with a single language code, but a series of codes, each embodying various amounts of information about the message, and each contributing to the accuracy with which the listener will be able to replicate the original thought. It is important for us to consider the nature of auditory and visual perception against this background, and against our knowledge of the general process of perception as has been suggested by Solley and Murphy [37, p. 18].

AUDITORY PERCEPTION AND THE SPOKEN MESSAGE

Let us examine the perception of the auditory stimulus within the framework of the perceptual model we have already discussed. We can divide the various stages into two major steps: (1) reception and identification and (2) perception. In this section, we shall consider the receptive identification step. Perception, which involves the attributing of meaning, will be discussed when we consider multisensory perception later in the chapter.

Reception

Before a person in a communication situation is ready to receive a speech signal, he must be motivated to do so. You are no doubt familiar with the experience of someone's trying to communicate a message to you when you are simply not interested in listening—the sort of situation that occurs when you are engrossed in an exciting detective story and someone calls you to dinner or, worse, suggests that you set the table. You are simply not prepared to receive the spoken message and will frequently protest that you did not hear the request. The motivation to listen is important, since it gives rise to auditory-perceptual expectancy. This constitutes the adoption of an appropriate auditory set of predictions, based upon our evaluation of the total communication situation. As a result, we direct our attention to the speech stimulus, which then becomes the figure. We have prepared ourselves to receive the acoustic aspects of the spoken message. The factors that affect this receptive process are particularly important to us, since the person with sensory or conductive deafness experiences a breakdown at this first stage of our communication model.

If the speech stimulus is to be received, *the acoustic power must fall within the limits of audibility*. Figure 5.2 shows the range of frequencies and intensities audible to a person with normal hearing. The lower limits of this auditory area are set by the threshold of audibility, while the upper limits are a function of the tolerance of the ear for discomfort caused by high sound-pressure levels. The distance between the threshold of audibility and the threshold of discomfort constitutes the intensity range within which speech sounds must fall to be of use. The effect of a hearing impairment is to reduce this area by raising the threshold of audibility. The problem is further aggravated in some types of sensori-neural deafness by the lowering of the threshold of discomfort. The implications that this has for aural rehabilitation will become clear when we talk about the use of amplification.

In Chap. 3, when we discussed the energy of speech, it was shown that the overall sound-pressure level of conversation averages about 65 decibels [11, p. 76]. This means that, for the most part, as a person with normal hearing, you listen to speech at a level 65 decibels above your threshold. You know from experience that you are quite capable of understanding speech at much lower intensity levels than this. It has, in fact, been demonstrated that if you listen carefully to simple, familiar, connected speech you will be able to understand correctly at only 24 decibels above your threshold [18]. It is not, therefore, essential to be able to amplify speech to a full 65 decibels above threshold in order to make the acoustic signal useful to a person with a hearing loss. In fact, quite frequently the loss is so severe that we may not have a range as great as 65 decibels between the thresholds of reception and discomfort. The 40-decibel range between the level at which speech becomes intelligible and the level at which we normally hear speech constitutes a part of acoustic redundancy without which aural rehabilitation would be considerably more difficult.

In addition to the necessity for the speech stimulus to fall within the auditory area, it must also be of an intensity greater than the acoustic noise in the environment. The figures we have mentioned with regard to the audibility of speech were obtained for subjects with normal hearing under conditions of quiet—that is to say, where room noise is less than 20-decibel SPL (30-decibel sensation level). For levels of environmental noise up to 20-decibels SPL, the speech reception threshold of subjects with normal hearing is not affected [20, p. 170]. If noise levels exceed this, then the threshold of reception will be raised progressively as the noise levels increase.

Physical Cues to Identification

To understand the auditory perception of speech we must first consider the physical properties of speech sounds that serve as cues to identification.

If you refer back to Table 3.2, which displays the relative intensity levels of English phonemes, you will see that a measure of the loudness of a speech sound relative to all other speech sounds makes possible the limitation of the phonemic units into which this speech sound might be placed. For example, there is evidence to show that /s/ and /ʃ/ can be distinguished as a class from /f/ and /θ/ on the basis of intensity alone [24]. Remember that the comparison of loudness between sounds is relative, not absolute. Your auditory mechanism is placing a given sound somewhere on a scale between the weakest phoneme, /θ/, and the strongest, /ɔ/. The raising or lowering of the overall intensity of speech does not normally affect the intensity relationship of the speech sounds to each other. A person with a long-standing hearing loss may have a different pattern of intensity relationships because the auditory impairment weakens some sounds more than others. If, however, the hearing loss is static, then the person's internal perceptual scale is also stable and will permit him to make judgments, even though the value of them may be reduced.

Just as the various phonemes differ in relative intensity, so does the relative duration of speech sounds vary. Table 5.1 indicates the average duration times for twelve vowels and dipthongs and fifteen consonants

TABLE 5.1. The Average Duration Times for Twelve Vowels and Diphthongs and Fifteen Consonants (After Crandall [7])

Phoneme	Duration	Phoneme	Duration
VOWELS AND DIPHTHONGS			
u	0.351	æ	0.294
i	0.341	ɔ	0.290
ɝ	0.331	ʌ	0.280
ou	0.325	ʊ	0.249
ɑ	0.306	ɛ	0.219
ei	0.305	ɪ	0.211
CONSONANT VALUES FOR TWO SPEAKERS			
ʒ	0.28 / 0.13	ʃ	0.18 / 0.17
s	0.27 / 0.19	f	0.15 / 0.30
z	0.24 / 0.22	g	0.12 / 0.10
j	0.22 / 0.14	b	0.12 / 0.19
v	0.20 / 0.25	tʃ	0.07 / 0.08
ð	0.20 / 0.18	k	0.07 / 0.08
d	0.13 / 0.10	θ	0.02 / 0.02
		p	0.02 / 0.04

obtained from a controlled speech sample by I. B. Crandall [7]. It is clear from these figures that the duration of vowel sounds is significantly longer than the duration of consonants, which permits an initial differentiation between these two categories. Furthermore, sufficient differences exist within each category to be able to further subdivide into groups of vowels and groups of consonants. However, you will observe that not every phoneme is noticeably different in duration from all others. We also know that the absolute duration of a particular phoneme for a given speaker varies with phonetic and semantic context. Stressed syllables, for example, are of longer duration than unstressed. Such variations are not accidental; they occur because a speaker causes them to occur; the encoding processes are perceptually known to the speaker and to varying degrees predictable by the listener. Although we have not been able to understand the exact nature of the duration code that we use so expertly, we are aware that it is an important contributor to speech discrimination, even though speech-sound identification cannot be made on the basis of duration alone.

The third major clue to speech-sound discrimination rests within the frequency spectrum. You are familiar with the form and structure of vowels and know that each may be characterized by the nature of its formants. It is generally recognized that F_1 and F_2 are of greatest importance in the perception of the quality of a vowel sound. It is these two formants that contribute the information we need to make a phonemic classification. E. Fischer-Jorgensen, in his discussion of new techniques being used in acoustic phonetics, explains that for a single speaker, and to a lesser extent for a group of male or female speakers, the decisive element in phoneme recognition from formant structure seems to be the actual frequencies at which the energy concentrations occur [10, p. 123]. However, a comparison of the vowel sounds produced by adult males, females, and by children indicates that the formant pattern for women is 17 per cent higher in frequency than that for men, while that for children is even higher. It appears, therefore, that the perception of the position of the formants relative to each other is also an important factor in our ability to understand the speech of different people.

When we consider the acoustic characteristics by which consonants are distinguished, we learn from the literature that they are recognized partly by frequency distribution of their energy and partly from the effect that they have on the spectrum of adjacent vowels. Turning once again to the helpful explanation of acoustic phonetics by Fischer-Jorgensen we learn that:

> The spectra of the consonants proper contain the cues for the distinction between various categories of consonants according to manner of production (e.g., stops, fricatives, nasals), and these differences are sufficiently clearly perceived when consonants are heard in isolation. On the other hand the differences between consonants according to place of articulation are to a great extent perceived by means of the influence exercised on the second (and partly third) formant of the adjoining vowel. There are also differences in the spectra of the consonants according to place of articulation, but except for voiceless fricatives these differences are not always sufficient for recognition. It is difficult to distinguish isolated stop explosions but the vowel "transitions" will often be sufficient for the auditory differentiation between b, d, and g, even if there is no explosion at all. [10, p. 126]

It has been explained in a previous chapter that speech consist of a continuous wave form. In order to be able to make evaluations of phoneme intensity, duration, and frequency spectrum, it is obviously necessary at some stage of the analysis of the auditory message signal to break down this wave form into a series of discrete phonemic units. We have just seen that the actual spectrum of a sound may be noticeably influenced by the sound generated by the movements of the speech articulators from the position of the previous sound and toward the subsequent sound. We also know that these transitions are important contributors to the recognition of consonants. The process of breaking down the sound wave into phonemic units cannot therefore be considered as analogous to a phonetic transcription, which provides us with a series of related but unconnected symbols. Each speech sound is intimately related to adjacent sounds by the transitions it shares. The transition belongs equally to the two sounds it links. The recognition of this fact is important, since it means that the transitional characteristics of a sound may be sufficient to enable the listener to identify the sound itself, even when it is distorted. In Table 5.2, which illustrates the principal frequencies present in English sounds, you will notice that /d/ and /b/ both contain the same amounts of energy at around 350 Hz and a second band at about

TABLE 5.2. Sensation Level and Frequency Characteristics of Speech Sounds (After H. Fletcher [11])

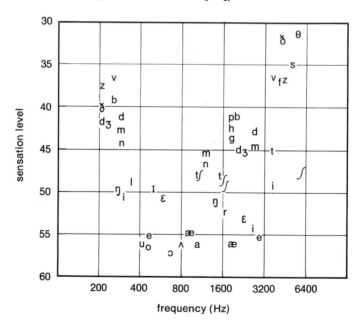

2800 Hz. Because of the similarity in the intensity and frequency of the lowest component of these two sounds, one might anticipate that it would be impossible to discriminate between them without being able to hear the differentiating second component. However, experiments have shown that one can differentiate between these two consonants on the basis of the transitional changes that they induce in the formant structure of the adjoining vowel [15, p. 72]. Additional transitional cues have been shown to rest in the duration of the transition and in the presence or absence of a silent interval between the steady-state stage and the transition. The contribution that the transitions make to intelligibility of other phonemes has been similarly demonstrated.

Here is sufficient evidence for us to assume that we do not have to hear all of the frequency components of a sound in order to be able to recognize it. It is important that you should understand this concept, since it constitutes the basis of the approach to auditory training that we shall develop in Chap. 7.

Our discussion of the factors involved in the recognition of speech sounds cannot be concluded without at least a brief reference to the controversial issue of whether or not motor-kinesthetic feedback plays a role in speech perception. This question involves the relationship that may exist between the articulatory, acoustic, and auditory stages of speech communication.

Research in experimental phonetics has shown that many of the distinctive characteristics that one hears in a speech sample become considerably less identifiable when heard in isolation or in a synthetic speech pattern that closely approximates the sound spectra of human speech. Studies have also shown that even a skilled listener may fail to recognize distinctive characteristics of phonemes if he is unaware that he is listening to a speech sound. On the basis of these findings, A. M. Liberman et al. [26] have suggested that the distinctiveness of a speech sound "is not inherent in the acoustic signal, but is rather added as a consequence of linguistic experience."

These findings have led several authors to suggest that speech may be perceived by reference to articulation [25, 26]. They maintain that it appears likely that the listener interprets the acoustic signal only after he has mimicked the articulatory pattern that he predicts gave rise to the acoustic signal he has received. This articulatory mimicry is often observed in an overt form in children who may appear to be mumbling when being spoken to. In adults, however, Liberman suggests that the process is in some way short-circuited. The sensations of the articulatory movements of speech production may in some way be represented by the corresponding neurological patterns in the brain. These serve to mediate between the acoustic stimulus and the final perception of speech.

It is important for us to reflect upon the implications that these suggestions may have upon our understanding of the speech and hearing abilities of people with hearing losses. It strongly suggests another instance in which we are unjustified in separating out any one particular process involved in the chain of events that constitute human communication. We have argued that vision and audition interact in a manner that produces an end result that cannot be predicted on the basis of data obtained from the two processes functioning in isolation. We need now, in the light of the theory of motor-kinesthetic speech perception, to consider the relationship between speech therapy for the hard of hearing and auditory-visual training. This relationship will be discussed in more detail when we are discussing the integrated multisensory approach to aural rehabilitation.

In addition to these cues to phonemic identification, information important to meaning is also conveyed by the stress patterns and rhythm of speech. Specific rhythmic patterns of speech are peculiar to particular languages; we learn them when we learn the language. When we listen to a person from another country who has recently begun to learn English, we often encounter difficulty in comprehending some of the things he says because he uses unusual stress patterns, both within words and within sentences. As a native of England, I observed, for example, that my students looked surprised and sometimes puzzled when I used the word "controversy," since I stress the second syllable, con-*trov*-ersy, rather than the first. Given the following three words, you are able to distinguish between them purely on the basis of the stress pattern.

argue   farmer   intent

In fact, the meaning of an isolated word or words often rests ultimately in the ability to identify the stress patterns.

con-tent   con-*tent*

in *sight*   *in*sight

Changing the stress patterns of the sentence can also change the meaning:

Where do you think you are going?

Where *do* you think you are going?

Where do *you* think you are going?

Where do you *think* you are going?

Where do you think *you* are going?

Where do you think you *are* going?

Where do you think you are *going*?

Changes in the inflectional pattern of the voice, that is in the rise and fall in pitch, also provide acoustic cues to meaning. My fourteen-month-old daughter is perfectly able to detect the question form on the basis of the inflectional pattern alone. She greatly enjoys shaking her head violently in a negative response to any question, even when she could not possibly understand the meaning, e.g., "Does 2 and 2 equal 6?"

DEVELOPMENT OF AUDITORY DISCRIMINATION

We have seen that the process of recognition is as much one of elimination of alternatives as it is one of a positive identification of the stimulus origin. Auditory discrimination consists in using the characteristics of a sound to differentiate between various auditory experiences. The cues that make this possible include variations in the frequency spectrum, the intensity, and the duration of the sound waves. These various cues serve to narrow down the choice of possible sound sources or, if we are concerned with speech, values of speech sounds from which final identification will be made. We have already emphasized that auditory perception does not function independently of the other pathways; we make predictions concerning what we will hear on the basis of sensory data reaching us through several sensory pathways and through associations between these and the memory of previous similar stimulus complexes.

At its simplest level, *auditory perception refers to the prediction of the nature of the sound-generating object on the basis of the auditory cues received from it, verified by associated sensory information, all occurring within an environmental framework.* The additional factors of other sensory information and environmental context are important, since either one or both of them is usually present in a perceptual experience. At this simple level of auditory perception, we are concerned with the ability to discriminate between sounds that differ considerably in their identifying characteristics, environmental sounds to which we refer as *gross sounds.* As adults with normal hearing, we consider it a relatively easy task to predict whether a sound originates from a watch, a jet airplane, a dog, or a piano. It is easy because the dissimilarity of the various acoustic signals severely limits the probability according to which we make our prediction. This probability is further limited by our familiarity with the sources that generate these sounds and with the environmental context in which they usually occur. We are so familiar with them that, once learned, the total sensory input cues generally provide a sufficiently high level of redundancy to permit us to predict correctly, and therefore to perceive, the sound source on the basis of the acoustic cues alone. However, there are gross sounds that we cannot encounter with sufficient frequency to permit such redundancy to occur. When faced with the auditory aspects of such sound sources out of context, we may have considerable difficulty in identifying them. I. M. Solovev, in discussing the role of environmental sounds states:

> In reality, the perception of the environment by means of hearing and listening to the surrounding world of sound provides a firm addition to the knowledge of the environment that is visually acquired. . . . We know whether a book or knife fell from the table in the next room. It is by means of sound that we recognize whether the book which fell was large or small or whether a tablespoon or a teaspoon dropped to the floor. In addition to size, the material from which the object is made, such as cardboard, wood, metal, glass, etc., can be recognized on the basis of sound. Several criteria of internal structure, such as the presence of empty space in an opaque object or the thickness of glass can be revealed by means of sound. [41]

The types of sounds we encounter, the frequency with which we encounter them, and the significance that they have for us are major factors in the determination of whether or not we will internalize the sound together with the other stimuli associated with it. The internal representation of such a stimulus complex constitutes our memory of it, our total perception. Sensory experiences to which we are unable to attach value, hence meaning, fail to be internalized. We do not perceive them since they have no value in our *personal* knowledge of the world. You will recall that the figure-ground phenomenon is greatly influenced by the anticipatory set of the individual. We perceive what we are prepared for, that which we are able through association to incorporate within our existing representation of our world, our schema or pattern, and to which we can therefore attribute meaning.

DEVELOPMENT OF AUDITORY PERCEPTION

How and why does the child with normal hearing learn to recognize sounds? At birth, the peripheral hearing mechanism is fully developed. The child hears; but as with von Senden's patients after cataract removal, the incoming stimuli, in this case auditory, are devoid of meaning. They are cues to nothing, since the child has no internal schema into which they can be fit, even if he were intellectually capable of the task. As the child develops neurophysiologically, the sophistication of the central nervous system increases, permitting him to process an ever-increasing complexity of stimulus configurations. His developing brain makes it possible for him to keep a very simple record of his experiences. It is simple because the manner in which he is able to apprehend things is, in itself, simple. Early experiences are little more than physiological in nature, with no cognitive associations, occuring in an all-or-nothing form. The child is hungry or satiated, warm or cold, threatened by a loud sound or unaware of it.

The increasing sophistication of the mechanism for processing sensory input and the associated increase in awareness of complexity of stimulus patterns impinging upon the organism gives rise to the need for, and stimulates, a rapid growth in the ability to discriminate. As soon as an organism becomes aware that an incoming stimulus complex differs significantly from those that have already been experienced and internalized, the restructuring of internal representations is necessary if the new stimulus complex is to be incorporated into the individual's experience and given meaning. This process may occur by the modification of the existing schemata or by the addition of a new one, associated with existing internal representations of experience, but sufficiently different to exist in its own right.

We can say then, that the growth in discrimination ability in all sensory channels arises as a combination of a growth in neurophysiological development and the pressures of a complex environment that places ever-increasing demands upon the individual. Joseph Church refers to these two factors as biological and experiential [3, p. 78]. He suggests that "theories which assume that ontogenetic changes in behavior are produced by maturational changes must take account of the possibility that many maturational changes are in turn induced by perceptual stimulation" [p. 30]. He goes on to say that "while some part of the change that occurs in infancy can be accounted for in terms of physical maturation, we know that maturation stands in a circular feedback relationship to experience—the things the organism does, feels, and has done to it" [p. 36].

Initially, the infant recognizes the stimulus complex by its gestalt, without awareness of its components. He is aware of new stimulus complexes by what they are not rather than by what they are, and then later by their overall pattern rather than by their specific components. This is an important concept, and we shall need to discuss it further in relation to its implications for various approaches to training visual and auditory perception.

The beginnings of auditory-perceptual development therefore involve, first, *an awareness of sound*, which results from an ability to internalize auditory stimuli and to integrate them with other sensory stimuli in order for a relationship between the child and the sound source to be established within a context. Mother's voice is recognized first in the context of her visual image, the warmth of her body, and the feel of her arms. Later, the auditory cue alone will provide sufficient information for recognition of mother. Second, auditory-perceptual development involves *an ability to discriminate between sounds* and, therefore, between sound sources. The initial discrimination is elementary. It involves a decision between "it is" or "it is not" mother. As the child's repeated contact with other sound-generating people or objects in situations that affect him increases, he has reason to differentiate between them in order to control his world. This requires internal representation of all sensory cues to the new experience. The child's auditory world consists of, for example, mother, father, bottle, squeaky toy, and several sounds in the "not-one-of-these" category. These latter sounds he is aware of, but is not yet sufficiently familiar with them to have completely internalized them together with their concomitant stimuli and associations. The library of internalized sound patterns and associations grows rapidly in the first year of life as the child becomes increasingly auditorily oriented. It has already been pointed out that sound cues play an important role in orientating the child in space, in providing him with information about his ever more complex world, and in protecting him from impending dangers or reassuring him that all is well.

This is the pattern of the early stages of auditory development in young children with normal hearing. The initially painstaking task of discrimination begins to grow easier as the child's brain learns to process the incoming information with greater and greater sophistication and ease. Auditory discrimination, which was first only possible between a few of the most dissimilar sounds, begins to be possible between an increasing variety of sounds and between those that differ less and less in acoustic structure. This occurs because of the auditory training that the environment continually provides the child with normal hearing—auditory training of which the hearing-impaired child is deprived.

The factors involved in learning to discriminate between gross sounds may be summarized as follows:

1. Awareness
2. Repeated exposure to the sound within a context
3. Predictable association of the acoustic stimuli with other sensory stimuli arising from the same sound source
4. Internal representation of auditory and other sensory impressions
5. Multisensory or gestalt recognition of sound-generating objects
6. Identification (prediction) of a sound source on the basis of its acoustic characteristics alone

DEVELOPMENT OF SPEECH-SOUND DISCRIMINATION

With a few exceptions, the normal child is born into a family in which speech constitutes the major form of communication. The child's parents presume that he, too, will develop the ability to utilize this form of communication. Since the infant's mother is herself very dependent upon the verbalization of ideas and, therefore, feelings, it is natural for her to talk both to herself and to the child when she is attending to the child's needs and when she is relaxed with him. In addition, the child will be exposed to varying amounts of verbal communication between parents and other siblings. He exists in a speech environment.

We have already concurred with Church's statement that maturation stands in a feedback relationship to experience. We may postulate, therefore, that the development of auditory-perceptual ability is heavily dependent upon the exposure to environmental sounds and speech sounds which takes place from birth. We must not neglect the importance of the role of this pre-verbal auditory experience. It is fascinating to note, for example, that even in birds, for some species, exposure to the singing pattern of the parent bird has been demonstrated to be necessary for the learning of the song of the species, even when it occurs before the young bird is itself physiologically ready to sing [43].

The same factors that we listed as being involved in the learning of gross sounds discrimination are valid in the learning of speech perception. The child must first become aware of speech. This awareness is closely related to the figure-ground phenomenon, which is in itself determined, to a large extent, by the ability of the individual to attribute meaning to certain stimulus complexes.

But figure-ground organization is dictated neither by stimulus intensities (except at disruptively high levels of contrast) nor by the formal organizational laws of Gestalt theory. Those objects, and those properties of objects, stand out which offer some relevance to the child himself, in terms of promise or threat or concrete action. Those things which are meaningless seem also to be beyond perception. The young infant is oblivious to the screaming sirens of the fire trucks that go racketing past, to the hubbub of the thunderstorm, to the clamor of the telephone or doorbell; but he may wail in distress when his mother sneezes in the next room. Here we are saying two things: that the child perceives only personally meaningful objects, and that what he perceives is not so much the objects as their meanings. [3, p. 4]

Meaning grows out of association, which results from repeated exposure to particular sensory stimuli in concurrence with other sensory stimuli.

The most meaningful person in a child's early life is its mother, one of whose characteristics is that she speaks. Since, as we have said, the child's early perceptions are in the form of a gestalt or holistic impression, for a child with normal hearing, vocalizations of the mother, both her singing and the words she speaks, will become as integral a part of the child's perception of her as will the visual image, the physical contact, and the way in which she handles him. The child is not initially capable of isolating, out of this gestalt, the individual components; this is a much later developmental behavior pattern. The reason the child pays attention to, and becomes aware of, speech is because it is an intimate part of his perception of mother. H. O. Mowrer has gone so far as to suggest that it is this identification of speech patterns with mother, combined with a normal autistic need in the child to recreate mother's image in her absence, that gives rise to early babbling and its modification to an ever more exact replica of mother's vocalizations [27].

Mother's contact with her infant is limited to its waking periods and the nature of her relationship limited by the needs of the child. One talks to a baby in a particular way and about particular things, especially in activities that involve the child and the adult. The vocabulary used by the mother is therefore fairly restricted by situational constraints that provide the necessary repeated contextual exposure to the sound patterns of certain words. For the most part, when mother talks to the child, she is with him, so that he receives the auditory stimulus together with the associated visual and tactile impression. These permit him to develop internal representations of the auditory and other impressions. When these have been developed, the child seems to be able to predict the meaning of certain spoken words on the basis of his total perception.

The spoken names of things are first given to him in the presence of the object. While handling a ball, he is told, "That's a ball. Isn't it a pretty ball? Throw mommy the ball"; or, "Where are your shoes? Let's put your shoes on. Here are your shoes. Let's put them on your feet. One shoe, two shoes." Out of these sentences the child focuses attention upon salient words. Certain words in a given situation become salient words because of the natural tendency that we have to stress them, because they are repeated more frequently than other words, and because they refer to objects and events within the perceptual experience of the child. Early speech perception therefore begins to occur in a situation in which redundancy is very high. The child's predictions are greatly aided by information that he has received through other senses and by the very limited alternative choices with which he is presented. As a result, he is likely to experience success, and the parents are likely to reinforce his attempts to identify things by their names. We say a child knows the name of something when he is consistently able to identify it on the basis of the spoken word alone.

This basic process continues to develop and to become increasingly sophisticated. It does so because the ability to make accurate predictions about one's environment and the people within it is greatly enhanced by the comprehension of speech. Even before he can use expressive speech as a means of directly manipulating his environment, he finds that his ability to discriminate between the words "cookie" and "milk," contained in a question asked by his mother, considerably speeds up the process of getting whichever he wants on a particular occasion. Accurate speech perception is therefore a rewarding process and encourages the child to refine and develop his skills in this behavior. His increasing ability to differentiate between more and more words and, therefore, between the objects and ideas to which they refer, causes him to become increasingly dependent upon speech as a source of information. The greater his skill, the better able he is to function under conditions of reduced redundancy. The child who is initially able only to discriminate a few words under conditions highly favorable to accurate prediction is ultimately able to identify complex ideas by spoken words received under markedly adverse listening conditions.

The Effect of Hearing Loss Upon Auditory Discrimination

An impairment of hearing that is present in a child at birth immediately results in a distortion of incoming auditory signals. The peripheral hearing mechanism is, in many ways, similar to a microphone of an amplifier. It serves as a sensing device capable of responding to changes in the pressure of the air around it. It is capable of transducing the energy in sound waves into an electrical wave form that embodies coded information directly correlated to the sound wave. We are able to describe the sensitivity of the human ear in the same way as we described the sensitivity of the microphone. Equal loudness curves derived by H. Fletcher and W. A. Mundson (Fig. 5.3) are

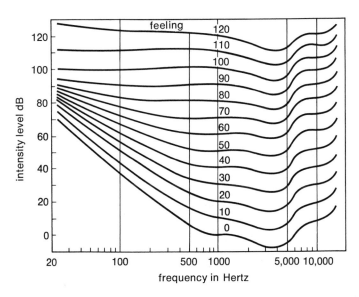

Fig. 5.3.   Loudness-level contours. These lines link points that may differ in intensity but that are equal in perceived loudness. (After Fletcher and Mundson [12]).

statements of the sensitivity of the ear at different sound-pressure levels
[12, p. 124]. From these curves we learn that, for input sounds of a sound-
pressure level of 50 decibels and above, the sensitivity of the ear is essentially
flat across the frequency range of 300 to 4000 Hz. At normal conversational
loudness, the normal ear does not favor some frequencies in the speech range
more than others. Neither the differences in sound-pressure level nor the
relative strengths of the formants in the various phonemes is affected by the
normal ear. This fact no longer holds true once the sensitivity curve of the
ear is changed by the presence of a hearing impairment. A hearing loss
always affects the overall loudness of the input signal; frequently it also
affects the perceived frequency spectrum.

Consider first a typical conductive hearing impairment (Fig. 5.4), which
reduces the hearing sensitivity relatively evenly across the speech frequency
range. Even though the sensitivity curve is evenly depressed, a reduction
in the loudness of speech affects the perception of some phonemes more

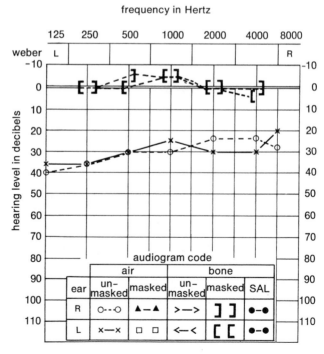

Fig. 5.4. Audiogram of a person with a typical conductive-type hearing impairment.

rapidly than others. This has been documented by Fletcher [11, p. 415–23]. He conducted a series of tests of speech perception for individual speech sounds. Using the average intensity level of normal conversational speech as a reference level, he derived articulation gain curves for each phoneme as a function of intensity. In other words, the graphs he derived showed the effect upon the accuracy of speech sound recognition (measured as a percentage) of progressively reducing the speech intensity. The results of these studies show that vowels are more easily recognized than consonants, with the exception of the vowel /ɛ/ as in "ten," which is exceptionally difficult, and for consonants /l/, /r/, /ŋ/, which are easily recognized. The sounds /s/, /θ/, /f/, and /v/ were found to be the most difficult to recognize. The voiced sound /z/, which is easily identified at normal conversational level, rapidly becomes extremely difficult to recognize when the intensity level is reduced. The vowels and dipthongs /i/, /ou/, /ɛ/, and /o/ are extremely resistant to loss of identifying qualities as a result of reduction in intensity. Finally, Fletcher points out that at normal conversational level the sounds /v/, /f/, and /θ/ together represent more than half the mistakes in recognition of fundamental speech sounds.

These findings indicate that, although a person with a relatively flat conductive hearing loss may not begin to notice difficulty until the impairment reaches a level of 35 to 40 dB (International Standards Organization), there will, in fact, be a loss of information conveyed by the acoustic signal. This results in a reduction of the overall redundancy of the message. We see evidence of this in the fact that a person with a progressive-conductive-type loss usually first notices difficulty in situations in which the redundancy of the message itself has already been reduced by adverse listening conditions. He finds difficulty, for example, in understanding lectures and sermons or conversation in a group. He may comment that he hears better when he has his glasses on or when he is able to watch the speaker's face. Paul J. La Benz has indicated the extent to which the loss of speech discrimination increases as a result of progressive reduction of intensity [23]. His findings are shown in Table 5.3. These assume that the loss is fairly flat in configuration. Note

TABLE 5.3.   Predicted Discrimination Scores for Subjects With Flat Conductive Audiograms (After LaBenz [23])

Average loss 500–2000 Hz (ASA*)	Discrimination score for phonetically balanced words	
	Hearing alone	Hearing and vision
20–30	75%	88%
40	40%	70%
50	10%	50%
60	less than 10%	20–30%

*American Standards Association

how the increased redundancy of sentences accounts for much better discrimination scores.

Although some sensori-neural losses may be as flat in configuration as the characteristic conductive loss, for the most part they tend to result in an uneven threshold pattern. Some frequencies, generally the higher ones, are more seriously affected than others. The sensori-neural hearing loss therefore results in a loss of sensitivity, coupled with an uneven distortion of the sensitivity of the ear to different frequencies. In attempting to understand the result that this may have on speech discrimination, remember that, with one or two exceptions, speech sounds possess three formants. The first and second formants are essential to recognition of the phoneme, while the third is not essential.

The sensori-neural hearing loss will reduce the sensitivity of the ear to certain frequencies. The resultant effect upon discrimination will depend upon the frequencies involved and the strength and frequency characteristics of the various formants of a given speech sound. The distortion of a phoneme may make its recognition impossible, or it may be sufficient to make the sound inaudible. Numerous research studies on the effect of frequency distortion on speech perception indicate that auditory discrimination for speech sounds is increasingly impaired as more and more of the frequency spectrum is eliminated. The degree of resistance to frequency distortion shown by phonemes varies quite noticeably. This is primarily a characteristic of the pattern of distribution of their sound energy. Fletcher points out, for example, that the sound /i/ as in "team" was correctly identified 98 per cent of the time when either the frequencies above or below 1700 Hz were eliminated [11, p. 415–23]. By contrast, however, the elimination of frequencies below 1500 Hz only slightly affected a listener's ability to recognize the phoneme. The exclusion of frequencies above 400 Hz made recognition practically impossible. Fletcher showed that, while the frequencies below 1000 Hz appeared to be important to the recognition of short vowels, those about 2000 Hz do not contribute very much to discrimination. Long vowels and the diphthongs appear to possess enough distinguishing characteristics in either half of their frequency range to make recognition possible when there is marked distortion.

The high frequencies were shown to contribute a very high percentage of the recognizable characteristics of fricatives. When frequencies above 3000 Hz were eliminated, the percentage discrimination for the sound /s/ was reduced to 40 per cent, for /θ/ to 66 per cent, for /z/ to 80 per cent, for /t/ to 81 per cent, and for /f/ to 85 per cent. Other speech sounds experienced less than a 10 per cent reduction in discrimination when frequencies about 3000 Hz were eliminated. A further incursion into the frequency spectrum, eliminating frequencies above 1000 Hz, again reduced the discrimination scores for consonants without, in general, seriously affecting vowel-sound discrimination. However, once the cutoff excluded frequencies above 500 Hz, the second formant in most vowels was seriously encroached upon and vowel discrimination dropped dramatically. Under this condition, vowel discrimination was sometimes poorer than the discrimination of some of the consonant sounds that were recognized by transition clues.

The data that we have available concerning the affect of frequency and amplitude distortion upon speech-sound discrimination has essentially been obtained by using subjects with normal hearing. It is clear from these findings that the result of such distortion is to reduce the amount of information carried by the acoustic signal as the number of speech frequencies eliminated and the degree of intensity loss increases. We have seen that not all speech sounds are equally affected by this, that in general vowels are more resistant to distortion than consonants, and that the fricative sounds are the most seriously impaired. However, we already know that speech discrimination is not dependent upon the auditory signal alone. The extent to which a person will be able to compensate for acoustic distortion of connected speech will be influenced by how well he can predict the missing components. Unlike the adult, or the child who acquires deafness after learning to speak, the child with a congenital deafness will be hampered not only by his ability to make use of the acoustic signal, but also because of the resulting impairment in the acquisition of language skills, which further reduces the redundancy of a message signal. In spite of the tremendous strides that have been made toward the provision of enriched experiences for the hearing-impaired child, a congenital hearing loss is still likely to result in an impairment of language, even though, in the case of moderate or mild hearing losses, this may only affect the understanding of the subtler aspects of communication.

The Effect of Hearing Impairment on Auditory Perception

It is not possible to make a general statement concerning the effect that hearing impairment has upon the individual's perceptual function, since numerous variables are involved. The severity and pattern of the hearing impairment is obviously of paramount importance. If the hearing loss is profound, the child will be deprived of all auditory input without amplification; thus, his experience of the world will not include awareness of sounds. The child will be deprived of the information that he would normally be able to obtain from environmental sounds; people or objects that do not fall within his visual field will be literally outside his immediate environment. For the deaf child, when the mother leaves the room, all contact with her is lost; he is unable to derive reassurance from hearing her voice and the sound she makes from performing her various household activities when in another room. Unlike those of us who have normal hearing, the person with a profound hearing loss is unable to predict what is occurring in the environment on the basis of the information carried by the auditory cues. For example, as I sit in my office writing this chapter I predict that a secretary is in the front office, since I can hear the sound of typing originating from that direction. I am also aware of the fact that someone is using a tape recorder in an adjacent therapy room and that the blackboard, which I requested to be mounted in one of the rooms, is being put up by the maintenance man.

Experience in working with very young deaf children who have profound congenital sensori-neural hearing losses indicates that in many cases the child has utterly no concept of sound. He develops no awareness of it, and so when he is first introduced to it through a high-powered amplifying unit, he will tend to reject it as something that confuses him and, therefore, impairs his ability to function. It serves as no more than an unpleasant distraction. For such children it is imperative that the teacher or therapist be clearly aware of the impact that amplification of environmental sounds, including speech, will have upon the child. She must be prepared for this rejection and be capable of working with patience in developing awareness of the sound and an understanding of its referential value at the introductory stages of auditory training.

The auditory-perceptual development of the child who has a severe hearing loss, but for whom amplification is not provided during the early years of life, may be similar in many ways to that of the child with a profound deafness. He may also fail to hear most of the environmental sounds at an intensity level at which sufficient information can be derived to make it meaningful. If he is able to hear some sounds he may demonstrate a better awareness of acoustic stimuli. He may show pleasure in listening to sound-making toys that may be partially audible when held very close to his ear. He may also have learned to derive some value from loud environmental sounds that he is able to associate with visual or tactile knowledge of a sound-making object. We can expect the severely hard-of-hearing child, therefore, to have had a modicum of experience in gross sound discrimination. The extent to which he will have incorporated this into his system of adjustment will depend upon the degree to which his residual hearing has made it possible for him to use the sounds he hears to identify things in the environment. Speech, on the other hand, may not have been heard as anything more than a faint mumbling. His inability to derive any meaning from this suggests that it exists for him only as a noise factor. When this type of child is fitted with amplification, the task of making him aware of environmental sounds and speech may be expected to be somewhat easier than it is when working with a profoundly deaf child. In addition, since there is probably considerably more usable residual hearing, the amount of information that amplification will make available to him is much greater. Increased meaning may, after a while, serve to establish a self-rewarding feedback situation.

For the child with a mild-to-moderate loss, the problem is not normally one of a lack of awareness, since a great number of sounds in the environment will have been audible to him. He may be expected to have developed a system of communication with his environment that will incorporate the auditory signal whenever it is loud enough to be utilized. Speech, however, by virtue of the fine discriminations that are involved, has probably never been clear enough or loud enough to be of real value to him. He has probably learned to derive cues from the stress and intonation pattern, and he may listen to the voice even though he is not able to understand the speech. Such a child may or may not be using the speech signal as a means of increasing the amount of information he is able to obtain about a situation. Careful evaluation of the child's communication system will need to be made in order to know at what level he is functioning and the nature of the training that he will need.

In all instances, we have presumed that these children have been deaf from birth and have not previously been provided with amplification. For the child who acquires deafness after speech inception, and for the adult, the problem is very different. In this case, the person is well aware of environmental sounds and has developed a communication system that depends heavily upon the use of audition for information. However, the hearing loss considerably decreases the redundancy of the auditory signal to the point at which the child or adult may no longer be able to comprehend speech in all communication situations. Amplification may compensate for this loss of redundancy by raising the signal intensity to adequate loudness level. However, we have seen that amplification does not provide a high-quality reproduction and compensates little for the frequency distortion imposed by the hearing loss. The hearing-aid user therefore will need training in associating the new sound patterns with his previous internal representations.

VISUAL PERCEPTION AND THE SPOKEN MESSAGE

The role of vision in helping the receiver to reconstruct and interpret the message has, to some extent, been covered in Chap. 4. We shall now consider in more detail the visual cues the listener may make use of and the nature of their contribution to communication.

General Background Cues

Many of you will have seen at least a televised performance of a ballet, in which a story is told completely through body movements. Recently, we have seen an increasing use of such nonverbal communication by certain movie directors. After a performance of the movie "Women in the Dunes" at the State University of New York at Buffalo, the University Film Committee decided that the visual impact of the film was so strong that for one performance a silent version would be shown. In their review of the movie they stated, "Kyoko Kishida's face is more expressive at these moments than any line of the dialogue." Such experiences leave us in little doubt that information can be and is transmitted in the visible nonverbal form. We may be less convinced that this takes place in a more everyday communication situation. One of the easiest ways to decide whether you utilize visual cues in a communication situation is to sit before a television set with the sound turned off. If, under these conditions, you are unable to obtain any information that might be used in an evalution of what the speaker might be saying, then you could conclude that vision is unimportant to communication. I suspect, however, that you will find that this is not the case. Among the things you might find that you had noted might be, whether the speaker was a man, woman, or child; his approximate age; his general appearance; and his manner of dress. You may be able to reach a conclusion concerning the type of person you are watching. Further information concerning his role in the situation will be obtained from the relationship he evidences with other people in the environment and from his general manner or conduct. We make all of these observations about a person who is engaged in a particular activity in a particular situation. The conclusions we reach may not hold true for another person in the same situation or for the same person in a different situation.

On the basis of our observations, we assign a role to the speaker. We are able to do this most easily when the person wears an easily recognizable uniform, a particular mode of dress, or is engaged in a particular activity, such as conducting an orchestra.

> The interpretation of mutual roles serves the purpose of clarifying the verbal, gestural and action messages that people consciously convey to each other. ... Those who are quick to recognize roles and are aware of the shifting nature of roles are at an advantage in dealing with social situations.
> [33, p. 72] (Fig. 5.5)

This is the type of awareness that E. B. Nitchie advocates we should attempt to develop in the hearing-impaired person [29]. He refers to it as "intuitiveness"; you will recognize it as the ability of the person to make accurate predictions on the basis of a minimal pattern of verbal, and nonverbal cues. J. Ruesch and W. Kees emphasize this process when they state:

> In the practice of communication we are continually assessing our material surroundings, making attempts at identifying others and their roles, their status, and their group membership, in order to arrive at a kind of diagnosis that will combine all these features into an integral pattern: *the social*

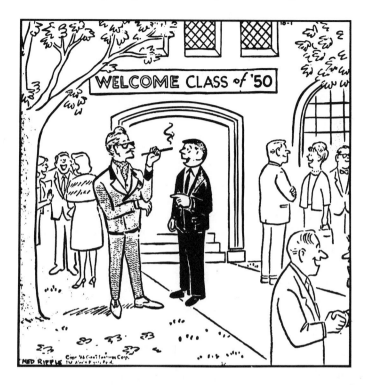

WELCOME CLASS of '50

"I'm trying to remember—did you major in geology or drama?"

Fig. 5.5.   "Those who are quick to recognize roles and are aware of the shifting nature of roles are at an advantage in dealing with social situations." From Ruesch and Kees [33]. (Illustration courtesy of General Features Corporation, New York.)

> *situation.* In the truest sense it is the social situation that determines the context and nature of any communicative exchange. [33, p. 37]

Or to quote R. S. Peters:

> We know what the person will do when he begins to walk toward the pulpit in the middle of the penultimate hymn or what the traveller will do when he enters the doors of the hotel because we know the conventions regulating church services and staying at hotels. [31, p. 7]

These same conventions also regulate the conversation of people and therefore considerably increase our ability to predict what may be said.

In summary, we can say that the contextual cues originate from:

1. The physical environment in which the message is communicated
2. The people in the environment
3. The relationship of the speaker to the people in the environment
4. The general appearance of the speaker, including his build, his age, and his type of dress

Cues Directly Related to the Message

Try now to recall what you noticed about the speaker himself while watching the television without sound. You will almost certainly agree that you observed visual cues that arose from his physical actions. If you consider these more carefully, you will recognize that they consisted of two types of cues:

1. Those that arise from an activity in which the speaker was engaged, or that are expressive of an emotion
2. Those that were clearly intentional gestures

Cues From Implemental Activities

Implemental activities, such as a person taking a wallet from his pocket, opening it, and removing three dollars, provide information against which we interpret the spoken message. Of more particular interest to us, however, are expressive movements that connote a particular emotion. These are primarily of an involuntary nature and may be scarcely noticeable as separate entities. We may, for example, find it quite difficult to say exactly which muscular actions are involved in conveying a look of puzzlement. Yet it has been demonstrated by several investigators that we are able to recognize such emotional expressions from photographs either of actors posing [4, 15] or of emotions elicited by authentic situations [8]. There is little doubt that we expect certain facial expressions to be associated with the emotion evoked by certain situations (Fig. 5.6). Therefore, when seen in context the visual cues help us to predict the verbal message and may considerably increase our accuracy in doing so. They increase the number of constraints and serve as a source of information upon which intersensory trial-and-check procedures can be carried out.

Gestural Cues

Gestures, unlike expressive movements, are made consciously and used in a communication situation. They may be made with almost any body

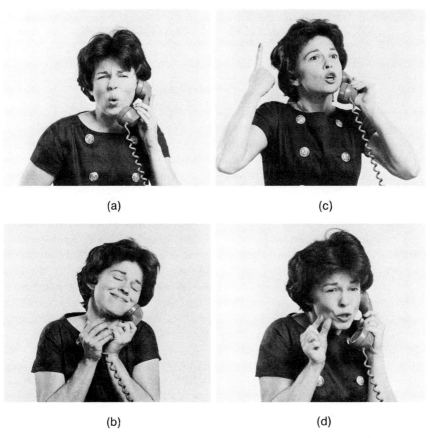

(a) (c)

(b) (d)

Fig. 5.6. Information is present in facial expressions and gestures: (a) learn estimate for fixing the fender; (b) learn husband still loves you in spite of the fender; (c) get out the vote; and (d) tell the store to send those *teeny-weeny* tomatoes for the party. (Courtesy of Ormond Gigli, Inc., New York.)

part, though we are most aware of those involving the head, face, shoulders, and hands and arms (Fig. 5.7). We recognize the significance of the nod of approval or disapproval, the protruded tongue, the shrug of the shoulders, the extended hand, or a raised hand in a classroom. Such gestures may serve as substitutes for the spoken word, though for the most part they accompany speech.

> Gestures are used to illustrate, to emphasize, to point, to explain, or to interrupt; therefore they cannot be isolated from the verbal components of speech. [33, p. 37]

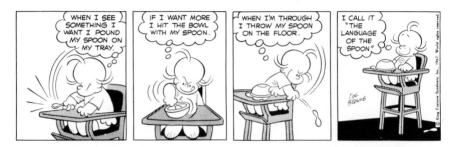

Fig. 5.7.   Gestures can often prove very meaningful. (Illustration courtesy of King Features Syndicate, Inc., New York.)

In normal conversational speech, gestures are used as signs. That is to say, the meaning of the gesture is closely related to the act itself. Such gestures are illustrated in Fig. 5.8. These serve the secondary function of augmenting or modifying the spoken message in some way. It is, however, possible for gestures to be given symbolic value. When this occurs, the meaning is arbitrarily given to the gesture, which now *stands for* the object, event, or idea, rather than being *an extension of it*. In such cases it is impossible to interpret the gesture unless you are familiar with what it stands for. The gesture is no longer a modifier of the word—it has replaced the word. This is how gesture is used by the deaf in a system of symbolic gestural communication that is misleadingly called sign language. Similar systems are used by bookies at a race track and by jobbers in the stock exchange.

Cues Arising Directly From the Spoken Message

Finally, we must consider the contribution made to speech intelligibility by the visible characteristics of the spoken message itself.

The organs of articulation that contribute most to the visible aspects of speech are as follows:

1. *The lips.* Cues to recognition may be derived from various degrees of lip rounding or spreading, ranging from the marked rounding that characterizes the production of the vowel /u/ as in *boot* and the /w/ in *wind*, to the spread lips for the vowel /i/ in *meek* (Fig. 5.9). Protrusion and lip rounding together help in recognition of the /tʃ/ in *church* and /ʃ/ in *ship* (Fig. 5.10).
   Cues to the bilabial plosives /p/ and /b/ and the bilabial nasal /m/ are obtained from observing the lips being brought together (Fig. 5.11). The contact of the lower lip and the upper teeth facilitates the recognition of the labial dental fricatives /f/ and /v/ (Fig. 5.12).

2. *The tongue.* Observation of the tongue position contributes valuable information to the recognition of such sounds as the lingual dental /θ/ and /ð/ in think and these, the /l/ in letter, the lingual alveolar plosives /t/ and /d/, and the lingual nasal /n/ (Fig. 5.13).

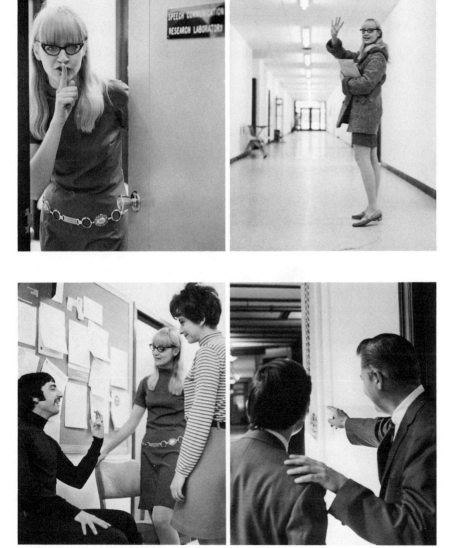

Fig. 5.8.   In conversation, gestures are closely related to the act itself.

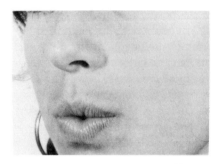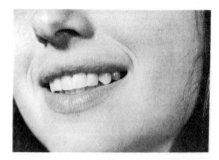

Fig. 5.9. The posture of the lips helps in the discrimination between /u/ or /w/ and /i/.

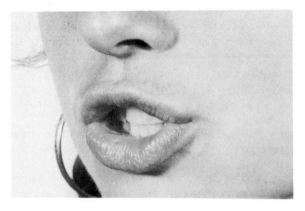

Fig. 5.10. Protrusion and rounding of the lips assist in the identification of /ʃ/ and /tʃ/.

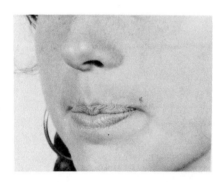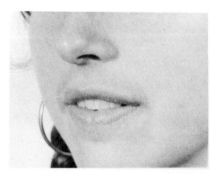

Fig. 5.11. The phonemes /p/, /b/, and /m/ are characterized by lip closure.

Fig. 5.12. The contact of the lower lip and the upper teeth facilitates the recognition of /f/ and /v/.

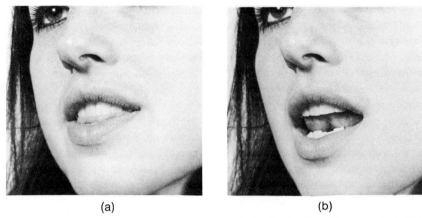

Fig. 5.13. Observation of tongue movement helps in the identification of (a) / θ /, / ð /, and / l / and (b) the sound groups / t /, / d /, and / n /.

3. *The jaw*. From observation of the degree of opening of the jaw, together with information about other articulators, we obtain cues important in the differentiation between vowels, for example, between /a/ as in *arm* and /i/ as in *him* (Fig. 5.14).

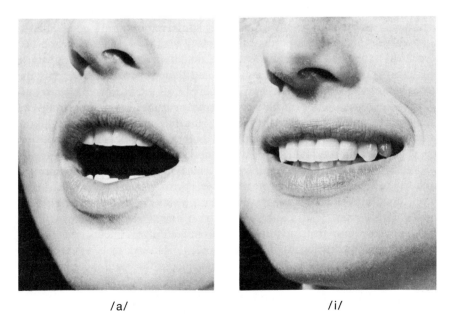

/ a /   / i /

Fig. 5.14. Differentiation between vowels is made on the basis of jaw opening and lip shaping. The contrast between [a] and [i] is shown here.

To the information obtained from these articulators we must add that contributed by the secondary movements of facial muscles associated with the articulation of certain phonemes discussed earlier (Chap. 4).

At this time we are only concerned with the amount of information conveyed by the visible aspects of speech when the auditory components are absent. In an attempt to obtain a little more information about this, we conducted a small project involving twenty college students with normal hearing. We found that when we asked them to recognize phonetically balanced monosyllabic words from visual cues alone, the mean score based upon 100 words was 7.0 words correctly identified. In other words, when visual perception of the spoken word provided the only source of information about the message, only 7 per cent of the material was correctly identified.

J. Utley administered her film test, "How Well Can You Read Lips," to 761 deaf and hard-of-hearing subjects [44]. The mean score obtained on the word-recognition part of the test was 6.9 words (19 per cent) of a possible total of 36. The words in this test were, however, not monosyllabic, but were selected from a test of the first 1,000 most frequently used words. They included a number of bi- and tri-syllabic words, which increased redundancy, and a score of correct was given on the basis of recognition either of the test word or of any of its homophenes. Even so, less than one-fifth of the words were recognized by experienced lip-readers.

If we view these results in the light of our understanding of the factors that limit the visual reception of speech, the low scores obtained through vision alone will not be surprising. The little information one is able to obtain from the visible aspects of the spoken message signal itself is derived from the revealing movements of the articulators. M. Woodward, whose findings we discussed earlier, demonstrated that when we receive only the visible cues to speech the most we can achieve, as far as consonant recognition is concerned, is to be able to classify them into one of six groups of homophenous clusters [45]. Further classification proved impossible on the basis of visual observation alone.

Another observation made by Woodward and supported by J. B. Brannon and F. Kodman, Jr., was that the visibility of movements was related to their place of articulation [2]. Mirror observation of your own speech will illustrate this relationship. You will notice for example that the bilabial cluster /p/, /b/, and /m/ and the lingual dental cluster /f/ and /v/ are far easier to recognize than the lingual alveolar cluster /t/, /d/, /n/, and /l/ or the lingual velar sounds /k/, /g/, and /ŋ/. It is, however, not true to claim that the relationship between visibility and place of articulation is on a one-to-one basis. Since the formative movements of the lingual alveolar fricative sounds /s/ and /z/ and the alveolar fricatives /θ/ and /ð/ occur at the same place of articulation as the /t/, /d/, /n/, and /l/ cluster (see Table 5.4), they should be equally hard to recognize. In fact they possess a high coefficient of visibility (1.0) bestowed upon them by the secondary revealing movements of the lips.

TABLE 5.4. Homophenous Clusters of Initial English Consonants (After Woodward [45])

(a)	p	b	m						
		f	v						
	m	w	r						
(b)	ch	dʒ	ʃ	ʒ	j				
	t	d	n	l	s	z	θ	ð	
	k	g	h						

TOTAL PERCEPTION

In this chapter, so far, we have studied some of the general principles involved in the process of perception. We have looked a little more closely at the aspects of the auditory and visual stimuli that contribute to the ability of the receiver to reconstruct the message-signal codes reaching him through various sensory channels. To facilitate our study of speech perception, we examined the auditory and visual components independently. You will recognize the artificiality of such a dichotomy. The integral relationship of sensory pathways in the process of perception has already been stressed.

The influence of sensory data received through audition upon the perception of data received through vision has been demonstrated among others by J. W. Gebhard and G. H. Mowbray [17] and later by T. Shipley [36]. They studied the effect that the rate of flutter of a clicking sound would have upon a subject's perception of the rate of flicker of a flashing light. They established both the critical flicker and the critical flutter rate. Critical flicker is the frequency at which a flashing light first appears steady, while critical flutter is the frequency at which a clicking sound appears to be uninterrupted. Intersensory interaction was then demonstrated by presenting a light at a given frequency at a specific rate of perceived flicker. Simultaneously the subject heard a complex sound set to flutter at the same frequency as the visual stimulus. The frequency of the auditory stimulus was then gradually increased and decreased. As would be expected, the rate of auditory flutter was perceived to increase or decrease accordingly; however, the surprising observation was that the perceived visual flicker rate also increased and decreased in the same manner, even though the physical stimulus was held constant. It is interesting to note that it was not found possible to reverse the procedure and modify the auditory perception by varying the visual stimulus. The experiment does, however, emphasize the role of intersensory-neural interaction.

We can, perhaps, understand how this can occur if we see it within the context of the interchannel trial-and-check process. The desire to achieve intersensory-perceptual agreement was so great that it produced what was really a misperception. Such interaction of sensory information also occurs between the olfactory (smell) and gustatory (taste) senses when you perceive the flavor of something you eat. You are familiar with this because of your experience with the reduction in the perception of flavor that often accompanies a cold. Perhaps less obvious to you is the relationship between color and taste [30]. I can well recall a meal I once had in Norway that proved unappetizing primarily by virtue of its complete lack of color. It consisted of boiled potatoes, boiled cod, and cauliflower in white béarnaise sauce, all served on white bone china. My artistic talents cried out for a bottle of ketchup!

We shall review more fully the research findings concerning the integration of visual and auditory information when we discuss the integrated approach to therapy in Chap. 9.

The process of total perception may therefore be seen as involving an internal restructuring of the symbolic representation of the situation, event, thought, or idea, which occurs in ones external environment. We do this by the use of data reaching us through our various sensory channels. In human communication we are concerned with the process of transmission and reception of a series of instructions. These carry information designed to permit the receiver to predict, with varying degrees of accuracy, the idea that the sender wished to communicate. This stage is concerned with comprehension, with information processing. It requires the ability to sustain recognition over a period of time. In this stage, words and nonverbal cues are stored in order to establish context to permit the occurrence of the probability analysis, which we discussed earlier (Chap. 4).

As the data comes in through the sensory pathways and travels up to the central processing area, different parts of it are analyzed at the various substations along the route [1, p. 338]. The information from all sensory modalities is then put into a common pool. The important question is now whether, as a listener, using your knowledge of structural, contextual, and situational probabilities, you have enough information within the pool to reconstruct the message.

For communication between individuals with normal hearing under favorable listening conditions, the amount of information in the pool is usually far greater than the minimum required to predict the message. The auditory pathway alone contributes more than enough for this purpose. The data contributed by the other sensory pathways constitutes the redundancy factor to which the receiver turns for additional information when the noise level in the system makes accurate reception difficult.

To reconstruct any particular message the person needs a certain minimum amount of instructional information. We have seen in our discussion of communication that it is possible to predict accurately a significant percentage of those instructions on the basis of limited information. We learned that the amount of data we need in order to predict the missing components varies with a variety of factors, which we listed in Table 2.2. If you obtain a minimum amount of information, it is immaterial through which channels it came.

The situation may be considered analogous to that which might occur if a group of three students wished to purchase a second-hand car. The reason they agree to pool their financial resources is that no one person has sufficient funds to purchase the car alone. The actual price of the car may be $600; the minimum needed to obtain it is a down payment of $150. It is most convenient to assume that each student contributed an equal sum toward the down payment, though it would be perfectly possible for the sum to be obtained by each student contributing different proportions. No matter how the contributions vary in proportion, providing a minimum of $150 is raised, the car will be obtained. If each of the students contributes $100 to the fund, then the additional $150 is in excess of what they actually require in order to take possession of the car. They may, however, need the additional money if they discover that the price has subsequently been raised or if they failed to allow for the sales tax. In this analogy, the salesman represents the receiver, the total cost of the car ($600) represents the total message, while the down payment ($150) represents the minimum information necessary to understand the essential aspects of the message. The three students, each contributing a sum of money to the pool, stand for the channels through which the receiver obtains his information. The difference between the amount of money the students absolutely have to contribute and the amount they actually have may be considered to be the redundancy factor that will be reduced if the noise in the system (unexpected sales tax) goes up. The important point to remember is that, just as in the analogy, it is perfectly possible in communication that the information arriving through a single channel is not sufficient for perception to take place. This does not, however, mean that this channel is not important. It may be that no one channel is contributing enough information to permit perception, yet when the various amounts of data from different channels are pooled, the total may be more than adequate to permit the reconstruction of the original message. It must again be stressed that the pooling of data is not a simple additive function as would have been the case in our analogy of the student's financial contributions to the group fund. The process is one of integration or blending. Each unit of information assumes a different value when combined with the other units. A single piece of a jigsaw puzzle may be meaningless alone, yet when fitted together with several other pieces, it not only adds information, it also modifies your perception of the other pieces and may suddenly acquire a meaning of its own, permitting perception to take place. If you now remove it and view it alone, you see it quite differently by virtue of what you know about its interaction with the other pieces.

This philosophy underlies the approach to rehabilitation that characterizes this text. We recognize that the hard-of-hearing person in many communication situations receives inadequate information through the auditory channel to permit him to accurately reconstruct the idea the speaker wishes to convey. Unfortunately it has been demonstrated that the visual channel alone does not convey enough information for it to serve as an alternative source from which that information may be derived. Our aim must therefore be to establish a program of rehabilitation that integrates all sources of information. G. A. Miller, in his chapter "The Perception of Speech," concludes:

> Perceiving speech is not a passive, automatic procedure. The perceiver contributes a selective function by responding to some aspects of the total situation and not to others. He responds to the stimuli according to some organization that he imposes upon them. And he supplements the inconsistent or absent stimulation in a manner that is consistent with his needs and his past experience. [28, p. 79]

We aim to provide the hearing-impaired person with a perceptual approach to communication that is more productive. Although during training we shall function to a great extent on a conscious level of behavior, ultimately the hearing-impaired person must incorporate these patterns into an unconsciously assumed communication behavioral set—what Church refers to a an "organismic mobilization." In subsequent chapters we shall consider how this may be achieved.

REFERENCES

1. Bocca, E., and C. Calearo. "Central Hearing Processes." in *Modern Developments in Audiology,* ed. James Jerger. New York: Academic Press Inc., 1963.

2. Brannon, J. B., and F. Kodman, Jr. "The Perceptual Process in Speech Reading." *A.M.A. Archives of Otolaryngology* 70 (1959): 111–19.

3. Church, J. *Language and the Discovery of Reality.* New York: Random House, Inc., 1961.

4. Coleman, J. C. "Facial Expression of Emotion." *Psychological Monographs* 63 (1949): 1–36.

5. Cooper, F. S., K. S. Harris, and P. F. MacNeilage. "A Motor Theory of Speech Perception." *Proceedings of the Speech Communication Seminar, 1962.* Stockholm: Stohckholm Royal Institute of Technology, 1963.

6. Cotzin, M., and M. Dallenback. "Facial Vision: The Role of Pitch and Loudness in the Perception of Obstacles by the Blind." *American Journal of Psychology* 63: 485–515.

7. Crandall, I. B. "The Sounds of Speech." *Bell System Technical Journal* 4 (October 1925): 586–626.

8. Dolanski, V. "Les aveugles possidentile les sens d'obstacles," *Année Psychologique* 31 (1930): 1–51.

9. Dusenbury, D., and F. H. Knaiver. "Experimental Studies in Symbolism of Action and Voice: I. A Study of Meaning in Facial Expression." *Quarterly Journal of Speech* 24 (1938): 424–36.

10. Fischer-Jorgansen, E. "New Techniques in Acoustic Phonetics." *Psycholinguistics,* ed. Sol Saporta. New York: Holt, Rinehart & Winston, Inc., 1961.

11. Fletcher, H. *Speech and Hearing in Communication.* New York: D. Van Nostrand Company, Inc., 1953.

12. Fletcher, H., and W. A. Mundson. *Hearing: Its Psychology and Physiology,* eds. S. S. Stevens and H. Davis. New York: John Wiley & Sons, Inc., 1938.

13. _____. "Loudness: Its Definition, Measurement and Calculation." *Journal of the Acoustical Society of America* 5: 82–108.

14. French, J. D. "The Reticular Formation." *Scientific American* 196 (1957): 54–60.

15. Fry, D. E., and E. Whetnal. *The Deaf Child.* London: William Heinemann, Ltd., 1962.

16. Fryda, N., and E. Philipzoon. "Dimensions of Recognition of Expression." *Journal of Abnormal Psychology* 66 (1963): 45–51.

17. Gebbard, J. W., and G. H. Mowbray. "On Discriminating the Rate of Visual Flicker and Auditory Flutter." *American Journal of Psychology* 72 (1959): 521–29.

18. Hawkins, J. E., and S. Stevens. "The Masking of Pure Tones by White Noise." *Journal of the Acoustical Society of America* 22 (1950): 6–13.

19. Hilgard, E. R. *Introduction to Psychology.* (2nd ed.). New York: Harcourt, Brace, and World, Inc., 1957.

20. Hirsh, I. J. *The Measurement of Hearing.* New York: McGraw-Hill Book Company, 1952.

21. Jacobson, E. "Electrophysiology and Mental Activities." *American Journal of Psychology* 44 (1932): 677–94.

22. Kohler, I. *American Foundation for the Blind Research Bulletin* 4 (1944) No. 14.

23. LaBenz, Paul J. "Potential of Auditory Perception for Various Levels of Hearing Loss." *Volta Review* 58 (1956): 387–402.

24. Lawson, Chester A. *Brain Mechanisms and Human Learning.* (The International Series in the Behavioral Sciences). Boston: Houghton Mifflin Company, 1967.

25. Liberman, Alvin M. "Some Results of Research on Speech Perception." *Psycholinguistics,* ed. Sol Saporta. New York: Holt, Rinehart & Winston, Inc., 1961.

26. Liberman, A. M., F. S. Cooper, D. P. Shankweiler, and M. Studdert-Kennedy. "Perception of the Speech Code." *Psychological Review* 74 (November 1967): 431–61.

27. Mowrer, H. O. "On the Psychology of Talking Birds." *Learning Theory and Personality Dynamics.* New York: Ronald Press Co., 1950.

28. Miller, G. A. *Language and Communication.* New York: McGraw-Hill Book Company, 1963.

29. Nitchie, E. B. *Lip Reading: Principles and Practice.* New York: Frederick A. Stokes Company, 1912.

30. Pangborn, P. M. "Influence of Color on the Discrimination of Sweetness." *American Journal of Psychology* 73 (1960): 229–38.

31. Peters, R. S. *The Concept of Motivation.* London: Routledge & Kegan Paul, Ltd., 1958.

32. Rice, Charles. "Human Echo Perception." *Science* 155 (February 1967): 656–64.

33. Ruesch, J., and W. Kees. *Nonverbal Communication.* Berkeley and Los Angeles: University of California Press, 1956.

34. Senden, Marius von. *Space and Sight.* The perception of space and shape in the congenitally blind before and after operation. London: Methuen & Co., Ltd., 1960.

35. Seward, J. P. "The Effect of Practice on the Visual Perception of Form." *Archives of Psychology* 20 (1931): no. 130, p. 72.

36. Shipley, T. "Auditory Flutter: Driving of Visual Flicker." *Science* 145 (September 1954): 1328–30.

37. Solley, C. M., and P. Murphy. *Development of the Perceptual World.* New York: Basic Books, Inc., Publishers, 1960.

38. Solomon, R. L., L. J. Kamin, and L. C. Wynne. "Traumatic Avoidance Learning: The Outcomes of Several Extinction Procedures with Dogs." *Journal of Abnormal and Social Psychology* 48 (1953): 291–302.

39. Solomon, R. L., and L. C. Wynne. "Avoidance Conditioning in Normal Dogs and in Dogs Deprived of Normal Autonomic Functioning." *American Psychologist* 5 (1950): 264.

40. _____. "Traumatic Avoidance Learning: The Principles of Anxiety Conservation and Partial Irreversibility." *Psychological Review* 61 (1954): 353–85.

41. Solovev, I. M. "The Significance of the Training of Hearing for the Development of Perceptual Activity in Deafmute Children in Russian Translations on Speech and Hearing." *American Speech and Hearing Association, Report No. 3* (March 1968), pp. 122–23.

42. Supa, M., M. Cotzin, and K. M. Dallenbach. "Facial Vision: The Perception of Obstacles by the Blind." *American Journal of Psychology* 57 (1944): 142–52.

43. Thorpe, W. H. *Learning and Instinct in Animals.* London: Methuen & Co., Ltd., 1956. See F. A. Beach, "Experimental Investigation of Species-Specific Behavior." *American Psychologist* 15 (1960): 1–18.

44. Utley, J. "A Test of Lipreading Ability." *Journal of Speech and Hearing Disorders* 11 (1946): 109–16.

45. Woodward, M. "Linguistic Methodology in Lip Reading Research." *John Tracy Clinic Research Papers* 6 (December 1957): 1–32.

46. Woodworth, R. S. "Reinforcement of Perception." *American Journal of Psychology* 60 (1947): 119–24.

CHAPTER SIX

Amplification and Hearing Aids

The type of questions asked about hearing aids by parents and teachers of hearing-impaired children and by adults who have purchased aids illustrate the many misconceptions that exist concerning the benefit that amplification can provide to a person with a hearing loss. An audiologist or teacher is frequently asked:

> For how long will Mary need to wear the hearing aid?
> Will the hearing aid improve my hearing to the point where I will be able to manage without it?
> Will my hearing deteriorate as a result of using the aid?
> Won't he become dependent upon the aid?
> Doesn't he hear as well as I when he's wearing the aid?
> He still doesn't seem to understand me even though he now has the aid.
> Why is his speech still not normal even with the aid?
> Will my baby learn to speak now that she has been fitted with the aid?
> Will she need to wear the aid at home as well as in school?

These questions are helpful in providing us with an indication of the type of information that the teacher or hearing therapist needs to have if she is to be able to provide meaningful counseling, information that this chapter and the next attempt to provide.

Perhaps the simplest question that we can ask pertinent to the topic of this chapter would be: What is a hearing aid? We can answer it quite simply by stating that *a hearing aid is any device capable of intensifying the sound reaching a person's ear (cochlea).* This intensification, more commonly referred to as amplification, may be achieved in two ways: (1) The sound energy may be concentrated at the ear rather than being permitted to dissipate across a wide area, or (2) energy may be added to the original signal.

MECHANICAL AMPLIFICATION

An example of the concentration of sound energy is provided by the added loudness that occurs if you cup your hands to your ear or listen to someone whispering into one of the cardboard tubes found in the center of a roll of kitchen paper or aluminum foil. This method of amplifying sound was one of the earliest used to aid hearing-impaired persons. The use of ear trumpets (Fig. 6.1), before the development of electrical hearing aids, was based partly on the principle of concentrating energy gathered over a relatively large area onto the small area represented by the ear piece. This is the same principle of amplification as that provided by the human middle-ear mechanism. In the ear, energy is gathered over the relatively large area of the tympanic membrane, or eardrum. This energy is then conducted across the ossicular chain and concentrated on the very small area of the oval window into which the foot plate of the stapes is inserted. The ossicular chain thus serves to match the low impedance of the eardrum to the high impedance of the cochlea and reduces energy loss.

In addition to the concentration factor, mechanical hearing aids utilize the phenomenon of resonance to concentrate the energy within the frequency

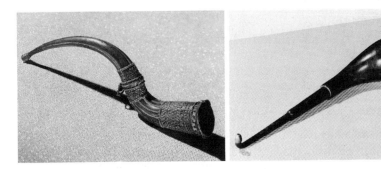

Fig. 6.1. Two artistically designed ear trumpets. (Courtesy of Zenith Hearing Aid Sales Corp.)

range most important to speech. The improvement in speech reception threshold provided by such instruments has been shown to be as much as 15 decibels [1, p. 268]. This may be sufficient additional intensity to make speech useful to a person to whom it might otherwise be just barely audible. Additional intensity is gained since the speaker generally speaks directly into the broad end of the tube, providing further concentration of sound energy.

Such devices are seldom used now, though local hearing-aid dealers say that they still occasionally find an older person who is able to derive benefit from a mechanical aid when they are unable to tolerate the use of an electrical one.

ELECTRICAL AMPLIFICATION

The principles of electrical amplification are obviously far more complex than those involved in mechanical amplification. It is not necessary for the hearing therapist to have a thorough knowledge of the electronics of the hearing aid. However, knowledge of the fundamental principles involved in amplification and a familiarity with the major components and controls of the hearing aid is important. It serves to eliminate the feeling of inadequacy that the therapist or teacher may otherwise feel when first encountering a hearing-aid user. It also encourages her to make better use of amplifying units, and it is essential to the counseling of the hearing-impaired person and his family in the most effective use of hearing aids.

Types of Electrical Hearing Aids

Hearing aids that utilize the principles of electrical amplification may be classified within three main categories:

1. Wearable aids
2. Portable desk amplifiers, referred to as auditory training units or speech training units
3. Group hearing aids

Wearable Aids

There are many types and makes of wearable hearing aids. These may be designed to be worn attached to an article of clothing, they may be built into the temple of a pair of glasses, they may be shaped to curve behind the ear, or they may even be designed to fit within the ear canal itself (Fig. 6.2). Obviously one of the most important factors that the manufacturers have

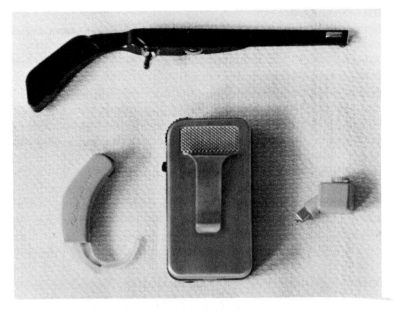

Fig. 6.2. The existing categories of wearable personal hearing aids. (Courtesy of Beltone Hearing Aid Co.)

had to consider in the development of wearable hearing aids has been the size of the instrument. The progress that has been made in this direction is very apparent if you compare the two aids shown in Fig. 6.3. However, even with the advent of the transistor amplifier, the size of an aid still remains a factor in determining both the amount of amplification that can be provided and the number of modifying features that can be incorporated. In general, it may be stated that, while the insert ear-canal-type aid may provide assistance to some people with mild losses, a moderate hearing impairment will require the use of a behind-the-ear model, a glasses aid, or one of the smaller body aids. Children and adults with severe or profound hearing losses generally benefit only from the more powerful aids worn on the clothing or in a special harness. We shall consider the factors that are taken into consideration in recommending a particular type of wearable aid when we discuss hearing-aid selection procedures.

Auditory Training Units

Auditory training units perform the same function as a wearable hearing aid, but since they are not as restricted by the factor of size, they are able to provide higher-quality sound reproduction. The range of frequencies to which the auditory trainer is sensitive is much greater than those of wearable

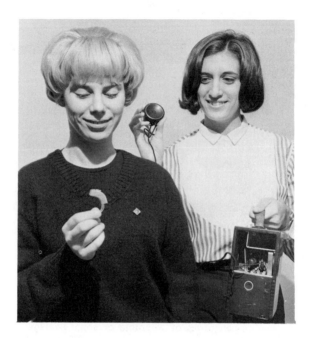

Fig. 6.3. Progress in hearing-aid design, 1921–1969. On the left is a contemporary hearing aid; on the right is a model of the first vacuum-tube hearing aid manufactured. The large table-model vacuum-tube instrument, patented by Earl Hansen in 1920, used a single vacuum tube. The instruments shown are from the hearing-aid museum at Kent State University, Kent, Ohio. (Courtesy of Kent State University.)

hearing aids. The maximum amount of amplification is also greater, and a wider range of tone-control settings are often available. In addition, the auditory trainer can be built to contain two entirely separate amplifying systems within one unit, providing true binaural or stereophonic sound reproduction, the advantages of which we shall discuss later. Auditory trainers are manufactured by a number of companies so that there are a variety of makes and models available. We shall be considering several representative types and will discuss the various features that should be considered when purchasing a unit. We shall leave our discussion of the most effective use of these aids until we consider, in the next chapter, the methods of auditory training.

Group Hearing Aids

Group hearings aids are, as their name implies, amplifying units that provide multiple outlets to provide high-quality amplification to a group of hearing-impaired children or adults. These units may be portable table-top models used by an itinerant teacher of the deaf or a hearing therapist, or they may be console units designed to drive many headsets and to incorporate a record player and a tape-recording-playback unit.

Before we consider these various types of amplifying systems, let us examine some of the components basic to them all.

Components of Hearing Aids

We have seen that hearing aids are amplifying units. All such units, whether they constitute large public-address systems or small wearable hearing aids, may be reduced to three basic components (Fig. 6.4). These are:

1. The microphone
2. The amplier
3. The speaker

We shall examine each of these three parts of the amplifying system to see what its particular function is and, briefly, how it achieves this function.

The Microphone

The purpose of the microphone is to change into electrical energy the energy carried by the sound waves. Since the frequency and intensity patterns of the sound waves represent coded information concerning the mes-

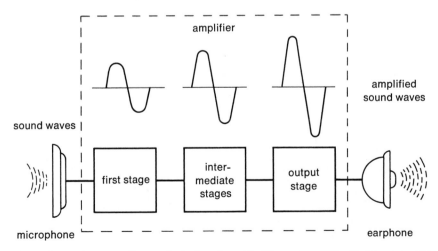

Fig. 6.4. Schematic diagram of a hearing aid. (Courtesy of Zenith Hearing Aid Sales Corp.)

sage, they must be duplicated as exactly as possible when they are changed into electrical form. How is this achieved?

We know that magnetized materials such as magnets, set up magnetic fields around them. These fields link together the north and south poles of the magnet (Fig. 6.5). When the north and south poles of the magnet are placed close to each other as occurs in a magnetic microphone, the lines of magnetic flux exist in the "air gap," and the loop, which constitutes the magnetic circuit, must always be completed. An electrical conductor is placed in the air gap perpendicular to the lines of flux. Unless we move the conductor, no change will occur in the magnetic field, and no current will flow. If, however, we connect the wire conductor to a complete circuit (as a loop containing a resistor), it is possible to induce a current flow by movement of the conductor perpendicular to the lines of magnetic flux. If the circuit is not completed, current will not flow, though a voltage will be induced in the wire.

The electrical current is actually the result of the movement of electrons within the conductor. This has been brought about by the physical movement of the conductor between the north and south poles of the magnet, thus converting (transducing) mechanical energy to electrical energy. The flow of electrons alternates in direction between the north and south poles. The direction of the current flow, which is determined by the direction of the movement of the wire conductor, also alternates. When the flow is toward the north pole, we say the current has *positive polarity*; when it is toward the south pole, the polarity is said to be *negative polarity*.

The amount, or intensity, of current induced is proportional to the rate at which the flux lines are cut by the moving conductor. The potential energy is expressed in *volts* relative to a reference voltage in the same manner as sound-pressure level is expressed relative to a reference pressure, which we may refer to as zero decibels. Variations in pressure are then expressed as plus or minus a given number of decibels. Similarly the reference voltage, zero volts, need not mean that no current is flowing; it simply represents a constant reference level of voltage that constitutes a steady state. Voltage amplitude is then expressed relative to this reference figure.

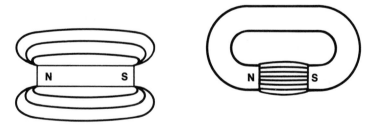

Fig. 6.5.   Lines of magnetic flux couple the north and south poles of the magnet.

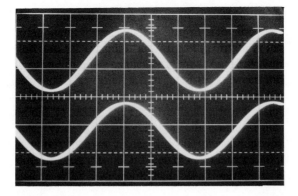

Fig. 6.6. A comparison of a pure-tone wave form and an alternating electrical wave form.

The number of times that the current flow reverses itself in a given time unit is determined by the number of physical movements of the conducting wire. Since the current flow is alternating in direction, the cycle, from the zero-volt reference level, through the positive and then the negative phase, back to the reference point, constitutes the *frequency* expressed in Hertz. Figure 6.6 illustrates graphically the positive and negative phases of this electrical cycle alongside the sinusoidal wave form of the pure tone. From this illustration it will be apparent how it is possible to achieve in the electrical wave an exact duplication of the intensity and frequency pattern of the sound wave. This transduction process is provided by the microphone. Reference to Fig. 6.7 will help you to understand the way in which it functions. From the diagram you will observe that two magnets are placed with the north and south poles opposite to each other. One set of poles are separated by nonmagnetic brass spacers, providing what is essentially one magnet with a north and south pole. The brass spacers hold in position a thin strip of metal, called the *reed*, which extends between the north and south pole of the magnet. Around the reed is wound a coil of copper wire, the leads of which run to the amplifier. Attached to the reed is a metal drive pin, the other end of which is connected to a diaphragm.

The diaphragm of the microphone consists of a thin sheet of metal foil stretched so that it is sensitive to changes of air pressure occurring when sound waves impinge upon it. The compression and rarefaction of the air molecules that are in contact with the metal diaphragm causes the diaphragm to move on either side of its position of rest. The movements are transmitted to the magnetized reed through the drive pin, causing changes to occur in the magnetic field. These changes are reflected in the molecular movement of the wire coil and result in the induction of a small alternating current. You will recall that we said earlier that an induced current results

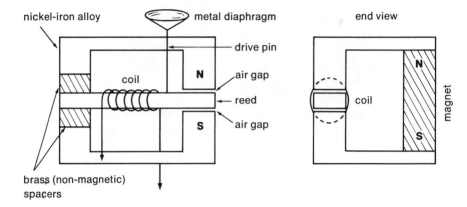

balanced armature microphone

Fig. 6.7. Schematic diagram of a microphone. (Courtesy of Zenith Hearing Aid Sales Corp.)

from the movement of a conductor within a magnetic field. In actual fact, in the microphone just described, the magnetic field moves through the coil, rather than the coil moving through the magnetic field. However, the end result remains the same.

The movement of the diaphragm is determined by the compression and rarefaction of the air particles. As the air pressure builds up, the diaphragm will be pressed inward; as the air pressure decreases the diaphragm will be relaxed and will move outward as rarefaction occurs. The resultant *induced voltage* follows this same movement, so that there is a relative shift toward the positive polarity during the compression stage, and a shift toward the negative polarity during rarefaction, resulting in the induction of an *alternating current* in the coil. The current will alternate at exactly the same frequency as the sound waves striking the diaphragm. If the intensity of the sound wave increases, then the backward and forward excursion of the diaphragm, resulting from the increased compression and rarefaction, will cause a greater movement of the reed, a more significant disturbance of the magnetic field, and therefore, an increase in the amplitude of the voltage induced in the coil.

The Amplifier

The amplifier constitutes the most complex part of a hearing aid. It contains transistors, resistors, capacitors, switches, and wires, each of which has a particular function. Since you will not be qualified to make any adjustments to these internal parts, there is no purpose in our discussing them. However, should you be interested in obtaining more specific information concerning how they function, an explanation of this basic technical information will be found in the text *Hearing and Deafness* [1, pp. 278–86] and in an excellent booklet entitled *Hearing Aids and Their Components* [20]. We shall consider the controls that operate the amplifier later in this section.

The Receiver

The earphone or bone-conduction vibrator of the wearable hearing aid, or the headphone of the auditory training unit constitutes the receiver. The acoustic signal that was picked up by the microphone and transduced into electrical energy is fed through the amplifier and then to the receiver. The function of the receiver is exactly opposite to that of the microphone. The microphone converts acoustic energy into electrical impulses, whereas the receiver serves to transduce those amplified electrical impulses back into acoustic energy. The receiver is therefore a sort of microphone in reverse, and its structure is almost identical to that of the microphone. Its basic components are a magnet, a coil, and a diaphragm. You will observe from Fig. 6.8 that two magnetic pole pieces are attached to a permanent magnet.

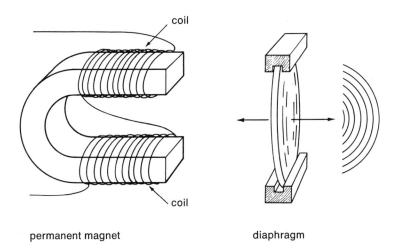

coil

coil

permanent magnet   diaphragm

Fig. 6.8. Representation of an output transducer for converting electrical energy to acoustic energy. (Courtesy of Zenith Hearing Aid Sales Corp.)

Around these pole pieces is wrapped a coil of fine copper wire, the ends of which are connected to a cord that runs from the amplifier. Mounted a few thousandths of an inch in front of the ends of the pole pieces is a very thin diaphragm of magnetic material.

The current from the amplifier travels to the coils wound around the magnetic pole pieces. In doing so, they cause changes to occur in the field of the magnet, alternately increasing and decreasing the magnetic pull of the current in the coil. In this way, the diaphragm is caused to be alternately attracted to and repelled by the magnet. This oscillating movement of the diaphragm sets up pressure changes in the air surrounding it, thus converting electrical energy into the physical energy of sound waves. The greater the intensity of the alternating current, the greater the changes in the magnetic field, resulting in a greater backward and forward movement of the diaphragm. Thus, the intensity of the electrical current determines the intensity of the pressure waves produced. The frequency with which the current alternates will determine the rate of oscillation of the diaphragm and, therefore, the frequency of the sound waves generated.

The sound waves that are emitted by the earphone are therefore theoretically duplicates of the sound waves that stimulated the microphone, except that they have been increased in their intensity by the amplifier. The bone-conduction receiver operates in exactly the same manner, except that the diaphragm is firmly attached to the plastic case, which is worn in contact with the mastoid process of the listener who receives the vibrations through bone conduction.

Very briefly, one may say that the microphone transduces the pattern of the sound waves into a similar pattern of electrical energy, the amplifier then makes these electrical impulses stronger, while the earphone transduces the amplified signals back into sound waves.

The Controls of the Aid

The Volume Control

All hearing aids are equipped with a volume control, often referred to as the *gain control*. It is by use of this control that the intensity of the signal leaving the receiver can be varied over a range of decibels. This is achieved by amplifying the incoming signal, the *input*, by a predetermined maximum amount known as the *maximum gain*. The gain is then attenuated, or reduced by the volume control to a desired level, by the introduction of a resistor, which is simply a poor conductor of electricity (Fig. 6.9). In the wearable hearing aid, the resistive element consists of a circular strip of carbon. A small metal arm attached to the revolving wheel of the volume

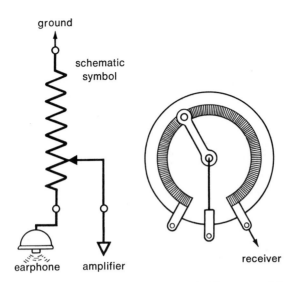

Fig. 6.9. Schematic diagram of a volume control. (Courtesy of Zenith Hearing Aid Sales Corp.)

control is moved around the carbon ring as the volume control is turned up. In doing so, the amount of carbon placed between a fixed terminal and the movable arm may be varied, thus varying the resistance to the current. If the current is required to pass through the complete arc of carbon, then almost all of it is attenuated. The schematic symbol on the left-hand side of the diaphragm in Fig. 6.9 shows that, as the volume control is moved, the amount of the resistor through which the signal travels, from point *A* to the arrow contact, varies. In this way, the overall amount of amplification or gain added to the input signal is modified. The rate of attenuation of maximum gain will vary from aid to aid. In the wearable hearing aid, the volume control may be marked by numerals or letters, or it simply may not be marked at all. Any markings on individual aids can only be used as rough guides to the intensity settings. The gain in decibels represented by turning up the control from one setting to the next cannot be assumed to be a constant factor, since the intensity growth is seldom linear. Battery power drainage also constitutes a factor influencing the consistency of the gain provided at a given setting.

In the auditory training units, the volume control is generally calibrated to provide attenuation levels that may either be read directly from the markings on the control or obtained from the specification sheets. This makes it possible to preselect a listening level, an advantage that is particularly valuable when working with small children.

Output Limiter

The development of transistorized amplifying circuits has made the provision of large amounts of gain a simple task. It is therefore essential for a hearing aid to incorporate a maximum acoustic output limiter. The term *maximum acoustic output* refers to the maximum acoustic energy that can be provided by the amplifier, regardless of the intensity of the original signal fed into it. If, for example, an amplifier has an overall gain of 50 decibels and a maximum acoustic output of 130 decibels, the output level of 130 decibels cannot be exceeded even if we feed into the amplifier an input signal of 95 decibels. Were the output not limited, an input signal of 95 decibels added to 50 decibels of gain would produce an output of 145 decibels.

The limiting of output is necessary to insure that high-intensity input sounds are not amplified to levels that exceed the listeners' threshold of discomfort and pain. The normal ear is sensitive to discomfort at approximately 120 decibels SPL above 0.0002 microbar, experiences tickle at 130 decibels, and feels pain at 140 decibels SPL. In some cases of deafness the presence of recruitment may markedly reduce the tolerance for high levels of amplification. The phenomenon of recruitment produces in the listener an unusually rapid growth in loudness once the threshold of hearing has been crossed. People with this condition frequently exhibit lowered thresholds of discomfort; that is, the threshold of discomfort is reached at a lower intensity level than normal.

Methods of Limiting Output

There are two methods by which the maximum acoustic output of the amplifier can be limited. The first is by a process of *peak clipping*. This involves the cutting off of peak intensities whenever they exceed the maximum output limit (Fig. 6.10). It has been conclusively demonstrated that the peak intensities of speech can be quite severely clipped without producing any significant loss of intelligibility [3, 14]. This is due to the fact that the vowel sounds, which are more intense than consonant sounds and which contribute less to intelligibility, reach maximum output levels first. Clipping the vowel peaks permits the overall gain to be turned up. Amplification of the relatively weaker consonants can therefore occur without impairment of vowel intelligibility. The spectra of speech sounds subjected to peak clippings has been shown to be only slightly modified by the process [15]. However, although intelligibility remains unaffected by moderate peak clipping, the quality of the sound is generally adversely affected. This can be compensated for by providing relatively greater amplification of the high-frequency components of speech sound than of the low-frequency sounds.

The second method of providing output limitation is by *compression*

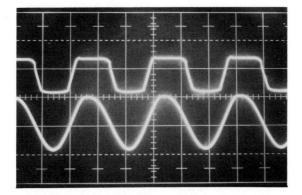

Fig. 6.10. The effect of peak clipping on the wave form of an acoustic signal.

amplification. This is achieved by an automatic electrical-circuit servo-system, generally referred to as the *automatic volume control* (AVC) or automatic gain control (AGC). When the intensity of the electrical signal at the final stage of amplification (output stage) exceeds a predetermined level, sufficient current flows through a feedback circuit to the first stage or first and second stages of amplification to influence its function in a manner that decreases the gain it provides. The intensity level of the electrical signal at the output stage that will induce this decrease in gain may be modified on a variable resistor similar to the volume control. In some aids it involves the choice of one of several control settings, each of which represents a feedback circuit offering a particular resistance to the feedback current. The current intensity must be sufficient to overcome the resistance before compression of the sound wave will occur. The control that determines this level is sometimes referred to as the *comfort-control.* The chart shown in Fig. 6.11 illustrates the compression provided by AVC at various levels of gain. You will see that for the full-gain curve, changes of 50 to 100 decibels of input intensity at the microphone (a 50 decibel increase) result in output changes of less than 10 decibels. This provides protection to the hearing-aid wearer. The compression action for stated gain levels below maximum is also shown. The effect of AVC is to permit restriction of the range of output levels, generated by a wide range of input sound intensities, within one-thirtieth of a second of the arrival of a sound-pressure level that exceeds the selected sensitivity of the AVC. The gain of the instrument has been reduced to prevent the signal from crossing the tolerance level. It takes one-tenth second for the gain to return to normal level when the input sound-pressure-level peak drops. We shall consider the use and value of this method of output limiting when we discuss hearing-aid use.

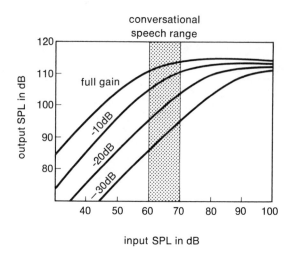

Output at 1000 Hz at various settings of the
gain control and with various input levels

Fig. 6.11. Signal compression of various degrees resulting from compression amplification at various levels of gain. (Courtesy of Zenith Hearing Aid Sales Corp.)

The Tone Control

Before we consider the way in which the tone control functions, it will be necessary for us to study the frequency response of an amplifying system, since the purpose of the tone control is to modify this response pattern. The frequency response refers to the sensitivity of the system, or parts of the system, to sounds of different frequencies. In our discussion of resonance in Chap. 2, it was explained that vibrators are more easily set in motion at some frequencies than at others. The frequencies around which a vibrator or an electrical system most easily vibrates are known as the resonant frequencies. In designing hearing aids, every attempt is made to reduce this resonance to a minimum, so that the system is fairly equally sensitive to sound across the range of frequency components important to speech intelligibility. If this is not achieved and resonant peaks occur, the electrical patterns and, therefore, the resultant sound-wave patterns produced by the vibrations of the diaphragm of the receiver, will differ from the sound-wave patterns picked up by the microphone before amplification. The difference will be heard by the listener as a distortion of quality, and the aid may be described as tinny, metallic, or booming.

The frequency-response curve is obtained by feeding into a hearing aid, or a hearing aid component, a pure tone of known frequency and intensity. This sound being fed into the system is known as the *input*. A measurement is then made of the sound that leaves the component or the system, a reading referred to as the *output*. The difference in intensity between the input and the output signal is the result of a component or system and is known as the *gain*. By repeating this procedure at each frequency, it is possible to plot a frequency-response curve showing the gain in decibels against the frequency. A typical frequency response of a hearing-aid microphone is shown in Fig. 6.12. The frequency response of a receiver can be assessed in the same manner. A typical curve for a wearable hearing-aid earphone is shown in Fig. 6.13. A frequency-response curve of an instrument is similar to a person's audiogram. It depicts for each frequency the amount by which the instrument amplifies the incoming signal. For an individual component, such as a receiver, it indicates its sensitivity to vibrations of different frequencies in the same way as the audiogram does for the ear. These frequency sensitivity curves show us how the pattern of amplification provided by the hearing aid may be varied according to its components. With a wearable hearing aid we do not have access to the microphone, so this will contribute a constant response pattern to the total system. However, it is well to remember that with the larger group-type hearing aids, if we connect to the system a microphone other than the one that was designed for it, we can no longer expect the amplifying systems to function in accordance with the specifications provided by the manufacturer. You may also find that, in addition to

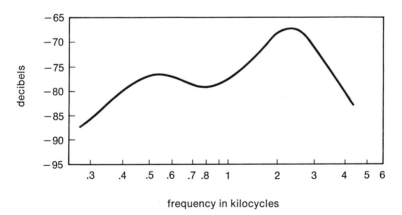

frequency in kilocycles

Fig. 6.12. A typical frequency-response curve of a hearing-aid microphone. (Courtesy of Zenith Hearing Aid Sales Corp.)

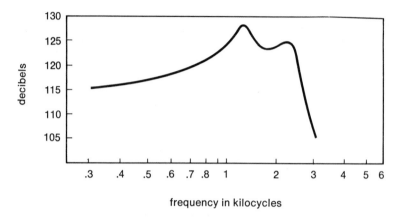

frequency in kilocycles

Fig. 6.13.   A typical frequency-response curve of a hearing-aid earphone. (Courtesy of Zenith Hearing Aid Sales Corp.)

having changed the frequency-response characteristics, we will also have changed the overall gain of the system because of an impedance mismatch between the microphone and the amplifier.

The receiver of the type of hearing aid worn in glasses or in a single behind-the-ear unit is, like the microphone, a built-in component not accessible to the user. The receiver of the body-type hearing aid, however, is quite accessible and can be easily detached and replaced with a different one. Since the receiver of the hearing aid also has frequency-response characteristics, it is perfectly possible to change the response characteristics of the total system by changing the receiver. This method of altering overall response characteristics is used with some types of body aids. It must also be recognized that the response curve will be affected by the coupling device used to feed the output signal into the ear canal. This includes any plastic tubing connecting the aid to an earmold, and to the mold itself.

The *overall frequency-response characteristics* of the aid, which represent the interaction of the response characteristics of its individual components, are determined in the same manner. Overall specifications typical of a wearable hearing aid are shown in Fig. 6.14.

The aim of the manufacturer is to provide a pattern of amplification that does not distort the input signal. However, although speech contains frequencies across a range from approximately 100 to 8000 Hz, good comprehension of conversational speech can be achieved providing one receives frequencies in the range 300 to 3000 Hz. For reasons of instrument size, the frequency-response characteristics of many wearable hearing aids (standard response aids) do not generally extend beyond this range. The fidelity

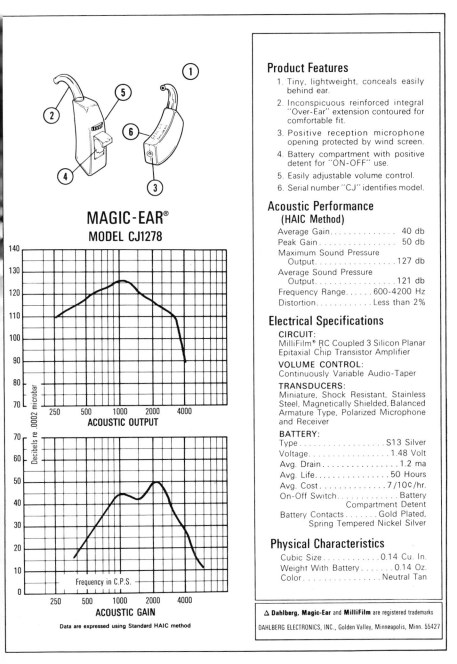

Product Features

1. Tiny, lightweight, conceals easily behind ear.
2. Inconspicuous reinforced integral "Over-Ear" extension contoured for comfortable fit.
3. Positive reception microphone opening protected by wind screen.
4. Battery compartment with positive detent for "ON-OFF" use.
5. Easily adjustable volume control.
6. Serial number "CJ" identifies model.

Acoustic Performance
(HAIC Method)

Average Gain	40 db
Peak Gain	50 db
Maximum Sound Pressure Output	127 db
Average Sound Pressure Output	121 db
Frequency Range	600-4200 Hz
Distortion	Less than 2%

Electrical Specifications

CIRCUIT:
MilliFilm* RC Coupled 3 Silicon Planar Epitaxial Chip Transistor Amplifier

VOLUME CONTROL:
Continuously Variable Audio-Taper

TRANSDUCERS:
Miniature, Shock Resistant, Stainless Steel, Magnetically Shielded, Balanced Armature Type, Polarized Microphone and Receiver

BATTERY:

Type	S13 Silver
Voltage	1.48 Volt
Avg. Drain	1.2 ma
Avg. Life	50 Hours
Avg. Cost	7/10¢/hr.
On-Off Switch	Battery Compartment Detent
Battery Contacts	Gold Plated, Spring Tempered Nickel Silver

Physical Characteristics

Cubic Size	0.14 Cu. In.
Weight With Battery	0.14 Oz.
Color	Neutral Tan

△ **Dahlberg**, **Magic-Ear** and **MilliFilm** are registered trademarks

DAHLBERG ELECTRONICS, INC., Golden Valley, Minneapolis, Minn. 55427

MAGIC-EAR®
MODEL CJ1278

ACOUSTIC OUTPUT

ACOUSTIC GAIN

Data are expressed using Standard HAIC method

Fig. 6.14. Overall characteristics of a behind-the-ear model hearing aid. (Courtesy of Dahlberg Electronics, Inc.)

with which the input signal will be amplified may be assessed by the flatness of the response curve. If the aid favors some frequencies while suppressing others, then frequency distortion will be present. Remember, however, that frequency distortion is assessed relative to normal hearing. In designing amplification systems to meet the needs of hearing-impaired persons it is recognized that in most instances the hearing-aid user will already be experiencing frequency distortion due to the greater loss of sensitivity to some frequencies than to others. The auditory-response curve is not flat to begin with. This may present a problem. If a flat pattern of amplification is used, frequencies that may be relatively unimpaired by the hearing problem will be amplified equally with those that are more severely affected. Thus, sounds that are heard at comfortable loudness without amplification become abnormally or uncomfortably loud, while the less audible sounds may still fail to be amplied sufficiently. It seems, therefore, reasonable to ask whether the selective amplification of sound energy in the frequencies where the hearing loss is greatest will improve the value of amplification in oral communication.

In 1947, H. Davis reported the findings of a study designed to provide information relative to this question [3]. The report, commonly referred to as the Harvard Report, indicated that the most effective amplification was provided by an instrument that possessed a flat response or provided moderate high-tone emphasis across a wide frequency range and that also incorporated true square-top peak clipping.

The findings of this study did not, however, resolve the controversy concerning the value of varying degrees of selective fitting. Both wearable hearing aids and auditory training units available today make provisions for the modication of the overall frequency-response pattern. We have already seen that for some types of aids it is possible to achieve this by changing the earphone. By replacing a receiver that has a relatively flat frequency response by one that has a high-frequency peak, we are able to produce a pattern of amplification that emphasizes the high frequencies. Similar modifications in the response characteristics of the receiver can be achieved by the use of small plastic inserts that fit into the nozzle of the earphone. These are designed to provide various degrees of reduction in the earphone opening, thus modifying the overall hearing-aid response.

The tone control of the hearing aid is designed to permit the selection of one of several specified response patterns within a single aid. The amplifier of the aid contains various circuits designed specifically to emphasize different frequency bands. The tone-control switch permits the user to select a particular tone-control circuit and in doing so to increase or decrease the relative amplification of the high, middle, and low frequencies. In this way, selective amplification of specific frequency bandwidths is possible. The selectivity is made possible by the use of capacitors and resistors in the circuit that vary in the efficiency with which particular frequencies are transmitted. For example, if a given circuit is more sensitive to high frequencies than low frequencies, the energy in the low frequencies will be reduced or attenuated considerably more than will the energy in the high frequencies. For a hearing-aid user who has a more severe loss in the high frequencies than in the middle or low frequencies, this makes it possible to turn up the overall amplification of the system to bring the high frequencies above this threshold without unduly amplifying the middle and low frequencies for which he has relatively good hearing.

SPECIFICATION DATA FOR WEARABLE HEARING AIDS

The purpose of our previous discussion has been to provide information on those aspects of amplification for which an understanding is considered essential to the effective utilization of amplification in training the hearing-impaired person. With a grasp of these general principles you will, it is hoped, be in a position to make better use of information about hearing aids that you may previously have been unable to understand or that, through unfamiliarity with the terminology, you simply did not attempt to read.

The most important source of information about a particular amplifying unit, whatever type it may be, is the *specification sheet*, commonly referred to as the *spec sheet*. These sheets should accompany every auditory training unit and are available for all models and makes of wearable aids. Following is a discussion of the information contained in these sheets.

Peak Acoustic Gain

The peak acoustic gain represents a reading in decibels of the *highest gain* provided by the amplifier *at any point* across the frequency range of the instrument. This measure is important since it may determine the maximum volume setting that the wearer may be able to tolerate. When the input sound contains high energy levels around the peak frequencies of the aid, amplification may result in an output level above the threshold of discomfort of the hearing-aid user, causing him to turn down the overall level of amplification.

Average Gain

The term *average gain* refers to the average of the maximum values, at 500, 1000, and 2000 Hz, measured when the volume control is set to provide maximum acoustic gain. The average gain provides a measure of the amount of amplification which will be added to the input signal across the range of frequencies most important to speech comprehension. From this figure we can tell whether or not a particular hearing aid will be able to provide an adequate amount of amplification for a person with a particular degree of hearing loss. The difference in the amount of acoustic gain that can be provided by a behind-the-ear aid, designed to help individuals with mild-to-moderate impairments, and a high-powered body-worn hearing aid may be as much as 35 decibels. For some people this may constitute the difference between hearing and not hearing speech.

Output

We spoke earlier of the need to limit the maximum acoustic output, both to protect the listener from discomfort and to insure against overloading the receiver, a factor that will produce distortion. The maximum acoustic output represents the average of the maximum saturated sound-pressure levels at 500, 1000, and 2000 Hz. This figure tells us the maximum intensity that the output stage of the amplifier will feed to the receiver or headphones before peak clipping will occur. Remember that the strength of the output signal is determined by both the input intensity and the acoustic gain at the particular volume-control setting being used. We can tell from the maximum output value whether an aid is designed to handle the intensity of output signals that we require for a particular hearing loss. For example, the maximum acoustic output for an insert hearing aid currently on the market is stated in the specification sheet as 106 decibels. This factor alone makes it unsuitable for persons with severe loss who require output values of up to 135 decibels.

Frequency-Response Curves

We have already discussed the nature of frequency-response curves. We have said that just as we plot the hearing sensitivity of the individual (audiogram), so do we also measure the sensitivity of the amplifying system at each frequency across the range of the instrument. Since this pattern of sensitivity is measured at the receiver, it is a statement of the sensitivity response of the total system. The standard frequency response is generally obtained at a lower gain setting than the maximum possible. By plotting this response curve on the graph at what would be the maximum gain setting, it is possible to read both the actual frequency-response curve and the relative gain provided by the aid at each frequency.

Signal-to-Noise Ratio

The fifth characteristic of amplifying units that we need to mention is the very important one of signal-to-noise ratio. All electrical systems necessarily generate a certain amount of internal electrical noise. Since the acoustic signal that impinges upon the microphone is converted into an electrical representation, the signal will exist against the background of this electrical noise. The relationship between the signal and the electronic background noise is known as the signal-to-noise ratio (S/N). For comprehension of speech under normal listening conditions, it is necessary for the signal to be stronger than the noise. The greater the signal-to-noise ratio, the greater the intelligibility of the speech and, therefore, the greater the redundancy factor.

In many amplifying systems the volume control is placed in the circuit immediately after the microphone-input stage, before the signal is amplified. The transistor at this input stage generates a certain amount of noise that will remain constant in voltage. When the amplification of the input signal is high, as would be necessary for a person with a severe hearing loss, the S/N ratio will also be high. If, on the other hand, the same hearing aid or auditory training unit is used by a person with only a mild hearing loss, turning down the volume control will reduce the intensity of the signal but will not reduce the noise level, which remains constant. This results in a decrease in the S/N ratio, which may affect speech intelligibility remarkably. In the construction of auditory training units, various circuit designs have been utilized in an attempt to overcome this. One of the newest methods used by one manufacturer has been termed "operational feedback." The specification sheets for this auditory trainer indicate a S/N ratio of 60 decibels measured at maximum SPL output, with a volume-control range of 46 decibels. The dynamic range—that is, the range of decibels over which the instrument will tolerate variations in input signal intensity without overloading—is given as 30 decibels minimum at the lowest volume setting.

Signal-to-noise ratio is an important factor in determining the intelligibility of speech under varying listening conditions. It may be that the specification sheets for an amplifier fail to state this. It is a factor on which information should be sought by anyone considering which instrument to purchase.

Distortion

Distortion is present when the output signal of the amplifying system differs in wave form from the original input signal. Such a difference reflects an undesired change in the relative intensity of the frequency components of the complex sound wave.

There exist four major forms of distortion. The first of these is *harmonic distortion*. This results from the addition of harmonic vibrations not present in the input sound wave.

The second type, *linear distortion*, occurs as a result of unequal amplification at different frequencies. This is apparent in a sensitivity curve that is not flat across the band of frequencies that one is amplifying.

Intermodulation distortion results from the fact that two pure tones occurring simultaneously give rise to an effect perceived in the form of a warble or beat phenomenon. If an amplifying system is subject to the presence of harmonic distortion, the interaction of the input signal with the harmonic distortion may result in the perception of a beating tone known as intermodulation distortion.

Finally, there exists the form of distortion that results from the resonant characteristics of the electrical and mechanical components of the amplifier. If these components are not adequately damped, they may give off sympathetic vibrations known as transients, resulting in *transient distortion.**

At this point you may be more than a little overwhelmed by technical data. You are probably finding difficulty in relating this material to the needs of the hearing-impaired person. It is therefore appropriate for us to consider how the clinical audiologist evaluates the need for a hearing aid and recommends a particular type.

Some Misconceptions About the Value of Amplification

In *The Affluent Society*, Kenneth Galbraith, writing about the persistence of certain inappropriate concepts in the field of economic theory says, "Because familiarity is such a test of acceptability, the acceptable ideas have great stability. They are highly predictable" [5]. He refers to these ideas as "conventional wisdom." They generally consist of concepts that have developed partly on the basis of factual evidence, partly on the basis of misinterpretation of the findings or observations. Although the information may at one time have been perfectly correct, the passage of time, the availability of new information based on research findings and experience, and the development of instrumentation may cause these concepts to become inaccurate at a later date. The fields of education of the deaf, audiology, and speech pathology abound with examples of conventional wisdom. We shall be much concerned in clarifying some of these misconceptions. It is not suggested that all members of our profession are misguided in their beliefs, but that there is a considerable time lapse between the development of new ideas or the availability of new information and its general acceptance by people working in the field, and an even larger time lapse before it is used by our colleagues in allied professions.

In considering the benefits that amplification may provide for a person with impaired hearing, we immediately encounter the surprisingly prevalent

---

*For a more complete examination of the topic of distortion the reader is referred to an article, "Sound Distortion in Hearing Aids," in *Fenestra*, No. 3 (July 1968).

belief that a person with sensori-neural hearing impairment (nerve loss) cannot benefit from amplification. This is quite falacious. I believe the misconception arises because it is often said that persons with conductive losses respond well to amplification since their problem involves only a loss of loudness. It is then erroneously reasoned that, because sensori-neural hearing losses frequently involve reduced auditory-discrimination ability, the simple amplification of sound for people with this type of loss will not improve the ability to understand speech. While it is true that people with conductive deafness do respond well to amplification, the need for them to resort to its use has been dramatically reduced by the advances made in the medical and surgical treatment of this kind of loss. *Most candidates for hearing aids are therefore people with sensori-neural deafness.*

The amount of help that amplification may give varies considerably from subject to subject. In view of the emphasis we have placed in previous chapters upon the integrative nature of preception, it is obvious that we cannot predict the benefit that amplification will afford purely on the basis of the audiogram, or even on the results of speech audiometry. Unfortunately, failure to recognize this not infrequently results in a person's being advised against the use of the hearing aid on the basis of his audiogram or his failure to show a definite improvement in auditory discrimination on standard clinical tests. It can no longer be maintained that there exists a particular degree of auditory impairment that can, as a rule, be considered too mild to necessitate the use of amplification. As R. A. Winchester points out:

> Formerly, when only the body-worn hearing aid was available, a good rule of thumb for the hearing aid consultant to follow was to limit the selection of hearing aids to persons showing a loss in a better ear of 30 dB [decibels] or more in the speech frequencies. It was stated that a hearing loss less than 30 db was not socially or vocationally handicapping and that the circuit noise level of the available hearing aid would be sufficiently disturbing to limit successful use. The remarkable technological advances in design of instruments has clearly demonstrated that such limitations no longer exist. Experience with the newer ear level model aids indicates that individuals with losses less than 30 dB may benefit significantly from amplification. *Therefore, concepts of hearing aid candidacy formerly held should be disregarded and every person with a non-remedial hearing loss complaining of a communication problem should be considered for hearing aid selection regardless of the extent of the hearing loss.* (Italics added.) [18]

At the other end of the scale, it may be equally strongly claimed that there exists no degree of hearing impairment, as measured by pure-tone auditometry, that is too great to exclude the value of extensive trial use of amplified sound. Maurice H. Miller says:

No set of unaided audiological findings should be considered sufficiently definitive to rule out the possibility of amplification. To use an extreme example, even if the patient shows no response at any frequency in either ear at the maximum output of the audiometer, the hearing aid should still be tried because the maximum saturation output of some conventionally worn body "aids" and a number of auditory training units and desk model hearing aids exceeds that of most audiometers and it is entirely possible for the patient to obtain some limited but important assistance from powerful amplification which may contribute to the total program of auditory rehabilitation. [17]

Hearing-Aid Evaluation

The above statements should not be interpreted as negating the value of audiometric and speech test results in the assessment of the possible benefit that might be derived from amplification. What they do emphasize is that we should not approach the question with a preconceived bias based upon the pure-tone and speech audiometric data.

We may ask, "What, then, is the value of a reliable audiogram in a hearing-aid evaluation?" It is helpful to read the audiogram on the basis of the amount of residual hearing rather than to concentrate one's attention on the amount of hearing that has been lost. After all, the aim of rehabilitation is to train the person to make the best use of his remaining hearing in communication. From a reliable audiogram we will be able to assess the amount of usable residual hearing. This is represented by the area between the subject's threshold of detection and the threshold of discomfort. We may also predict how much amplification will be required to raise the intensity of speech sufficiently above the listener's threshold to make it useful to him. In Fig. 6.15, for example, we observe that the subject has an average loss of 35 decibels in the speech-frequency range of 500 to 2000 Hz. Subtracting 35 decibels from an assumed maximum tolerable output of 135 decibels, we are left with 100 decibels of usable residual hearing. A hearing aid that is selected will need to provide only a fairly low level of gain to overcome the 35 decibels of attenuation that the patient's ear is imposing upon the input speech signal of an average intensity of 60 decibels for conversational speech. If we add this 65 decibels input to the 35 decibels of gain, we arrive at an output figure of 100 decibels, which is well within the range of the patient's tolerance for loudness. A second audiogram, shown in Fig. 6.16 evidences an average loss in the speech frequencies of 80 decibels. Subtracting this figure from the tolerance level of 135 decibels, we find that our range of usable residual hearing for this person is no more than 45 decibels. If we were to amplify speech input by 85 decibels to compensate for the attenuation resulting from the hearing loss, we would find that conversational speech (60 decibels) when passed through

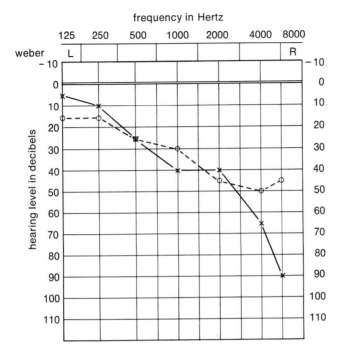

Fig. 6.15. Audiogram of a person with a wide dynamic range of residual hearing.

the hearing aid, would produce an output level of 145 decibels, which is above threshold of pain. In this case, it is clear that a high-gain hearing aid will be needed. If, however, we were to provide an 85-decibel gain, output limitation would result in peak clipping of the speech signal, causing a deterioration of the quality of what is heard. Although average conversational speech intensity is 60 to 65 decibels SPL, peak components often exceed this level and will be more severely clipped. Any resonant peaks in the response curve of the aid will cause further distortion, since speech-frequency components that coincide with them would be clipped first. Such information will help us to understand the limits within which amplification may be expected to afford help.

In addition to the information concerning the amount of residual hearing, the audiogram will also provide an indication of the relative distribution of the residual hearing across the frequency spectrum. Another piece of traditional wisdom tells us that it is not possible, or is at least very difficult, for a hearing aid to compensate for a high-frequency-type hearing loss. This used to be the case when hearing aids consisted only of the body type. The fact that this aid had to be worn on articles of clothing caused a great deal of low-frequency clothing noise to be generated. The amplification of this

158   Amplification and Hearing Aids

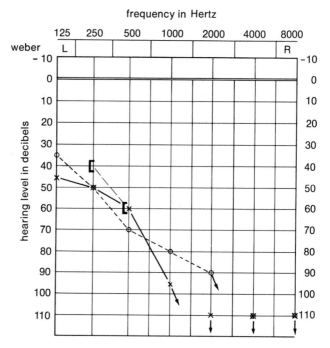

Fig. 6.16. Audiogram of person with a limited range of usable residual hearing.

noise across the range of frequencies for which the user had good hearing for the most part prevented him from enjoying the benefits of amplification of the higher speech frequencies. Further complicating the problem was the unfavorable effect that arose from wearing the aid on the sound-absorbent human body, which provided a baffle effect. These two difficulties have, to a great extent, been alleviated by the development of various types of ear-level hearing aids. Using one of these aids with an appropriate earmold means that many people with high-frequency hearing losses, who were previously unable to benefit from amplification, are now successful hearing-aid users.

Speech Audiometric Data

Having evaluated the pure-tone audiometric results, you should then turn to the information concerning the ability of the person to utilize what residual hearing he has. The pure-tone audiogram is an analytic statement of the person's hearing at threshold levels. It does not convey information about his ability to receive and analyze the complex signals that constitute speech. Unlike pure-tone tests, speech audiometry is a measure of above-threshold (supraliminal) function, a much more sophisticated hearing process. Two basic measures are provided by speech audiometry: *the Speech Reception Threshold* (SRT) and the *Speech-Discrimination Score* (PB)*

The SRT indicates the level of intensity at which the listener is correctly able to repeat 50 per cent of a list of two-syllable words that have equal stress on each syllable (spondee words). This is the point at which, when the individual is receiving only the auditory aspects of the message signal, hearing becomes useful to him as a means of following the gist of what is being said. Below this intensity level he is generally receiving too little information to be able to reconstruct correctly the idea that the sender wishes to convey. In people with normal hearing and in cases of deafness showing a minimum loss of speech discrimination, the speech reception threshold may be expected to correlate fairly closely with the average of the three speech frequencies, 500, 1000, and 2000 Hz. If it fails to do so, then we have reason to suspect either that one of the two measures is inaccurate or that we are dealing with a person experiencing a marked loss in discrimination function. A comparison of the speech reception threshold and the discrimination score obtained on monosyllabic words should give further indication as to which of these two possibilities is responsible for the disparity. For a person with normal hearing operating under favorable listening conditions, we need only to raise the intensity level of the speech sample by 10 decibels in order for the person to obtain a 90 per cent or greater score on phonetically balanced monosyllabic words. Clinically, we raise the intensity level by 40 decibels when testing speech discrimination. The clinical evaluation provides the discrimination scores obtained at 40 decibels above the subject's SRT. The speech reception threshold and discrimination scores are usually given both for the left and right ear individually, and binaurally as obtained in a free field—that is, when the sound is fed into the room through a speaker rather than directly through headphones. From these scores we may assess the maximum discrimination that the person is able to achieve on a controlled speech sample presented under favorable listening conditions. The independent assessment of each ear will show us which ear offers the greatest potential auditory discrimination for amplified speech. This is important in deciding in which ear the aid might best be worn. The free-field score gives us a basis against which we can make comparisons between the scores obtained with the subject wearing different hearing aids and those obtained without amplification.

The clinical hearing-aid evaluation also involves a test of speech discrimination in noise. This is obtained by presenting spondee words at a level 5 decibels above the speech reception threshold. A background of wide-

*PB refers to phonetically balanced monosyllabic word tests in which the phonemes of English are represented in the list in the same proportion as they occur in normal conversational speech.

spectrum noise is then introduced and increased in intensity until the subject is able only to correctly identify 50 per cent of the spondees. When this level has been assessed, the noise is then increased until his ability to repeat the words has been completely obliterated. By subtracting the level of the noise from each of these two measures, one may obtain the minimum and maximum speech-to-noise ratios.

Tolerance for Loudness

Finally, a measure of tolerance for sound is obtained by asking the subject to indicate when a gradually increasing sound stimulus, which may either be white noise or recorded conversational speech, causes definite discomfort. This is done first without a hearing aid and then with the various aids under test. By subtracting the speech reception threshold from this discomfort threshold figure, we obtain the subject's *dynamic range for speech*. It is this range that delineates the area of usable residual hearing.

Selecting an Aid

It has been traditional for hearing-aid evaluations to involve the assessment of these various measures of hearing performance for several different hearing aids. These aids are selected to approximate the amount of amplification and frequency emphasis that is suggested by the pure-tone audiogram and by the pattern of sounds missed in the speech-discrimination test. The aids that will be recommended must provide overall improvement in speech communication. One of the measures that will be used in determining this will be the degree of improvement in the aided SRT. This improvement should be achieved without an associated decrease in speech discrimination, either in silence or in noise, and should not decrease the wearer's tolerance for normal environmental sounds. It seems that many students feel that an improvement in the speech-discrimination score is impossible to achieve. We shall discuss this in the next chapter. It will suffice to say at this point that it is not unreasonable to hope for such an improvement in auditory discrimination if an appropriate pattern of amplification has been provided.

In addition to the formal test evaluation of the benefit provided by the various hearing aids, the audiologist frequently includes in the clinical session a subjective evaluation by the hearing-aid wearer of the benefit provided by the aid in actual environmental listening conditions. This sometimes means a visit to a local coffee shop or a short conversation held against the ambient noise present in the reception room of the clinic.

The whole question of the formal evaluation of hearing aids is one that causes many audiologists a great deal of concern. The value of such time-consuming and tiring procedures has been questioned in the literature by a number of authors. James Jerger, in reviewing research published in the *Journal of Speech and Hearing Research* in 1966 [10] (most specifically that of Yantis, et al. [19], and in other writings [11, 12]), observes that these research findings suggest that the use of monosyllabic words, such as those in the PB word lists, does not detect very substantial differences between hearing-aid performance and that, therefore, the suitability of such tests in clinical evaluations is highly questionable. He suggests that differentiation between the performance of aids can only be obtained if materials are carefully constructed to require the listener to discriminate meaningful material against a competing speech message. It was found that this means of testing was more effective than the use of PB words. He made the following provocative and rather courageous summary of research findings.

> It looks as though the best hearing aid for anyone is the best hearing aid for everyone. This is a severe blow to the philosophy of conventional hearing-aid fitting. Many audiologists have long accepted as axiomatic the notion that there is a single best aid or group of aids for any particular individual and that there is some other best aid for a different individual. This belief is the cornerstone of hearing aid selection. Not so, says research. There is no evidence favoring the idea and much evidence against it. It doesn't seem to matter what the type or degree of loss. Some hearing aids do better than others, and the best ones are best for everyone. If you found that hard to accept, consider the finding that differences in the physical characteristics of aids are most important for young patients with mild flat conductive losses and good PB discrimination, and least important for older patients with severe sloping sensory neural losses and poor PB discrimination. Is nothing sacred?

It is observations such as these made by Jerger that cause concern among audiologists responsible for making recommendations concerning the selection of a hearing aid. On the other hand, for the hearing-aid clinician or teacher of the deaf, these statements, if true, are in fact encouraging. What they say to the therapist is that, regardless of the exact nature of the hearing aid that the child or adult is wearing, providing it is strong enough to provide adequate amplification and is judged appropriate by an audiologist or competent hearing-aid representative, the therapist may be confident that she is working with as good an amplifier as might have been selected had the wearer been submitted to a series of sophisticated comparative tests. One thing that is clear from the research is that time invested in counseling the person to make optimum use of the hearing aid, including training in auditory discrimination, is the most effective means of improving the use of residual hearing. This gives the therapist confidence in working with the subject. She may concentrate her efforts now on the actual task of improving auditory perception and verbal communication ability without having to be unduly concerned whether or not she has the specific aid for a person with a specific pattern of hearing loss. This is particularly important when young children are concerned.

Hearing-Aid Evaluation With Children

Formal testing cannot easily be undertaken with children. Providing the child has sufficient verbal language, it is usual to make an assessment of the aid based on the improvement in the child's ability to respond to spoken directions when amplification is provided. It is also possible to compare the unaided and aided thresholds for various sounds of known intensity and spectrum. Using play, audiometry comparison may be made of the unaided and aided thresholds for pure tones fed into a free field. A warble tone is used to avoid the effect of standing waves. These techniques, however, provide at best a rough measure of the value of amplification rather than specific comparative data about various aids. Even more than with adults, the successful selection and adjustment of hearing aids for young children must depend not only on careful evaluation of clinical test results, but also upon observations made during a trial period of auditory training. During this time, the child will be helped to adjust to the aid and to utilize the auditory cues that the aid makes available to him. His responses during this period are more likely to be accurate indicators of the benefit that he derives from the hearing aid than any information that we obtain in a formal clinical setting.

A comprehensive discussion of the various procedures evolved for evaluating the effectiveness of hearing aids will be found in the American Speech and Hearing Association Report No. 2, *A Conference on Hearing-Aid Evaluation Procedures* (September 1967).

TYPES AND COSTS OF HEARING AIDS

There are on the market today four types of wearable hearing aids. These are the *body aid*, which is worn on the person's clothing, and three types of ear-level aids: the *eyeglass aid*, the *behind-the-ear aid*, and the miniaturized *in-the-ear hearing aid*. Within each of these categories are to be found a wide variety of makes and models providing various amounts of gain and different frequency responses, and additional features, such as a telephone pickup circuit. A detailed discussion of the various aids is beyond the scope of this text. We shall, however, consider the basic features and the types of losses that representative aids for these four categories are designed to accommodate.

The Body Hearing Aid

The price of the body hearing aid varies considerably. The minimum may be expected to be somewhere around $75, possibly a little less. Most body aids currently cost between $190 and $230, with the more powerful aids costing as much as $250 to $350. Manufacturers generally state a suggested retail price only, so the actual cost may vary somewhat from dealer to dealer.

Because of the relatively large size of the body aid compared to the other categories of aids, it is possible to design this type of aid to provide high levels of amplification and a wide frequency range for people with severe hearing impairments. Some of the design features that may be incorporated include a power control independent of the volume control, permitting the maximum power output to be set at one of several discrete levels, a greater variety of tone-control settings, and the inclusion of a telephone pickup circuit.

The receiver unit of the body aid, unlike those of the ear-level aids, is not housed within the same case as the microphone and amplifier, but is attached to an earmold. It is connected to the amplifying unit by a cord. The accessibility of the receiver makes it possible to modify the overall response characteristics of the aid by the use of different receivers that affect the frequency-response pattern for each tone-control setting. It is almost invariably this type of hearing aid that is worn by young children with severe losses. Figure 6.17 provides the specification data and frequency-response curves for an actual hearing aid. These specifications provide you with all the information concerning the characteristics that the manufacturer claims for this particular model. You will note that two types of batteries may be selected. The mercury cell provides the longer life with a slightly higher estimated battery cost per hour. The various measures of gain and output for the two batteries are specified separately, as are the figures for the two earphone receivers that may be used with this model aid.

The Y5R receiver is designed for moderately severe to severe lossses (85 to 95 decibels re: ISO standards). The average acoustic gain with the Y1 earphone is 74 decibels with an average output of 140 decibels, as compared to an average gain of 71 decibels and an output of 139 decibels with the Y5R receiver. This aid is therefore perfectly capable of amplifying average speech (65 decibels) to the level of 135 decibels, which is also within the limits of maximum output. The maximum power output can be internally modified by the use of a four-setting power control that provides flexibility for accommodating individuals with lower tolerance levels. The most noticeable effect of changing the earphone is seen in the resultant modification of the overall frequency-response curves. The frequency range for the Y5R earphone extends from 310 to 4000 Hz, while the range for the Y1R earphone is 350 to 3400 Hz. The effect of the high-frequency emphasis tone-control position is evidenced for both earphones, but note how the use of the Y1R earphone increases this emphasis even further.

One of the most recent modifications in body hearing aids is the development of low-frequency emphasis that is well below that which is cus-

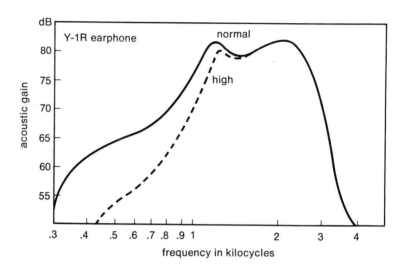

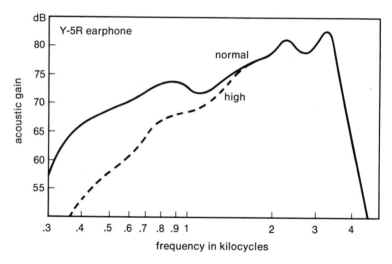

Data are expressed using standard H.A.I.C. method

Using 2 "N" cells (or ZN-2 pack)			Using 2 ZM-401 Mercury cells (or ZM-101 pack)	
Y-5R Earphone	Y-1R Earphone		Y-5R Earphone	Y-1R Earphone
82 dB	82 dB	Peak acoustic gain	79 dB	79 dB
71 dB	74 dB	H.A.I.C. average gain	68 dB	71 dB
139.5 dB	147.5 dB	Maximum acoustic output	137.5 dB	145.5 dB
139 dB	140 dB	H.A.I.C. average output	137 dB	138 dB

Fig. 6.17. Specification data and response curves for a body aid. (Courtesy of Zenith Hearing Aid Sales Corp.)

2.0 oz.	Weight with battery	2.36 oz.
8.0 ma.	Battery Drain (standby)	6.8 ma.
32 hours	Battery life	88 hours
78/100¢	Battery cost per hour (est.)	1.25¢

H.A.I.C.	*Controls:*	*Features:*	*Serial Numbers*
Frequency Range	Volume control	6 transistors, 3 diodes	(stamped on
Y-1R earphone:	OFF-HI-TEL-MIC	Push-pull output for	battery
350–3400 cps	Power control	greater battery efficiency,	compartment),
Y-5R earphone:	in battery	more distortion-free	first three
310–4100 cps	compartment	performance.	digits: 840
		Telephone pickup coil.	
		Automatic TEL-MIKE	
		switch (in Phantom	
		Phone ROYAL REGENT only)	

Fig. 6.17. (Continued)

tomarily provided. These aids extend the range of sensitivity so as to make it possible to provide amplification in the very low frequencies. Examination of specification sheets for standard wearable hearing aids indicates that, almost without exception, they do not provide amplification below 300 Hz. The justification for this rests in the fact that frequencies below this level do not normally contribute important information to the correct discrimination of speech. Since environmental noise is to a great extent concentrated at the low end of the frequency scale, amplification of these components detract from intelligibility under normal listening conditions. However, children with severe hearing losses who show no response to sound at 1 KHz or above appear to benefit in the development of normal vocalization and subsequent speech production from the amplification of frequencies down to as low as 100 Hz.

Many of the children enrolled in schools for the deaf have what may be termed residual hearing. For them, audition extends over only part of the speech range of frequencies. In such cases, low-frequency hearing is present, but there is a total loss of hearing for frequencies over 500, 1000, or 2000 cps [cycles per second]. The usual body-worn hearing aid is inappropriate for these more severely impaired children because it reproduces little or nothing within the child's range of hearing, but expends its energy over several octaves to which they are completely deaf. Given a conventional hearing aid, a child in this group may have less than one octave bandwidth available to him, namely 300–500 cps, the lower limit of his hearing aid to the upper limit of his hearing. [16]

One of the aids in this category is the model shown in Fig. 6.18. Such aids as this are now manufactured by a number of hearing-aid companies.

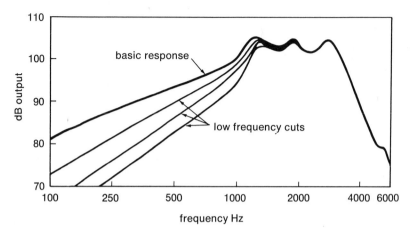

Fig. 6.18.   Tentative specification data for a low-frequency emphasis aid. (Courtesy of Radio Ear Corporation.)

The Behind-the-Ear Aid

Suggested retail prices for the behind-the-ear type of hearing aid fall in the range of $195 to $330. The advantages it offers are the complete elimination of the problem of clothing noise, a marked reduction in size compared to the body aid, and the placement of the microphone at ear level.

The aid is contoured to the ear and may be worn quite comfortably by either men or women. Women are often delighted to find that an appropriate hair style may completely conceal it. It used to be true that this type aid was unsuitable for use by children; however, we now see an increasing number of youngsters with mild-to-moderate hearing impairments who have demonstrated that the behind-the-ear model can be successfully used even by primary-school-aged children. It is not uncommon for true binaural amplification to be achieved by the use of two such aids, each adjusted to meet the needs of the ear to which it is fitted.

The degree of sophistication of the behind-the-ear models has increased considerably over the past few years. Typical of this class of aid is the model shown in Figs. 6.19 and 6.20. A separate on-off volume control is usually standard equipment, permitting the aid to be turned off without changing the required gain level. This eliminates the need to readjust the volume setting each time the instrument is turned on. Also available is the telephone circuit, which eliminates the external microphone, thus cutting out environmental noise when the wearer uses the telephone. Some more expensive models incorporate two sound openings, permitting the microphone to be stimulated by sound waves approaching from the front and from the rear.

The Glasses Aid

The glasses-type hearing aid (price range $195 to $350) incorporates the amplifying unit into the bow of a pair of glasses for the hearing-impaired

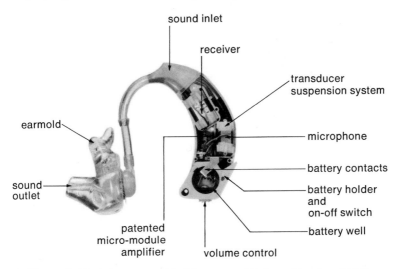

Fig. 6.19. A behind-the-ear model. (Courtesy of Beltone Hearing-Aid Corporation.)

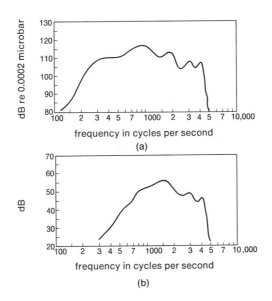

Fig. 6.20. Specification for aid shown in Fig. 6.19. (Courtesy of Beltone Hearing-Aid Corporation.)

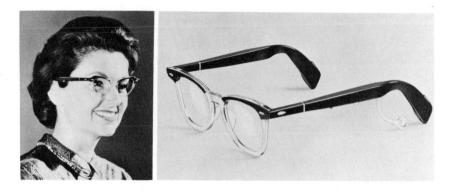

Fig. 6.21.   A typical glasses-model aid. (Courtesy of Zenith Hearing Aid Sales
Corp.

person who would like to use an ear-level aid but would find the behind-the-
ear type of hearing aid difficult to use because he also needs to wear eye-
glasses. Like the behind-the-ear model, the eyeglass hearing aid is generally
suited to people with mild-to-moderate losses. The degree of severity of
hearing loss for which this type of hearing aid is suitable has increased considerably over the past few years, so that models are now available that are
capable of providing amplification for people with hearing losses averaging
up to 75 decibels (ISO standards). This type of aid may easily be worn either
monaurally or binaurally and may incorporate both automatic volume control and telephone pickup circuitry. The microphone and the receiver are
housed within the glasses temple. A short length of tubing connects the hearing aid to the individual earmold worn by the user. Figure 6.21 illustrates
an eyeglass hearing aid being worn. The specifications for this model are
shown in Fig. 6.22. This model is designed for moderately severe losses
averaging 75 decibels (ISO standards). The average output is 129 decibels
with an average gain of 49 decibels across a frequency range of 420 to 4200
Hz. This provides for the amplification of normal conversation to a level of
approximately 110 decibels. The response characteristics may be modified
by varying the diameter of the plastic tubing to the earmold or by modifications of the earmold, as is discussed later in the chapter. The microphone
opening is situated in a forward position to provide improved pickup of
sounds from the front while reducing sensitivity to sounds from behind the
wearer. This model also incorporates a telephone induction coil to eliminate environmental noise while the user is on the phone. A slightly less
powerful model designed for losses of 60 to 65 decibels (ISO) has an average
gain of 42 decibels and an acoustic output of 109 decibels. This model
affords the wearer the advantages of automatic volume control.

The In-the-Ear Hearing Aid

A great deal of controversy has in the past centered around the in-the-ear type of hearing aid. When they first became available on the market,

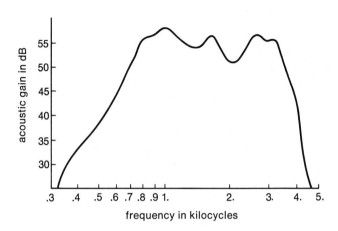

Data are expressed using standard H.A.I.C. method.

with ZS41 *silver-oxide battery*	(Tests made with 1½″ of #13 tubing)	*with ZM41* *mercury battery*
58 dB	Peak acoustic gain	53 dB
49 dB	H.A.I.C. average gain	44 dB
130 dB	Peak acoustic output	129 dB
125 dB	H.A.I.C. average output	123 dB
1.55 volts	Battery voltage	1.35 volts
75 hours	Battery life (est.)	100 hours
47/100¢	Battery hourly cost (est.)	35/100¢

H.A.I.C. frequency range—420 to 4200 cps
Features: Micro-Lithic® circuitry, 8 transistors, push-pull output
Telephone induction coil—EMBASSY-T
Spare battery compartment in matching temple
Controls: Continuous volume control
On-Off switch in battery compartment
TEL-MIKE switch—EMBASSY-T
Serial Numbers begin: Black 86—Mink 87 (EMBASSY-T)
Black 96—Mink 97 (EMBASSY)

Fig. 6.22. Specifications for aid shown in Fig. 6.21. (Courtesy of Zenith Hearing Aid Sales Corp.)

the quality of the units came under criticism as did much of the advertising with which they were associated. It was felt that the limitations of acoustic gain and frequency sensitivity placed upon the aid by its size were not clearly spelled out in the advertising material. As a result, many people came to believe that it was no longer necessary for a person with a hearing loss to wear one of the larger model aids, that the hearing problem could be well accommodated by the use of the inconspicuous in-the-ear type model. Attitudes toward this type of aid have, however, modified as further improvements have been made in its design and as the limitations of the type of losses for which it is appropriate have become more widely recognized.

The in-the-ear model fills an important gap in the range of available aids. It provides a useful amplifier for individuals with mild-to-moderate losses that do not necessitate a great deal of acoustic gain, or a wide frequency bandwidth, or special frequency emphasis. It is particularly appropriate for the person who needs to use a hearing aid in some situations but not in others, who would in the past have constituted such a borderline case that he might have rejected the use of the more conspicuous behind-the-ear model. It is likely that with future developments this type of aid will become increasingly versatile and will provide distinct acoustic and cosmetic advantages over the other ear-level aids. The price of the in-the-ear hearing aid is similar to that of the available behind-the-ear aids, falling in the range of $290 to $330.

The model shown in Fig. 6.23 is representative of this type of aid. The specifications are given in Fig. 6.24. This instrument weighs only one-eighth ounce and is no more than eight-tenths inch long, five-tenths inch wide and three-tenths inch thick. Using a silver-oxide battery for maximum

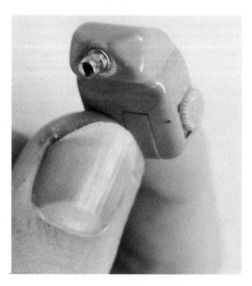

Fig. 6.23. A typical insert-type aid. (Courtesy of Radio Ear Corporation.)

power, the average gain is 30 decibels across a basic frequency range from 430 to 4400, with a maximum output of 115 decibels re: 0.0002 microbar. The gain represented by the range of frequencies most important to speech discrimination (500 to 2000 Hz) is noticeably higher than the average gain. This factor, together with the gradual rise in sensitivity with frequency to meet the needs of the gradually sloping loss, provides the model with considerable versatility. The basic sensitivity curve may be modified by use of insert fillers to accommodate more sharply falling audiograms. A custom earmold is obviously essential for use with this type of aid, though stock tips are available for demonstration and trial purposes.

Binaural Amplification

One of the biggest decisions that the potential hearing-aid user with a bilateral hearing loss must make is whether or not he should invest in binaural amplification. Let us first make clear that a true binaural amplifying system consists of two completely independent amplifying units, one for each ear. Unfortunately, the term binaural hearing is sometimes used to refer to a single wearable hearing aid in which the output is fed, by way of a Y-shaped cord to each ear. Some table-model amplifying units incorporate a control that permits the relative output at each of the two phones to be varied. Although this may make it possible for the user to balance the loudness level in each ear, he is still hearing the results of only one input signal. In fact, Ira J. Hirsh, in reviewing some experiments conducted with binaural hearing aids, went so far as to suggest that splitting the single input signal and feeding it to both ears may, under certain conditions, result in interaural inhibition, a condition in which the patient shows a poorer discrimination of speech in noise when using both earphones than he does when the input is fed to only one [8]. The role of binaural amplification is not, therefore, simply to balance loudness levels. Its advantages must be understood in the light of the knowledge of auditory localization and discrimination of speech against conflicting noise stimuli.

Auditory localization of sound sources is achieved by comparison of the differences in the time of arrival, the intensity, and the phase of the input signals arriving at each ear. The diameter of the average head is approximately eight inches. This distance is sufficient to result in a measurable difference between the phase of the sound wave as it strikes the ear nearest the sound source and its phase as it stimulates the ear farthest away. Similarly, the extra distance that the sound wave travels from one ear to the other accounts for a slight loss in the intensity and arrival time of the signal, a difference that the brain is capable of detecting and measuring. Two independent input microphones are therefore essential to the comparison of these signals.

The ability to utilize the auditory cues begins to show itself between the second and fourth month of life, when the infant first begins to search

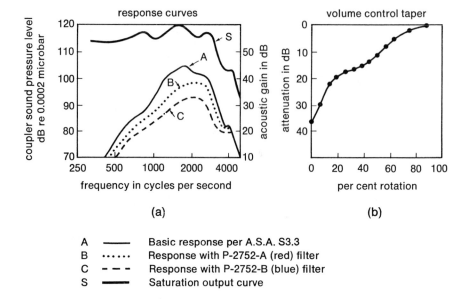

(a)   (b)

A ——— Basic response per A.S.A. S3.3
B ...... Response with P-2752-A (red) filter
C – – – Response with P-2752-B (blue) filter
S ▬▬▬ Saturation output curve

General: This Radioear model is a very small in-the-ear aid with above average gain and output for this type of hearing aid. It nestles snugly in the ear and is very inconspicuous. Either custom or stock earmolds can be used.

Size: .83″ long by .56″ wide (exclusive of volume control knob) by .38″ thick.

Weight: 3.6 grams (about ⅛ ounce) with battery.

Battery: Type S-312 silver-oxide or type 312 mercury battery.

Current Drain: 1.3 milliamperes (nominal) with silver-oxide battery; 1.0 milliamperes (nominal) with mercury battery.

Microphone: The microphone is a tiny balanced-armature type with high sensitivity. It is shielded to reduce electromagnetic interference, and is shock mounted and sealed into a compartment that is separated from the rest of the assembly.

Amplifier: The amplifier utilizes ultrasmall individually tested discrete components. A new construction technique eliminates printed wiring. All soldering is to slotted terminals firmly riveted to a glass-epoxy chassis plate. The complete 3-stage transistor amplifier provides all the gain that can be utilized.

Volume Control: A very tiny but rugged volume control is used. It has a neoprene seal to prevent entrance of moisture.

Fig. 6.24. Specifications for aid shown in Fig. 6.23. (Courtesy of Radio Ear Corporation.)

Battery Switch: The battery switch is an integral part of the volume control and has low resistance, long-life contacts made of silver. Turning the volume control counterclockwise to its "OFF" position, automatically disconnects the battery from the circuit.

Receiver: The "reproducer" is a tiny balanced-armature unit that is carefully shock and vibration mounted.

Case: The case is made of durable tough Tenite II with a carefully selected color to make it inconspicuous in the ear. Flesh color is standard; mocha is available on special order. The case is tightly sealed to prevent entrance of moisture, with only the battery compartment exposed.

Earmolds: The aid is shaped to utilize fully the space available at the entrance of the cana, but without any over-sized portion to be forced uncomfortably into the small section of the canal. This is accomplished by using either a custom or stock earmold beyond the angled part of the case. A snap-on nub and mating earmold ring is provided for all types of earmolds that will be used.

Gain (HAIC & USASI) Average: 30 dB using silver-oxide battery with volume control full on. Typical peak gain is 45 dB.
Subtract 4 dB when P-2752-A Filter is used.
Subtract 8 dB when P-2752-B Filter is used.
Subtract 8 dB when Mercury battery is used.

Output (HAIC & USASI Average): 115 dB re.0002 microbar with silver-oxide battery.
Subtract 4 dB when P-2752-A filter is used.
Subtract 8 dB when P-2752-B filter is used.
Subtract 2 dB when Mercury battery is used.
Frequency Range (HAIC & USASI Method of Computation:

Frequency Range (HAIC & USASI Method of Computation:
480-4400 cps basic response (curve A)
470-4500 cps range with P-2752-A filter (curve B)
430-4800 cps range with P-2752-B filter (curve C)

Distortion: Typically 4.5% measured with volume control full on; 65 dB input; average of 500, 700, and 900 cps). Distortion is lower at reduced volume control settings.

Fig. 6.24. Specification data (continued).

for sound sources by turning his eyes, and later his head. This ability achieves a high degree of sophistication in the adult with normal hearing. Deprived of visual cues, as we frequently are on a temporary basis when in a group situation, our perception of the direction of a sound source is dependent upon auditory localization. In Chap. 5 we discussed the role that hearing plays in our perception of space. In a group speaking situation, this localization function plays an important role in permitting us to follow the conversation as it jumps from one speaker to another. It tells our eyes where to look for the additional information that we receive through the visual channel. Without these auditory cues to localization, it would take a fraction of a second longer for us to locate the speaker who has taken up the conversation. Although this time lag may represent only a short interval, it is sufficient to deprive us of what might be important information. For the person with normal hearing the natural redundancy of speech is, under normal listening conditions, sufficient to compensate for this, so that it is possible for us to follow a conversation even when we are not able to see the speaker, though it is a situation in which we generally do not like to find ourselves. For the hard-of-hearing person for whom the redundancy of the speech signal may be considerably lower, the relative importance of immediate localization of the speaker and the consequent availability of additional visible clues may be vital to comprehension.

Even more important to the person with reduced auditory communication ability is the role that binaural hearing plays in improving speech discrimination against noise. Hirsh has stated that:

> The threshold of intelligibility for speech in the presence of noise is lower when the sources of speech and noise are separated spatially than when they are together. Between the least favorable (both sources together) and the most favorable (speech on the side and noise in front) conditions, the masked thresholds of intelligibility for normal hearing subject differed by about 10 dB. It was also shown that this difference, which was due to spatial arrangement of the sound sources, was not so large (if it existed at all) when the head was immobilized, or when only one ear was used. In other words, cutting down on a normal listener's ability to localize, either by preventing head movement or by preventing binaural listening, reduced his ability to separate the sources of speech and noise in apparent space and consequently reduced his ability to understand speech. [9, p. 240]

This is exactly the situation that occurs when a person is provided with a monaural hearing aid. Through the monaural system of the aid, sounds will be perceived as originating from the same position in the auditory field. In situations in which the signal-to-noise ratio is highly favorable, as when the hearing-aid user is talking to one other person in good environmental listening conditions, the speech redundancy may be sufficiently high to compensate for the limitations of monaural hearing. When, however, the signal-to-noise ratio is reduced by virtue of competing speech stimuli in a group situation or by such environmental sounds as that of a typewriter or radio playing, the hearing-aid user may experience a considerable loss of speech comprehension due to the fact that he lacks the ability to clearly differentiate between figure and ground.

The experimental evidence appears to be strongly in favor of the use of binaural hearing wherever there exists a binaural loss with useful residual hearing in both ears. The subjective evaluation of hearing-impaired people wearing binaural aids almost always confirms these conclusions. Hearing-aid users who have switched from the use of monaural to binaural aids frequently list, among the improvements that they notice, such factors as better comprehension of speech in noisy situations, greater ability to follow conversational speech in group situations, better hearing of speech at a distance, and more natural sound reproduction. It would be well to note, however, that because of the nature of the clinical tests that we traditionally use it is not always possible to demonstrate a clear improvement in the speech reception threshold or discrimination score using standard test procedures. There are still many aspects of speech perception that we are unable to quantify in a clinical test situation. It is for this reason that we should evaluate very carefully the subjective reactions of the wearer, particularly when these are made over a trial period during which auditory training is provided. This subjective improvement has been referred to by Frank Kodman as "ease of perception" [13]. This term appears to be sufficiently vague to permit us to include it in many subjective responses that we are yet unable to clearly differentiate, yet at the same time the use of it indicates that there does, in fact, exist something that is important to good hearing that goes well beyond the auditory processes involved in simple reception and discrimination.

CROS and BICROS

One of the most recent developments that has occurred in the use of ear-level hearing aids is the use of a system that has been labeled by some as a bi-unilateral hearing aid. The research in this area has been primarily the work of Dr. Earl Harford at Northwestern University [6, 7]. It is designed to meet the needs of people whose hearing loss falls in one of two categories that were previously difficult to assist by the use of amplification. These two categories are (1) those people with a unilateral hearing loss and (2) those with a bilateral hearing loss in which one ear is, for any reason, not suitable for the provision of amplification. This includes those that show very little usable residual hearing, low tolerance for loudness, or a chronic middle-ear infection.

The bi-unilateral fitting has been developed by Harford in two ways. The first and simplest system is designed to meet the needs of the person with a unilateral hearing loss and involves the routing of signals picked up by a hearing aid mounted behind the bad ear across the head, by way of a headband carrying an electrical wire, to a hearing-aid receiver at the good ear. Harford has referred to this as *contralateral routing of signals* (CROS). The system is simplified when the hearing-aid user wears glasses, since the microphone can be installed in the temple of the glasses on the side of the bad ear. The electrical contact wire runs through the glasses frame to an earphone mounted in the opposite temple by the good ear. The ear canal of the good ear remains open. Sound thus enters this ear by the normal hearing route but is augmented by the sound picked up by the microphone positioned at the bad ear and fed into the normal ear by means of a small plastic tube connected to the earphone. In this way the good ear is able to receive what is essentially a form of bilateral hearing, even though there is no hearing in one ear.

A further modification of this technique has been reported by Harford [6]. In the modified approach, a person with a bilateral hearing loss, but with only one ear showing usable residual hearing, is fitted with a hearing aid in the better ear, while an additional pickup microphone is situated close to the opposite ear. The sound energy transduced by this microphone is then fed back to a mixer unit that combines the signals before amplifying them and feeding them into the one usable ear. This type of amplification has been called *bilateral contralateral routing of signals* (BICROS).

Application of the principle of cross routing signals was provided by Otarion Electronics Corporation who, in 1955, introduced the first crossover eyeglass aid. They have subsequently eliminated the use of frame wiring by the use of coin-silver contacts between the temples and the front frame. This company now manufactures not only CROS and BICROS air-conduction glasses aids, but also a bone-conduction glasses model for use by persons with up to 20-decibel bone-conduction losses with an air-conduction loss across the frequency range of 500 to 2000 Hz of between 30 to 70 decibels. Many other manufacturers now produce a CROS BICROS hearing aid as a result of its wide application.

Once again it would appear from clinical reports concerning this type of amplification that the standardized tests do not necessarily indicate a significant improvement over the more conventional amplifying systems. However, subjective evaluation by the users of these aids strongly indicates that they do provide a great deal of benefit to people who previously had not been able to derive satisfactory benefits from the conventional-type aid.

THE APPROPRIATE HEARING AID

The ultimate purpose of a hearing-aid evaluation, whether it is carried out in the office of a hearing-aid dealer or in the community or university hearing clinic, should be to provide the individual with the hearing aid most likely to result in the greatest improvement in the person's ability to utilize his residual hearing in communication.

We have seen that the selection of an appropriate hearing aid purely on the basis of the configuration of the audiogram has not been demonstrated to be an effective method. Even careful comparison of the person's ability to discriminate speech with and without the aid may prove an inadequate measure upon which to predict how well the person may utilize the aid in his normal activities. Hearing-aid evaluation must not, therefore, be considered to constitute a reliable scientific procedure. It is still, and will probably remain, as much an art as a science. It requires of the audiologist the ability to combine the implications of test results with the implications of the subjective evaluations that he can obtain from the person who needs the aid. The potential user will have his own set of criteria. These will include how he thinks amplified speech and environmental noise ought to sound, the type of aid he is willing to wear, and the amount of money he can invest in the aid.

The question, "Which is the appropriate hearing aid for this person?" cannot, therefore, be categorically answered. One can, however, lay down certain minimum requirements that are applicable to each and every individual who is considering wearing a hearing aid.

The first of these requirements is that the aid must provide sufficient gain as to be able to reach the residual hearing that the person possesses. Do not misunderstand this to mean that there is a minimum amount of threshold improvement that must be evidenced before an aid will be recommended. For some severely deaf children the amount of amplified sound energy that exceeds their threshold of hearing may be relatively small; however, this small amount may constitute valuable additional information that, when combined with information received through other senses, will result in an improvement in their communication potential, not demonstrable when the auditory pathway alone is used. On the other hand, we have also mentioned that there is no maximum amount of amplification that ought to be required before a hearing aid might benefit a subject. There is little point in providing a high-gain hearing aid to a person who has so much residual hearing that only a mild amount of amplification is necessary in order to permit him to communicate without difficulty. Our first criterion can be restated: *The amount of gain provided for the individual should be appropriate to the degree of residual hearing demonstrated.*

Second, *the hearing aid should provide a degree of output limitation that insures that at no time will the amplified sound cross the individual's threshold of discomfort.* This is particularly true when fitting persons who give evidence of a decrease in tolerance for high-intensity sound. It is in this respect that an understanding of the output-limiting devices such as peak clipping and automatic volume control is important.

Third, *the frequency range of the hearing aid should be such that it provides adequate amplification across the range of frequencies represented by the person's residual hearing.* When that residual hearing exists primarily in the low frequencies, then consideration must be given to the selection of an aid specifically designed to be capable of picking up and amplifying these frequencies.

Fourth, *the aid should possess a wide dynamic range.* You will recall that this refers to the capability of the aid to pick up and amplify the weaker environmental sounds as well as to be able to reproduce the higher-level sounds without distortion and without exceeding the threshold of tolerance.

This requirement of absence of distortion should hold true for all levels of input sound pressure. Both the output control and the elimination of the frequency distortion at high input levels are most efficiently obtained when the aid is equipped with the automatic volume control.

Fifth, *the aid should have a wide signal-to-noise ratio* so that soft speech sounds are not masked by electrical noise in the amplifier.

The above requirements concern the capabilities of the aid itself. In addition to these, it is important that the audiologist ascertain the individual criteria by which the potential hearing-aid user will decide whether or not to wear the aid. The success indicator must be that the subject actually wears the aid rather than that he accepts the recommendation to purchase one, since many people who purchase aids do not subsequently use them. The task of the audiologist is, therefore, not only one of advisement, but through the rehabilitation program, it is one of persuasion. In subsequent chapters we shall examine the question of adequate counseling of the hearing-aid user, his immediate family, and in the case of children, of the appropriate school staff members. It is important that you should constantly remind yourself that the evaluation and recommendation for the use of amplification is not an independent unit. It is essential to the success of any such program that this measurement stage be carefully related to the total rehabilitation program.

THE EARMOLD

The earmold of a hearing aid must be considered as an integral part of the amplification, since an inappropriately designed mold may seriously impair the fidelity of the amplification that has been provided by a high-quality hearing aid. It has been stated in one publication [21]:

> It is quite probable that the earmold is the most neglected component in the chain of hearing aid performance. The most careful selection and adjustment of the hearing aid for the hearing impaired person's loss can be largely nullified by a poorly fitting earmold resulting from a carelessly made impression or the efforts of an inexperienced laboratory technician or both.

The earmold is an exact copy of an impression that was made of an individual person's ear. It serves two purposes: to couple the receiver of the hearing aid to the individual's ear and to transmit sound from the receiver to the eardrum.

Almost all hearing-aid earmolds are now custom made. They are divided into two major types: the *standard mold* and the *tube-type mold*. Illustrations of these may be seen in Fig. 6.25.

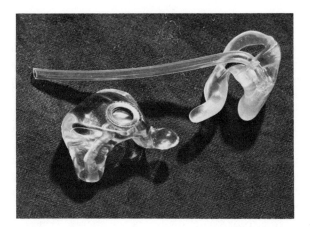

Fig. 6.25. The two major types of earmolds: the standard and tube-type mold.

The Standard Mold

It will be seen that the standard mold has the earphone clipped directly to it and that it inserts into the ear canal. This reduces the amount of energy loss between the amplifier and the eardrum. The best result is obtained when the length of the mold canal is sufficiently long to carry the sound around the natural bend in the external auditory meatus. Care must be taken in obtaining the impression since occasionally the attempt to meet the criterion of length results in a mold in which the canal is made too long. The result is discomfort or even pain as the movement of the temporo-manibular joint squeezes that portion of the ear canal against the mold. Because the standard earmold results in the least amount of energy loss, this type is imperative for use with severe hearing losses and is strongly recommended for moderate losses. It is essential for use with children. The standard mold may be obtained in either a rigid or a flexible plastic material or a combination of both, in which the base of the mold is hard plastic while the canal insert is flexible. Because young children are notorious for losing earmolds, and because failure to cooperate sometimes makes it difficult to obtain a satisfactory impression of the ear, stock earmolds are now available for children from six months to twelve years of age. Such molds are cheaper than custom-made molds, are invaluable in schools or nurseries where a mold may suddenly have to be found for a child who has lost his own, and are convenient for those situations in which one would like to provide a child with an aid on a trial basis.

In traveling from the receiver through the earmold to the eardrum, the acoustic wave form may change as a result of the sound-carrying characteristics of the mold. Knowledge of the effects that various earmold structures have upon the sound waves has made it possible to control certain conditions in such a way as to increase the transmission of certain desired frequencies. The characteristics of the standard earmold may be varied by shortening or lengthening the drill hole or by decreasing the diameter of the hole. A more commonly used method involves the insertion of tiny plastic filters into the earphone nozzle. These serve to reduce the diameter of the opening. The resultant attenuation factors for the various color-coded inserts are predictable. The use of earmold modifications to change the overall frequency response is exemplified by the acoustic-modifier earmold manufactured by Zenith (Fig. 6.26). In this mold, the canal portion has been almost completely eliminated, while the remaining canal opening has been enlarged to permit the maximum resonance of high frequencies. Two sound channels link the exterior flat surface of the earmold with the enlarged canal opening. Each of these channels is covered on the exterior surface by thin fabric disks, which serve to dissipate low-frequency energy. This type of mold is specifically designed for persons with steeply falling losses above 500 or 1000 Hz, and for persons with sensori-neural losses with low noise tolerance. The criteria recommended by the manufacturers for evaluating this type of earmold is a comparison of the aided-discrimination score in quiet using a standard earmold with the discrimination score obtained when using the acoustic modifier. Where possible the same comparison is recommended in noise conditions.

The Tube-Type Mold

The tubing-type earmolds, suitable for people with mild to moderate hearing impairments, are essentially cosmetic devices. By using a length of hollow plastic tube to connect the earmold with the earphone, the earphone may be worn in a less conspicuous position than when it is clipped directly to the earmold. Plastic insert filters may be used with the tube-type mold to modify frequency characteristics, which may also be modified by varying

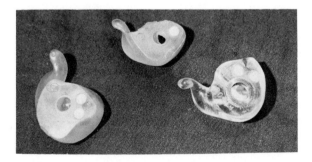

Fig. 6.26.   The acoustic–modifier earmold. (Courtesy of Zenith Hearing Aid Sales Corp.)

the diameter of the tubing. Unfortunately, the cosmetic improvement is often achieved at the expense of a loss in intensity of the output sound. The lengthening of the tube results in an increase in the loss in intensity and an increase in the distortion of tonal quality. The high frequencies are particularly affected. Since these are most commonly the frequencies for which the hearing-aid user requires the greatest amount of amplification, this type of mold may result in quite a significant decrease in the amount of improvement available to the user. Certain problems may arise in wearing an earmold, and these will be considered in the next chapter when we discuss the use and maintenance of hearing aids.

AUDITORY TRAINERS

Of all the available systems of amplification for use with the hard-of-hearing, the wearable hearing aid still has by far the most general application value. It is a completely portable unit that can be taken into almost every situation that a child or adult may encounter. Within the range of available aids we have seen that they vary considerably in size from those models which insert into the ear canal to the larger units which must be worn on the clothing. We have seen how this increase in size occurs as the wearer makes greater demands upon the aid for high levels of amplification, wider frequency response characteristics, better signal-to-noise ratios, and other features. On the first page of this chapter we defined the hearing aid as any device capable of intensifying the sound reaching the person's ear. Out of this range of amplifiers, we have selected for discussion those which are applicable for use by hearing-impaired people. The nature of our definition emphasizes that there exists no essential difference between wearable hearing aids, auditory trainers, and group hearing aids. These units differ only in the degree of efficiency with which they are able to faithfully amplify sound, the degree to which we are able to modify and control that amplification, the mobility with which they provide the individual, and the specific nature of the task for which each unit is designed.

For these reasons, the pattern of organization directing this discussion is dominated by the one factor of portability. Having discussed the completely portable hearing aid, we will now consider those hearing aids, often referred to as auditory training units, which are much larger but which still may be considered for the most part individual units and moderately portable. Finally we will consider the much larger and more static group-type unit.

Auditory Training Units

The early auditory training units suffered from the limited knowledge of electronics at the time. They consisted only of "hard" wire units in which the child's headphone cord was plugged into the desk and the teacher's microphone was plugged to the amplifier. Wired auditory trainers attempted to provide the necessary fidelity of acoustic reproduction, but they confined the movement of the child and teacher. This restriction imposed limitations on the teaching activity. Next appeared the desk-type auditory trainers, which came in both the monaural (one microphone and amplifier for each ear), binaural (a separate microphone, amplifier, and volume control for each ear), and the pseudo-binaural (a microphone and amplifier split between two ears). The child could carry the desk-type auditory trainer from place to place. However, as the child moved away from the teacher, the sound pressure level did not remain constant. This variation of sound pressure would also hold true for the hearing aid that a child was wearing. Therefore, the loop induction system evolved to meet the all-important requirements of high-quality amplification, constant sound-pressure level, a favorable en-

Outline of Evolution of Auditory Trainers

HARD WIRE TRAINERS: Teacher and child wired in

    monaural
    binaural
    pseudo-binaural

DESK-TYPE TRAINERS

WEARABLE TRAINERS

    monaural
    binaural
    pseudo-binaural

LOOP INDUCTION SYSTEMS: Auditory trainers or hearing aids used

    monaural
    binaural
    pseudo-binaural

LOOP INDUCTION SYSTEMS
WITH WIRELESS MICROPHONE: Auditory trainers or hearing aids used

    monaural
    pseudo-binaural

FM SYSTEMS

    binaural
    pseudo-binaural

vironmental signal-to-noise ratio for each child, and a maximum of mobility. The loop induction system freed the child within the classroom, but the teacher was still wired. In order to free the teacher, an optional FM wireless microphone transmitter has been incorporated into the loop systems which may be monaural or pseudo-binaural. The most recent developments are the complete FM wireless auditory training systems that provide the necessary fidelity, good environmental signal-to-noise ratio, constant sound-pressure level for each child, and mobility for both the teacher and children, outdoors as well as indoors. Monaural and binaural FM auditory training systems are available.

The manufacture of these auditory training units is not confined to companies who manufacture hearing aids. Until recently there were relatively few companies producing auditory trainers; however, the number has grown rapidly during the last few years so that the teacher has now available a wide range of makes and models from which to choose, some of which are illustrated in this section. Regardless of the make of the unit, its purpose and basic means of achieving it will always be the same. The purpose of the portable auditory trainer is to provide high-quality amplification across a wide frequency range up to an intensity level just below the threshold of discomfort, while permitting various degrees of modification to be made in the gain function, the frequency sensitivity curve, and the maximum output level.

Although it is possible to purchase auditory training units that provide pseudo-binaural amplification, as has already been explained, this falls far short of the true binaural system. Except in cases in which there is only usable residual hearing in one ear, the true binaural system is always preferable.

The Desk-Type Auditory Trainer

Three models of the desk-type auditory trainer are used to represent this type of unit (Fig. 6.27).

The Master model, a binaural auditory trainer, constitutes the most complex unit. Observe that the three controls are duplicated, indicating two entirely independent amplifying units. The two microphones are not visible in the photograph but are built into the amplifiers at the sides of the unit. The seven-inch separation, which represents the length of the unit, is sufficient to permit the ear to make the figure-ground separation, which we have seen is one of the important advantages of the binaural hearing. On this model the gain control, labeled in the illustration *gain-dB*, also provides the on-off switch. This control permits the user to determine the amount of amplification that will be given separately to the input signal being picked up by each microphone. The intensity of the signal reaching each ear may

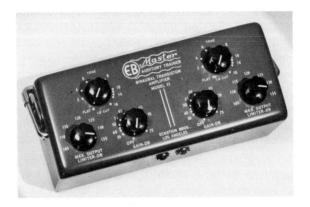

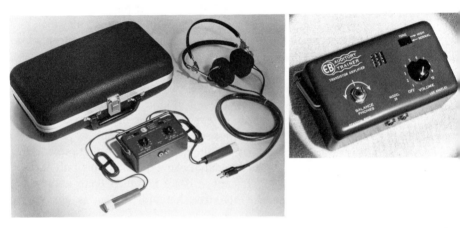

Fig. 6.27. Three models of desk-type auditory training units. (Courtesy of Eckstein Brothers.)

therefore be determined independently. An approximation of the amount of amplification that will be necessary may be made from the pure-tone audiogram. With this unit, the amount of amplification can be varied continuously across the range of 30 to 75 decibels; the settings marked in 5-decibel steps indicate points along this continuum. Remember that the 75 decibels is gain to the input signal. If we add this to the average intensity level of normal conversational voice (65 decibels re: 0.0002 microbar), we achieve an output level of 140 decibels SPL, which is up to the normal threshold of pain. Additional gain over and above a level of 75 decibels would therefore be of questionable value, since the individual would not be able to tolerate it.

With a potential output of up to 140 decibels, it is obvious that we will need to limit the maximum output of the unit. This is done by the control labeled *maximum output limiter-dB*. As we have seen, this represents the maximum intensity level that the amplifier is capable of reproducing, regardless of the intensity of the input signal and the gain-control setting. It is therefore possible to modify the maximum output level so that, with a constant input of 65 decibels and a constant gain setting of 70 decibels, the potential output of 135 decibels can be reduced in 5-decibel steps down to 105 decibels simply by the appropriate setting of the maximum output limiter. It must, however, be pointed out that in using this control we introduce a certain amount of additional distortion due to an overloading of the amplifier. As has already been explained, this may seriously reduce the information content of the acoustic signal. The maximum output limiter on any auditory training unit should therefore be set at the maximum possible level that the individual person is able to tolerate. Where possible, it is better to reduce the gain in decibels than to reduce the maximum ouput. However, in some situations a high gain level may be desirable to pick up the softer speech sounds, but the maximum output may have to be limited in order that the auditory trainer does not amplify environmental noise, such as a banging door or a book being dropped, beyond the level of the individual's tolerance.

The tone control is basically the same as the tone controls that we have discussed on the wearable hearing aids. It differs only in the degree of sophistication. As was explained, the tone control does not emphasize particular frequencies but, rather, de-emphasizes others, permitting the overall gain to be turned up, thus producing a relative emphasis of certain frequency ranges. You will observe in the photograph that the settings are labeled "flat, 2,4,6,8,10,14,18, and low-cut." These figures represent points on a variable attenuator designating the number of decibels of attenuation per octave for frequency components below 1200 Hz. Thus, if a gain setting of 65 decibels is used and the tone control is set at 6 decibels, the amount of amplification that is provided one octave below 1200 Hz (i.e., at 600 Hz) will be 65 dB minus 8 dB, or 57 dB. One octave below this, at 300 cycles, a further 8 decibels will be deducted, providing an amplification level of 49 decibels, while at 150 Hz, the amount of gain will be 40 decibels. Any intermediate amount of gain reduction can be chosen by setting the tone control to a level between those positions marked.

The second of the three models illustrated in Fig. 6.27 is a less sophisticated version. It, too, is a binaural unit with two controls, an on-off volume control, marked simply as settings rather than in decibels, and a two-position frequency-response selection switch labeled *tone*. This switch replaces the more sophisticated tone control on the first model shown. It permits the person to choose between a flat frequency response and a high-frequency emphasis.

The last model depicted represents the least-expensive nonstereophonic desk-type hearing amplifier with a volume control, a frequency-selection switch or tone control, and a balance control to balance the loudness level of the signal coming from the single microphone that is observable in the center of the unit.

The basic cost of these units, with accessories included, is approximately $300, $275, and $130 respectively. Each of the models may be worn either with dynamic earphones, with individual earphone receivers that clip onto the user's personal earmold, or with a lightweight, under-the-chin-type headset with phone-insert-type cushions.

It has been shown that it is possible to achieve high-quality amplification in a wearable unit without sacrificing the high fidelity offered by an efficient auditory trainer. Figure 6.28 shows a binaural auditory trainer that has been reduced to wearable size, weighing only 6 ounces. It provides true binaural hearing through separate microphones, amplifiers, and volume controls for each ear. When worn with earphones, it has a flat frequency response from 300 to 5300 Hz, well beyond the range of a conventional aid. The maximum output is 130 decibels, with an average acoustic gain of 60 decibels. Especially notable is the very high signal-to-noise ratio of 60 decibels, measured at maximum SPL output. The unit may also be worn with a hearing-aid earphone (insert receivers) and earmold, though this reduces the amplification of high frequencies to a maximum of 4000 Hz. With the hearing-aid phone, the maximum output is 140 decibels, with an average gain of 60 decibels. The unit also operates on long-life rechargeable

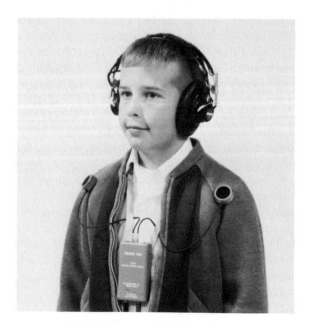

Fig. 6.28.   A wearable auditory training unit. (Courtesy of H C Electronics, Inc.)

batteries that markedly cut operating costs. Surprisingly, this binaural trainer, with cushioned headsets, costs less than a powerful body aid that provides only monaural amplification.

Group Auditory Trainers

Three major requirements of amplifying systems designed for use with hearing-impaired subjects are (1) that they provide high-fidelity reproduction, (2) that they permit each individual to control the level of gain he is using, and (3) that they do not restrict the wearer in mobility.

The use of the individual hearing aid, while providing the necessary mobility, makes it difficult to maintain a constant average-input intensity level as the child moves around the room. Furthermore, the fidelity of the conventional wearable hearing aid is, for the most part, inferior to that provided by group amplifying systems. Not only is the loudness level of the teacher's voice likely to be decreased in certain positions in the room, but more important, since the microphone of the aid is sensitive to all sounds in the room, the signal (teacher's voice)-to-noise (environmental sounds) ratio may be severely reduced as the separation of the signal source and the microphone increases or as the aid is brought in close proximity to a loud ambient sound source. Therefore, in teaching situations that depend upon the ability to provide a group of children with high-quality amplification, the teacher must turn to the group hearing aid, which provides the necessary fidelity of acoustic reproduction and permits the individual child to control the amount of amplification that the input signal is given.

This class of instrument may be represented by the trainer depicted in Fig. 6.29. It consists of two independent channels with separate amplifiers, microphones, and extension outlets for up to 20 headphones. The master output lead from the amplifier is fed to a series of student control boxes, each equipped with an independent gain control for the left and right earphone. In this way, the amount of attenuation provided to the maximum output originating at the amplifier may be determined according to the individual needs of each of the 20 students. In addition, the auditory trainer permits binaural extension microphones that may either be ceiling mounted or mounted on a floorstand, as shown in the diagram of a typical classroom in Fig. 6.30. In addition to the stereo microphone output, it is possible to use a four-speed record player to amplify either mono or stereo records.

The auditory training unit (Fig. 6.31) is representative of the large nonportable-type group auditory training units. The specifications state that the frequency response of this unit emphasizes the frequencies most useful to speech communication by providing a flat response from 300 to 3500 Hz, with a fall off of approximately 10 decibels at 100 Hz and, in the high frequencies, 3 decibels at 5000 Hz and 6 decibels at 10,000 Hz. The manufacturers justify this attenuation of the low and high frequencies by pointing out that, while these frequencies would not contribute to any improvement in speech communication, they do tend to provide amplification of ambient room noise in the low frequencies and to make the instrument susceptible to high-frequency squeals at the other end of the frequency range. The manufacturer's literature specifies that the instrument has output controls calibrated between 100 and 140 decibels sound-pressure level. This control works in conjunction with a gated compression-amplification system that is essentially an automatic volume control. The volume control for the console is adjusted by means of a magic eye that serves to provide a visual indication of the start of the compression circuit. This permits one to adjust the input control so that the peaks of normal voice or music just begin to activate the automatic volume-control circuit. The individual output setting for each ear of each child in the group then insures that, regardless of the input intensity at the microphone, the compression amplification will not permit the output at any particular headphone to exceed the value that has been set for it.

This trainer has three separate microphone-input connections with individual sensitivity and mixing controls, which provide for various combinations of microphone use. For example, the teacher may choose to wear a collar microphone while using an overhead-boom microphone on each of the other two channels, or the teacher's collar microphone may be coordinated either with two roving desk microphones or with a wall-boom microphone and a floorstand microphone. In addition to the phonograph and microphone inputs, connections may also be made to radio and television.

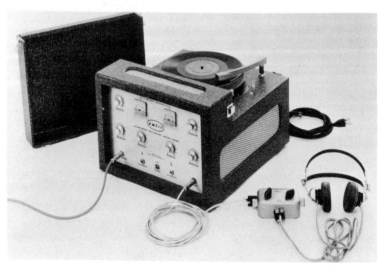

Fig. 6.29.   A transistorized group auditory training unit. (Courtesy of Ambco Electronics.)

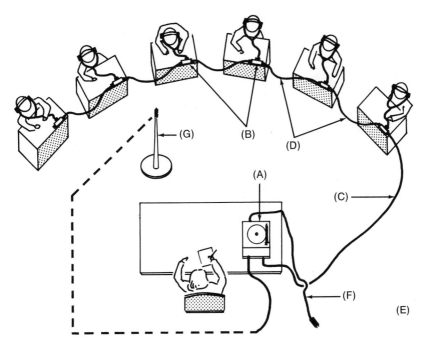

(A) Binaural amplifier or control unit (1450), located at teachers desk. May be installed in any other convenient place.

(B) Student control boxes (1451), each equipped with dual volume controls for individual student sound level adjustment.

(C) 12-foot-long interconnecting cable (1457), connects control unit (1450) to first student control box (1451).

(D) 4-foot-long interconnecting cables, connects student control boxes.

(E) 25-foot-long microphone cable, connects control unit to ceiling-mounted microphones.

(F) 8-foot-long AC cord, equipped with adapter where grounded 3-conductor wall socket is not available.

(G) Ceiling-mounted microphones (floorstand is optional). For the ceiling-mounted microphones we recommend a height of approximately 7 feet above floor level.

Fig. 6.30. Typical classroom layout for use of an auditory trainer. (Courtesy of Ambco Electronics.)

Loop Induction and Radio-Frequency Amplifying Systems

In teaching situations that depend upon the ability to provide the child with high-quality amplification, the teacher has turned to the group hearing

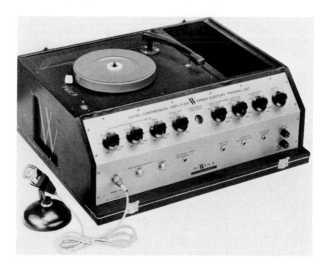

Fig. 6.31. Group auditory training unit. (Courtesy of L. L. Warren, Inc.)

aid as an alternative. This type of aid, as we have seen, provides the necessary fidelity of acoustic reproduction, permits the child individual control
of the amount of amplification that the input signal is given, but confines his
movements to the limits imposed by the length of the cord from his desk to
the headphones. This restriction immediately imposes limitations on the
type of teaching activity that the teacher may use. In general, lessons must
be somewhat formal in nature. The children usually sit in a small group
around the unit, unplugging the headphone connections whenever they
need to leave their desks to come before the group or work at the blackboard. Teachers sometimes arrange for an extra outlet to be provided at the
blackboard, but this is inadequate because of the lack of continuity resulting
from plugging and unplugging connections and because the individual intensity needs of each child cannot be accommodated.

   Two systems have attempted to meet the all-important requirements of
high-quality amplification, a constantly favorable environmental signal-to-
noise ratio for each child, and a maximum of mobility. These are the *loop
induction system* and the *FM (frequency modulated) auditory training
systems*.

Loop Induction Amplification

   The loop induction system of amplification differs from the conventional auditory trainer in that the output from an amplifier, instead of being
fed directly to a receiver, is fed into a loop of wire that circles the classroom.

The sound waves are picked up by the microphone and transduced into electrical current in the normal way. The signal is then strongly amplified and fed into a loop of wire that runs around the entire room. The flow of current within this wire causes a magnetic field to be set up within the room. The individual will be able to pick up the signal if he has a receiving unit capable of responding to changes in the magnetic field and transposing them into electrical energy that may then be amplified and transformed back into acoustical energy by an earphone. Since the strength of the magnetic field within the room should be a constant, the strength of the signal should not vary significantly in various positions in the room.

The regular body aid is sensitive only to sound-pressure variations; it does not respond to changes in the magnetic field in the room. However, if the instrument is fitted with a telephone pickup circuit, then it will be sensitive to variation in the magnetic field, since the telephone circuit is designed to respond to the very small magnetic variations within the telephone receiver.

In order to insure that the current supply to the loop is strong enough to activate the telephone circuit of a personal hearing aid, a power amplifier is used to amplify the input signal from a microphone or from another input source such as a tape recorder, a phonograph or television.

The great advantage of this system is that it is not limited by the number of headphones that the amplifier will drive, but only by the number of people capable of moving freely within the magnetic field. Since there is no longer any direct physical connection between the receiver and the amplifier, amplified speech may be received equally well anywhere within the magnetic field. Furthermore, since the external microphone of the aid is cut off when the telephone circuit of the hearing aid is activated, the signal-to-noise ratio remains a constant factor regardless of the distance between the microphone and the receiver.

By speaking into the microphone at a distance of a few inches, the system insures that a favorable environmental signal-to-noise ratio exists and the vowel sounds are not emphasized out of proportion to the consonant sounds, as tends to occur when the level of voice intensity is increased.

In addition to the flexibility of movement in teaching techniques that the loop system provides, it has the advantage of not requiring the purchase of expensive training equipment or of limiting the number of children who may participate. For this reason, it lends itself for use not only in the classroom, but also in halls or gymnasiums and even in private homes, where additional loops are installed.

When the loop system was first used, it was not possible for the child to pick up both the signal originating from the loop induction system and the sound of his own voice, which of course would not be fed into the loop system. Aids have now been modified specifically for use with loop induction systems. These provide three-position switches that permit the child to select either the normal external microphone circuit; the loop circuit, which excludes the microphone completely; or a loop and microphone setting, in which the child is able to pick up both the loop induction signal and the sound of his own speech. The setting that will be selected will, of course, be determined by the nature of the communication activity taking place.

Unfortunately, in addition to the advantages there are quite naturally disadvantages to this system. One of the biggest is the problem created by what is known as *overspill*. This occurs when there is more than one induction loop system working in a school building. The term overspill describes the situation in which the induced magnetic field in one classroom is strong enough to set up the same magnetic field in adjacent classrooms. Thus, when two systems are in operation, it is possible for a child also to be hearing the activity that is going on in the next room. It is difficult enough for a child to compete with the normal ambient noise of his own classroom; to find himself faced with a competing signal provided by the lesson that is going on in the next classroom can prove to be a highly disturbing experience. There are a variety of ways of reducing a spill over, though it is not necessary for us to discuss these in this text. It is, however, important to recognize that this problem does still exist.

When used with the child's personal hearing aid, the loop induction system is also limited by the quality of each individual child's hearing aid. The system can obviously be no better than the personal hearing aid with which it is used. The variation in the condition and fidelity of children's hearing aids is so great and varies so frequently that this does present quite a serious limiting factor. Furthermore, since it utilizes the body-worn hearing aid, it is, with few exceptions, confined to the provision of monaural amplification, a limitation that we have already discussed. The loop system can, however, be used with some desk-model auditory trainers. However, the advantage of mobility is obviously lost when a desk unit is used. The possibility of using a wireless microphone with the induction loop increases its flexibility to some extent. This application has been exploited by one manufacturer whose monaural RF induction loop system utilizes a fixed master control and loop installation with fully wearable student receivers that are powered by rechargeable batteries. The option of a wireless microphone permits the teacher freedom of movement, though the students must stay within the boundaries of the loop.

An additional feature is that the auditory trainer can be used in conjunction with a system they refer to as the *Learning Loop*. A pressure-sensitive tape is placed on the walls of the classroom and serves as an antenna to fill the room with the radio signal carrying the spoken word transmitted through a teacher-controlled transmitter-amplifier. This amplifier permits six programs to be presented simultaneously. In this way, the children may be listening and watching a film or television program, while the teacher adds her own commentary through a neck microphone, with a floor microphone available to pick up the responses and questions of the other children in the class.

The pupil receiver may be used either with headphones or with a personal earmold. Attached to each set of headphones is a boom microphone with adjustable sensitivity, a useful asset in training a child to moderate his voice level. When wearing insert receivers, a clip-on microphone is used as the child speaks, and his voice is amplified and fed to his headphones. The teacher may also plug a microphone into a student's unit to permit personal communication without disturbing the other children in the class.

Therefore, we can say that, although the loop system does provide for a greater degree of mobility of the children and a greater potential for flexibility of teaching, it still does not completely satisfy our requirements for a highly effective system of amplification. For this reason, manufacturers are beginning to explore the potentials of direct radio-frequency amplification as a means of better meeting the amplification needs of the hearing-impaired child.

Frequency Modulated Systems

As with the loop induction system, the frequency modulated system of amplification differs only from the standard methods in the way in which the signal is sent from the amplifier to the receiver. We have seen how the loop induction system attempts to provide mobility by using a magnetic field to convey the signal from the amplifier to the receiver. We have talked about the advantages and disadvantages of this system. The frequency modulated system attempts to provide the advantages of the loop induction system without the disadvantages. It uses radio-frequency waves to carry the information in the same way as a radio and television station broadcasts a signal that can be picked up by anyone with a radio receiver, providing they are within the limits of the maximum distance that the radio transmitter can reach. This distance is purely a function of the strength of the signal being broadcasted.

The classroom teacher is fitted with a transmitting unit that transduces the audio-speech signal into radio waves. These are then transmitted into the environment. Since the teacher's microphone requires no cable or cord to a control console or amplifier, she enjoys complete mobility. Because of this mobility the FM unit, unlike the loop system, may be used anywhere the children and teacher go—on a visit to the library, traveling on a bus, visiting the zoo, or playing in the playground. The children wear what is essentially a small radio receiver that picks up the radio signal being transmitted by the teacher and transduces it back into an audio signal at a headphone or at a small receiver clipped to a personal earmold.

Although FM transmission may be subject to external interference from a local radio station on or near its frequency, it does reduce the problem of overspill from adjacent classrooms, while also providing for the use of more than one transmitter in the same room, since a multiple of frequency channels are available for transmission. Currently available radio-frequency auditory training systems permit the use of up to 20 separate channels without interference.

One wireless auditory trainer (Fig. 6.32) has an on-off switch and a three-position tone switch for low-, medium-, and high-frequency emphasis. It has a built-in microphone with a wind-blast filter to permit its use in outside situations. This microphone permits the signal originating from the teacher to be mixed with the microphone signal, picking out the child's own voice and amplifying it to a loudness level appropriate to the child's needs. Separate controls permit the intensity of the signal reaching each ear to be adjusted according to the particular problem of hearing loss of the child. It must be recognized, however, that this is pseudo rather than true binaural hearing. The unit is battery operated, the battery being fully rechargeable. The manufacturer's literature shows the frequency-response curve for the overall system to be 70 to 10,000 Hz. The output is listed as 125 decibels with headset and 135 decibels with ear inserts (re: 0.0002 microbar). The total cost of one complete student unit is listed as $325 and of the teacher unit, $375.

Another wireless unit evolved from the desk-type binaural auditory trainer, which was reduced to the wearable binaural auditory trainer (Fig.

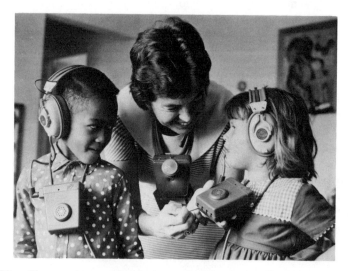

Fig. 6.32.   Classroom use of the Acousta. (Courtesy of Acousta and Alberquerque Hearing and Speech Center.)

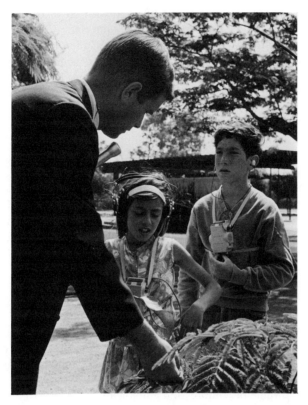

Fig. 6.33. The flexibility of teaching activities made possible by the use of FM amplification is illustrated here. (Courtesy of H C Electronics, Inc.)

6.32). In an attempt to meet the needs of mobility for the teacher and children, indoors or outdoors, provide binaural amplification, favorable environmental signal-to-noise ratio, high-quality fidelity, and a constant sound-pressure level, an FM receiver has been added to this unit, and a sophisticated FM microphone transmitter has been designed for the receiver. This model incorporates a separate volume control, microphone, amplifier for each ear, and power on-off and microphone on-off switches (Fig. 6.33). The FM transmission of the teacher's microphone transmitter is split between both amplifiers for the child's needs. The child can listen to the FM transmission and binaural amplification together or separately. For FM only, the child turns off the microphone switch and listens only to the teacher. For binaural only, the teacher turns off the microphone transmitter and the child turns on the microphone switch. If the teacher desires to have only a portion of the children listen to the FM transmission, she instructs the other children to pull out their colored plug-in module and turn on their binaural micro-phones. Further, if one child moves to another classroom, he unplugs the colored plug-in module matching his teacher's microphone, turns on his binaural microphones and listens to environmental sounds as he goes to the next class, then upon reaching the next class, he plugs in the colored module matching the other teacher's microphone. All microphone transmitters have an audio input for a tape recorder, record player, etc.

The FM auditory training system incorporates automatic noise rejec-tion. The transmission emits an inaudible tone, along with the carrier frequency, that is between 88 and 92 MHz in the educational bandwidth as allocated by the FCC (Federal Communications Commission). When the microphone-transmitter is turned off, the student receiver turns off and will not receive white noise. If an outside interference comes into the area, the student's receiver will not receive it when the teacher's microphone is off because his receiver will only turn on when it receives the basic frequency plus the inaudible tone. The manufacturer states that the overall frequency response is 300 to 5300 Hz (± 3 decibels) with the headphone and 300 to 4000 Hz (± 3 decibels) with the hearing-aid earphone. The output is 130 decibels SPL on the headphones and 140 decibels SPL on the hearing-aid earphone attached to a personal earmold.

This chapter has been based upon the assumption that, in order to make maximum use of amplification in aural rehabilitation, the teacher or therapist must have a basic understanding of the nature of amplification and a famil-iarity with the acoustic characteristics of amplifying systems. An under-standing of the value of compression amplification over peak clipping, of the importance of the extent to which frequency or gain characteristics can be modified, and of the implications of the signal-to-noise ratio and distortion factor go a long way in facilitating the choice of equipment. Unfortunately, however, such knowledge does not resolve the problem of dependence upon the specification sheets provided by the manufacturer. The manufacturers of the acoustic equipment are faced with the same problem of quality con-trol that faces the manufacturer of any product. The specification sheet represents an ideal that they would like to feel their equipment lives up to. Comparisons of the actual performance of amplifying systems relative to the specifications indicates the presence of a credibility gap. Teachers and thera-pists working with hearing-impaired children or adults have long been aware of this problem, but until recently there appeared to be no solution for a person not located in an institution capable of making its own analysis of equipment.

Fortunately, a number of professional people in California determined to provide comparative information pertaining to various aspects of commer-cially available amplification systems for use with the hearing-impaired [4]. The project was established by the California State Department of Education in conjunction with the San Diego Speech and Hearing Center. The study was developed under the direction of Donald F. Krebs of the Speech and Hearing Center and was funded by a federal grant awarded under the provisions of Title VI-A, Elementary and Secondary Education Act, 89-10, as amended. Utilizing the services of a variety of consultant staff members, the team subjected to careful examination most of the commercial amplification systems currently available—a total of 22 units. The data obtained includes a report on the acoustic response of the units covering acoustic gain, output, frequency-response characteristics, harmonic distortion, tone-control variability, uniformity between channels, control calibration, and compression attack and recovery time where appropriate. Response curves are provided to document the findings for each instrument.

In addition to the acoustic data, independent evaluation was made of quality assurance, which includes such factors as reliability, durability, practicability, portability, and maintainability. Finally, an educational evaluation was conducted by experienced teachers of the deaf, supervisors of instruction, administrators, consultants, and audiologists. The purpose of this evaluation was to assess the suitability of the various amplifying systems under study for the instructional programs for deaf and severely hard-of-hearing children enrolled in existing programs in California. The factors included in the survey an assessment of the physical features, quality of the system and components, acoustical performance, and educational suitability for different types of children and programs.

The results of this project, reported in a publication, *Educational Amplification Response Study*, by the San Diego Speech and Hearing Center, 8001 Frost Street, San Diego, California 92123, provide the reader with what is currently the only objective evaluative data by which it is possible to compare the performance of different types of amplifying systems on the basis of tests carried out on an objective basis. The document permits the reader to become familiar with many aspects of auditory training units that would remain unknown to him if he depended only upon the manufacturers' specification sheets. It serves the prospective purchaser in exactly the same way as do the various consumer guides that have been reporting to the general public on other manufactured products for a number of years. It would not be fair in this text to select certain of the manufactured items for the purpose of illustrating the type of data available within the report.

In general, reading the report must lead one to conclude that we are not justified in placing unqualified confidence in the specifications provided for us by the manufacturer. In many instances it was found that the actual performance data obtained did, in fact, concur with the claims made by the manufacturer. In many other instances, however, wide discrepancies were found, both with regard to the acoustic characteristics and with regard to the quality-assurance criteria. For example, some instruments were found to have poor uniformity of frequency response due to marked deviations from the desirable flat pattern, others exhibited a poor uniformity between separate stereo channels, while in some models the amount of harmonic distortion present was found to be high. Quality-assurance evaluation produced evidence in some instances of poor soldering and wiring, poor arrangement of parts, making servicing and replacements difficult, or the use of case and mounting frames considered highly vulnerable to damage. The educational survey revealed such problems as generally unsatisfactory workmanship on some of the external parts of an instrument, inflexible and uncomfortable headbands, poorly cushioned earphones, the unsuitability of microphone stands, and the limitation placed on mobility by the fixed position of student controls on junction boxes.

Data such as these are invaluable in making a decision concerning which type of currently available equipment one should purchase. It would seem that this first attempt at comparative qualitative evaluation of instruments used in educational training of the hearing-handicapped person should therefore be given every possible support. It should be insured that periodic studies of this nature should be routinely made and the data published, perhaps, by the professional organizations representing hearing therapists and teachers of the deaf. In the foreword to the report Krebs states, "This report is the first of what is hoped will be a series of publications dealing with electronic training systems." We should insure that this hope is realized.

To conclude this chapter let us attempt to summarize the basic points that we have made. We have paid particular attention to the topic of amplification since this constitutes one of the most vital aspects of a program of auditory rehabilitation. For a person with a hearing loss, the amount of residual hearing that can be designated as usable is primarily determined by the extent to which the sounds of speech can be raised above the person's auditory threshold. A person who with a hearing aid may now be functioning perfectly adequately in society may, if deprived of amplification, be quite unable to continue as an integrated member of the community. We have seen from our discussion that the term amplification today refers almost exclusively to electrical amplifiers. In the field of auditory rehabilitation we classify these under the terms hearing aids, auditory training units, and group aids. However, the principles underlying each of these types of amplifiers are fundamental. The same principles hold true for the tiny in-the-ear hearing aid as they do for the large group-type aid. We have considered the way in which sound waves are transduced into electrical wave forms that closely resemble the acoustic wave-form pattern, and the way in which these may be amplified and then once again transduced by the receiver into an acoustic wave form, which ideally should closely approximate the original sound-wave pattern. It has been explained how exact duplication of the original wave form at all stages of amplification is difficult to achieve, particularly when the amplifying system must be reduced to a wearable size. The further we reduce the size of the unit, the more difficult it becomes to faithfully reproduce the input signal. We have seen that this distortion factor is essentially a function of the sensitivity of the various components within the system. We have also explained how this apparent disadvantage may be capitalized upon to some extent by modifying the sensitivity curve of the system so as to add relative emphasis to those frequencies for which the listener shows a loss of sensitivity in the hearing mechanism. The limitations of this form of selective amplification have been pointed out.

In addition to our discussion of the general principles underlying amplification, we have discussed the various categories of amplifiers used in rehabilitation of hearing-impaired people. In general, we have adhered to the traditional categories of the wearable hearing aid, the wearable auditory training unit, the desk-type auditory trainer, and the group aid. In addition, we have considered two of the more recent modifications, namely the loop induction system and the FM auditory training system. No attempt has been made to review the various models available within each category; rather a representative of the category has been used to illustrate the advantages and limitations of the particular type of amplifier being discussed and to expose the reader to the basic specifications that will be available for specific models.

The question of selection and evaluation of wearable hearing aids has been briefly touched upon. A strong plea has been made that we differentiate between those things that we do on the basis of an accumulation of carefully evaluated data, and those that we do because they are part of the conventional wisdom of our profession. There is every justification for a pragmatic approach to aural rehabilitation; however, we must be careful to constantly evaluate what we are doing and to discover through experimentation and critical inquiry the underlying principles upon which pragmatic success occurs.

The overall purpose of this chapter has been to provide the reader with a better understanding of the tools with which he will be working in order that he may have greater success in shaping the life of the hard-of-hearing person through a more meaningful and, therefore, more effective program of aural rehabilitation.

REFERENCES

1. Davis, H., and R. Silverman. *Hearing and Deafness.* New York: Holt, Rinehart & Winston, Inc., 1961.

2. Davis, H., et al. *Hearing Aids: An Experimental Study of Design Objectives.* Cambridge, Mass.: Harvard University Press, 1947. Frequently referred to as

the "Harvard Report," this is a technical report of experiments conducted at the Psycho-Acoustic Laboratory under contract with the Office of Scientific Research and Development.

3. _____. "The Selection of Hearing Aids." *The Laryngoscope,* 56 (1946): 85–115, 135–63. A reprinting in full of report "PNR–7" issued December 31, 1945, by the Psycho-Acoustic Laboratory, Harvard University, Cambridge, Mass. It includes a theoretical analysis of the general problem of "fitting" a hearing aid and a critique of several fitting procedures.

4. Griffing, Barry L., and Gordon M. Hayes. *Educational Amplification Response Study.* Monograph no. 1. Project director, Donald F. Krebs. San Diego: San Diego Speech and Hearing Center, 1968.

5. Galbraith, Kenneth. *The Affluent Society.* 2nd ed., rev. Boston: Houghton Mifflin Company, 1969.

6. Harford, E. "Bilateral CROS Two-Sided Listening with One Hearing Aid." *Archives of Otolaryngology* 84 (1966): 90–96.

7. Harford, E., and Elizabeth Dodds. "The Clinical Application of CROS: A Hearing Aid for Unilateral Deafness." *Archives of Otolaryngology* 83 (1966): 455–67.

8. Hirsh, Ira J. "The Relation Between Localization and Intelligibility." *Journal of the Acoustical Society of America* 22: 196–200.

9. _____. *Measurement of Hearing.* New York: McGraw-Hill Book Company, 1952.

10. Jerger, James. "Annual Review of JSHR 1966." *Journal of Speech and Hearing Disorders* 32 (1966): 107–11.

11. Jerger, J., C. Malinquist, and C. Speaks. "Comparison of Some Speech Intelligibility Tests in the Evaluation of Hearing Aid Performance." *Journal of Speech and Hearing Research* 9 (June 1966): 253–358.

12. Jerger, J., C. Speaks, and C. Malinquist. "Hearing and Performance and Hearing Aid Selection." *Journal of Speech and Hearing Research* 9 (March 1966): 136–49.

13. Kodman, Frank. "Attitudes of Hearing Aid Users." *Maico Audiological Library Series* 2, no. 7.

14. Licklider, J. C. R. "Effects of Amplitude Distortion on the Intelligibility of Speech." *Journal of the Acoustical Society of America* 13 (1946): 429–34.

15. _____. "The Intelligibility of Rectangular Speech Waves." *American Journal of Psychology* 61 (1948): 1–20.

16. Ling, Daniel. "Implications of Hearing Aid Amplification below 300 Cps." *Volta Review* 66 (December 1964), pp. 723–29.

17. Miller, Maurice H. "Clinical Hearing Aid Evaluation." *Maico Audiological Library Series* 3, Part I, no. 7.

18. Winchester, R. A. "When Is a Hearing Aid Needed?" *Maico Audiological Library Series,* no. 12.

19. Yantis, P. A., J. P. Millin, and Irving Shapiro. "Speech Discrimination in Sensori-Neural Hearing Loss: Two Experiments on the Role of Intensity." *Journal of Speech and Hearing Research* 19 (June 1966): 178–93.

20. Zenith Hearing Aid Sales Corporation. *Hearing Aids and Their Components.* Chicago: Zenith Hearing Aid Sales, Inc. n.d.

21. ————. "The Custom Earmold." *Special Performance Bulletin,* no. 8 (June 1960).

CHAPTER SEVEN
Auditory Training

The practical application of the concept of auditory training dates back as far as 1805 when Jean Marc Gaspard Itard, at the Paris Institute for the Deaf, began to experiment in teaching auditory discrimination to deaf children. Arnold Toynbee and Max Goldstein in the nineteenth century also showed an awareness and concern for the value that might be derived from some form of auditory training. However, without the existence of the audiometer, the first of which was not developed until the early part of this century, the possibility of defining the limits of usable residual hearing was severely limited. Even when a child was shown to respond to loud speech or environmental noises, the amount of success that it was possible to achieve through auditory training without electrical amplification was not encouraging. Residual hearing did not provide for a viable system of communication. It was not until after the Second World War, when the personal hearing aid became widely available, that the possibility of retraining hearing as the major communication pathway became feasible for many hearing-impaired children and adults.

Numerous authors have attempted to define the term auditory training. R. Carhart refers to it as "the process of teaching the child or adult who is hard-of-hearing to take full advantage of sound cues which are still available to him" [4, p. 373]. E. Whetnall uses the term to imply "the application of conditions which reproduce for the deaf child as nearly as possible the conditions by which the normally hearing child learns to hear and talk" [27, p. 217]. Auditory training is seen by E. Wedenberg as "a procedure directed at systematic and individual exploitation of the existing hearing with a certain suppression—but only stressed in the beginning—of the visual sense" [26]. J. C. Kelly considers it a procedure aimed at improving awareness, discrimination, and retention of speech sounds [12, p. iv].

Other writers have avoided defining the term, concentrating instead upon a statement of the major aims. C. V. Hudgins suggested four major objectives [10]:

1. The development of auditory speech perception.
2. Better speech, which includes greater intelligibility, more natural voices, and rhythmic speech.
3. A broader and more flexible language development.
4. Acceleration of the general education program as a result of improved communication skills.

In the booklet, *The Use of Residual Hearing*, T. J. Watson defines five goals [25, p. 29]:

1. Greater understanding of the spoken language of others.
2. More rapid development of the use of language by the child and its extension in the direction of normality.
3. Better speech by the child in terms of voice quality, articulation, and rhythm.
4. Higher attainments in scholastic subjects, especially in basic skills.
5. Better social and emotional adjustments through the provision of a direct link, however tenuous, with other people and the world at large.

Although most writers agree that residual hearing should be thoroughly exploited, there is some disagreement as to whether auditory training should exist as a separate rehabilitative procedure. Watson states, for example:

> The term auditory training will from hence forth be dropped since it implies a "training of hearing." As has already been pointed out, this is the rock on which so much of the earlier work was founded. Attempts through formal exercises either to improve hearing or to improve the use made of residual hearing, when they have focused attention on hearing alone have either failed or have just not justified the time and effort spent on them. It is therefore emphasized that this use of residual hearing is part of a multisensory approach to development in education. It is not a subject for which separate time needs to be set apart, except for some occasional short periods when listening is emphasized more than looking. If such a description of the use

of residual hearing is accepted, then it is evident that it will be used in the main as an adjunct to lipreading. It will, in fact, be exposure to sound, but it will be planned and systematically directed exposure with improvement in auditory perception as a possible by-product. [25, p. 30]

Watson is writing with regard to children with relatively little usable residual hearing. The attitude toward auditory training expressed by those concerned with the rehabilitation of children and adults with less severe hearing impairments is somewhat different as exemplified by Carhart's position. He advocates the use of specific auditory training procedures for the improvement of speech perception. He includes among these the development of awareness of sound, differentiation between gross sounds, drill practice for discrimination between dissimilar speech sounds, and finally, fine auditory discrimination between phonemes with similar acoustic structure.

Using the model of communication that we have developed within this text, it is possible for us to agree, at least in part, with the approach represented by both of the above authors. We have argued that communication involves the ability to make predictions on the basis of multisensory cues, the most important of which, in a normal conversational situation, are transmitted through the auditory channel. While we recognize that the attributing of meaning to sensory stimuli involves the act of total perception, we also acknowledge that a sensory pathway is capable of acting at least semi-independently. We would therefore concur with Watson's statement that the "use of residual hearing is part of a multisensory approach to development in education." Watson's emphasis on the visual channel, with audition as an adjunct to lipreading, may be realistic for the profoundly deaf child, but it is untenable as a rehabilitational procedure for children with usable residual hearing. We accept the concept of training the student in the use of residual hearing within an educational framework; however, we also agree with the point of view presented by Carhart, that the child or adult can benefit from specialized training in auditory discrimination. The flaw in Watson's argument rests in his assumption that auditory training attempts to improve the child's hearing. The purpose of auditory training is not to improve hearing, but to improve communication. Our approach emphasizes the increase in the total flow of information rather than the dominance of a single sensory pathway. In many instances the success of auditory training may only be measurable in terms of total perception. Speech discrimination by hearing only may be impossible to attain.

DEFINITION AND AIMS

The following definition has therefore been made broad enough to encompass the concept of hearing as more than a unitary process. It is seen to be a part of an integrated experience: *Auditory training constitutes a systematic procedure designed to increase the amount of information that a person's hearing contributes to his total perception.* Note that the definition is equally applicable to the child or adult and that it covers all degrees of hearing loss.

It is suggested that the general aims of the therapist should be the following:

First, he must *explain to the person with a hearing loss (or in the case of a very young child to his parents) the nature of his auditory and communication problem.* It frequently occurs that a person enters a program of rehabilitation without even a rudimentary understanding of the nature of his difficulties. The effect of a prior explanation by an otologist or audiologist was probably nullified by the limited time that could be spent in consultation and by the anxiety generated at the time by the diagnosis of deafness. Rehabilitation should therefore begin with a simple, concise explanation of the person's problem as it has been evaluated. This should include an honest appraisal of the prognosis for improved communication and, where appropriate, a discussion of the social, educational, and vocational implications of the hearing loss.

Second, he must *provide an understanding of the approach to aural rehabilitation that will be used.* It is important that the individual be motivated by a sense of purpose in his program of rehabilitation. He should know what he is aiming toward and the steps he will take to reach his goal. No activity should be participated in without an understanding of its purpose. In this way, the therapist and the student work together to achieve for the student the common goal of improved communication.

The following are the specific goals for auditory training:

First, *to develop an awareness of sound and its referential function.* This stage is necessary for young deaf children for whom the provision of amplification makes sound audible for the first time. We should realize that when we first amplify sound for the hard-of-hearing child or adult he is faced with a new or at least a different auditory experience. The environment suddenly bombards him with sounds that previously were either inaudible to him or very soft. They are now made relatively loud. Those that were previously inaudible are strange and perhaps even frightening; those that were soft are now quite loud, and they sound different. If amplification is to be accepted by the child or adult, he must be taught to make use of the sound patterns he is receiving. The young deaf child may first need to be taught that many objects have auditory characteristics as well as visual and tactual ones. Most severely deaf children who have not previously worn an aid will have learned to depend upon vision and touch as their primary means of receiving information. Before these children can be taught to listen and discriminate between auditory stimuli, they must be provided with a reason for doing so. As with the normal child, this reason must be the awareness that auditory discrimination provides more specific information about the environment and that sound permits him to relate to it more successfully. Similarly, the hard-of-hearing adult will need immediate training with the aid to help him to recognize the relationship between the amplified sounds, including those of speech, and his previous auditory experiences. He will need to restructure his perception of auditory experiences.

Second, *to develop, as far as possible, a mobilization toward auditory stimuli.* We have seen how from birth onward the child with normal hearing begins to incorporate auditory sensations into his internal schema. Although he is receiving multisensory stimulation, it is the auditory and visual pathways upon which he depends most heavily for information. In the earliest years of life he develops habits of listening and looking.

The child with defective hearing, on the other hand, deprived of useful auditory information, comes to depend heavily upon the visual pathway. Even a child with usable residual hearing may find that the sound he hears cannot be relied upon as an adequate source of information; he may therefore turn to vision and touch as the major channels of information. Thus, the hearing-impaired child develops a communication system in which hearing plays, at best, a weak supporting role. If we are to be successful in training the child to incorporate auditory information, made available through amplification, into the common pool of sensory information, we must develop in him an auditory mobilization. Listening must become as much a part of his behavior as watching.

Third, *to teach the person to discriminate sounds under conditions of decreasing redundancy.* When we discussed the development of auditory discrimination, we pointed out that the child first learns the auditory characteristics of sound-generating objects at the same time as he experiences the object through his other senses. Similarly, in speech discrimination the child learns first to comprehend the meaning of words spoken in the presence of the objects or events to which they refer. After repeated exposure the child learns to recognize the word without the presence of the object and then, later, in the presence of competing stimuli. The difficulty of the conditions under which he will be required to achieve this will vary considerably. The auditory training program should recognize this and should aim to train the person to be capable of comprehending speech under a variety of conditions of variable difficulty.

Reference to improvement in speech and language skills, educational attainment, and social and emotional adjustment have been omitted, since these cannot justly be considered the immediate aims of auditory training; they constitute what we hope will prove to be desirable behavioral changes resulting from improved communication.

Preparing for the Training Session

We have finally reached the point in our discussion at which we may turn our attention to the practicalities of the training situation. Many of you will have experienced the sickening feeling that arises when you are not sure how you will occupy an impending 40-minute therapy session. "What on earth shall I do today?" The situation deteriorates after the session has been in progress for a while. You sneak a look at your watch for the nineteenth time only to find that there still remain ten more minutes. "Well Johnny," you say with a smile, "you've done so well today that I'm going to let you go early!"

Such situations reflect inadequate preparation. Good therapy of any sort is dependent upon a feeling of self-confidence by the instructor. This arises from the following:

1. Knowing what you wish to achieve.
2. Having a plan of action designed to produce the desired results.
3. Having the appropriate tools and materials available.

The Physical Environment

The first practical consideration that the therapist faces is where auditory training may be given. Reading some of the written material on the topic of aural rehabilitation may lead you to conclude that auditory training cannot be given unless one has available a sound-isolated or, at least, a sound-treated room. Naturally, a therapist would like to be able to work under the optimum conditions; however, this is not always possible, nor is it essential.

The three most important factors to be considered in the evaluation of potential therapy space are as follows:

1. The amount of acoustic noise within the room when it is empty.
2. The reverberance of the room.
3. The number of potentially distracting stimuli.

Room Noise

The noise level in the room is important since in the beginning we aim to provide the person with the most favorable listening conditions. Acoustic noise will serve both to distract attention from the stimulus sound and also to mask it. A list of acceptable noise levels for various types of rooms under average conditions was compiled by V. C. Knudson and C. M. Harris from empirical values based on their own experience [13]. The figure that they recommend as an acceptable ambient* noise level for an unoccupied class-room is 35 to 40 decibels SPL. In a study which I made of noise conditions in empty school classrooms in normal public schools [21], the average ambient noise levels were found to be approximately 15 decibels greater than the maximum level recommended by Knudson and Harris. On the other hand, in six sound-treated classes for the hard-of-hearing, housed in normal schools, the noise levels fell within the recommended limits (Table 7.1).

TABLE 7.1. Mean Values of Ambient Noise in Occupied Classrooms in Four Types of School Environments (After Sanders [21])

Type of School	Mean Value of Room Noise in Db Re: Sensation Level	Standard Deviation
Kindergarten	69	8.5
Primary school	59	6.2
High school	62	8.1
Special classes for the hearing-impaired child	52	4.7

Ambient noise can be divided into that which enters the room from outside and that which is generated within the room. Most of the noise in the above-mentioned study was found to occur as a result of overspill from adjacent occupied classrooms. This type of noise is critical, since the possible reduc-tion of noise within a room will be limited by the level of the noise when it is unoccupied. The amount of overspill was found to be greatest when the adjacent rooms were occupied by kindergarten or first-grade children, and least when occupied by the upper grade levels. This reflects the fact that noise levels in kindergarten and first-grade classes were found to be of the order of 10 decibels higher than those for the upper grades. It is notable that even among the schools situated in busy city environments, in only two instances was street noise shown to be a major source of disturbance. In both cases, these schools were located at a major road junction. J. E. John, in *Educational Guidance for the Deaf Child,* reports that in a classroom in such a school a noise level of 60 decibels, obtained with the window opened 20 inches, was reduced to 46 decibels when the window opening was only one-fourth inch [11, p. 172]. Therefore, when selecting a room for auditory training, if possible, some consideration should be given to the factor of noise originating from adjacent rooms and from outside the building.

Internally generated noise in a room used for individual or group audi-tory training should not present a major problem, since few children or adults are involved. Attention should nevertheless be given to the reduction of the noise that may occur from the sound of footsteps on a hard-surface floor,

*The term "ambient" simply means surrounding or environmental.

from the grating of desks or chairs when they are moved, and to the noise made by the activities participated in by the students.

It is surprising to realize how much noise everyday activities create. In the Department of Audiology and Education of the Deaf at the University of Manchester, England, investigations were made of noise levels produced by normal classroom activities [11, p. 174]. It was shown, for example, that the simple act of writing on the blackboard by an experienced teacher generated approximately 45 decibels of sound measured at a distance of 9 feet from the board. The intensity of the teacher's speech at the same position was only 10 decibels higher. Such a poor signal-to-noise ratio would have a serious effect upon the discrimination ability of a hearing-impaired child. A great deal of noise energy extends into the speech-frequency range; thus, when we amplify speech, we amplify the noise. Furthermore, the energy in noise is concentrated in the lower frequencies where the child is likely to have more residual hearing; the result tends to be a masking of speech. Even if speech remains intelligible, the redundancy factor is considerably reduced, making listening a more demanding task. Communication becomes more difficult and more tiring.

Reverberation

Reverberation refers to the "persistance of sound in an enclosed space as a result of multiple reflections after the sound has stopped." It results from the reflection of sound waves from nonabsorbent surfaces. As J. E. John explains:

> The reverberation time of a classroom is usually more than a second, and since a syllable takes about a quarter of a second to say, reverberation by a masking process renders speech less intelligible. In a three-syllable word, for example, the last syllable may only be heard against a background of strong reflections of a second syllable and weaker reflection of the first. The intelligibility of speech depends mainly on consonants which are made up of high frequency sounds and are much less powerful vowels. Both of these characteristics of vowels and consonants contribute to the masking, for absorption takes place chiefly at the higher frequencies, and the weaker consonants are swamped by the comparatively powerful vowel reflection. This effect is clearly shown in results of tests of the intelligibility of speech which have been carried in conditions of reverberation. In such experiments listeners make far more errors in consonants than in vowels [11, p. 169].

Figure 7.1 indicates the effect that John found reverberation to have upon the intelligibility of speech test material for listeners with normal hearing as a variable of the distance between the speaker and the microphone. The recorded speech sample was presented to the listeners at selective loudness levels through a group hearing aid.

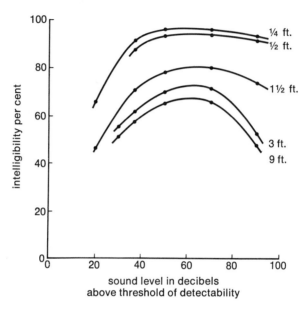

Fig. 7.1.   Graph of intelligibility per cent and sound level in decibels above the threshold of detectability. (After John [11].)

These findings illustrate for us the importance of keeping the distance between the speaker and the microphone as short as possible—at least during the early stages of auditory training. We may also conclude from this that we should use caution in predicting from sources obtained under highly favorable listening conditions how well a person will be able to discriminate speech when he uses his hearing aid under everyday listening conditions.

The same chapter contains a report on a study of the intelligibility of a single speech sample recorded in two rooms identical in size and shape. The first room represented an average school classroom, with plaster ceilings and walls and lineoleum on the floorboards. The second room had been treated with acoustic tiling, reducing the reverberation time. In the experiment, the distance between the speaker and the microphone was kept at a constant 9 feet. When the two recordings were played to a group of listeners with normal hearing, it was found that the speech recorded in the untreated room was practically unintelligible. It is pointed out in the report that the subjects with normal hearing did not experience difficulty in understanding the speech sample when they listened to it in the untreated room, although the same speech was almost unintelligible when picked up by a single microphone and recorded. This is not difficult to understand in view of what we have said in Chap. 6 regarding the comparative effects of monophonic and stereophonic listening. It is not difficult to imagine how much more serious a limitation reverberation places upon a hard-of-hearing person wearing a monaural hearing aid. Yet in a survey of 50 relatively newly erected classrooms for the teaching of deaf children, H. Thomas found that the reverberation time varied from 1.3 to 3.4 seconds, far above the 0.5 seconds recommended for rooms in which hearing aids are to be used [24, p. 64/3].

Realistic auditory training programs must therefore include under our fifth aim, "To teach the person to discriminate sounds under conditions of decreasing redundancy," experience in listening to speech presented under conditions that vary both in the ambient noise level and in the reverberation time of the room.

The extent to which a therapist or teacher is able to be selective in the type of physical facilities available to her is generally very limited. It is an unfortunate fact that many hearing therapists in the public schools find that in some situations the available space is beyond modification. Therapists are known, on occasions, to have to work in hallways, store rooms, or janitor's offices. You may, however, be more fortunate and find yourself with a separate room, such as a music room, library, or school nurse's office. Similarly, teachers in schools for the deaf may find that a separate room has been set aside for auditory training and, in many cases, will already have been partially or completely sound treated.

Presuming that you need and are able to make certain modifications in a room, you will wish to know what might be reasonably practical to attempt. If you are in a school for the deaf or in a school system that has a sufficient number of hard-of-hearing children grouped together to justify a request for a room for the purpose of giving special treatment, quite effective results can be obtained at relatively low expense by the use of sound-absorbent tiling. Naturally, professional advice should be sought concerning the type and amount necessary to achieve a minimal level of desired absorption. Specifications concerning the coefficients of absorption in the various types of manufactured materials, and guidance in their use, are available from several sources. In general, it has been found that, if anything short of complete sound treatment is to be used, the absorption material should be distributed in patches rather than concentrated upon one wall. Particular attention should be paid to the treatment of surfaces directly opposite such highly reflective materials as plate-glass windows or wall-mounted blackboards.

Where it is not possible to undertake such extensive treatment, a certain amount of absorption can be obtained by hanging heavy drapes, particularly if they are hung in such a way as to stand away from the wall. In a large room used for other purposes, an enterprising teacher might easily design and make, or have made, an auditory training booth consisting of two or three portable wooden screens covered with acoustic tiling. Alternatively, one might drape with two or three blankets the large, movable notice boards found in many schools. The effectiveness of treating in this way a very limited part of a large area is recognized by the telephone company in the construction of the small wall-mounted booth designed to sound treat a small area around the telephone and the head and shoulders of the speaker (Fig. 7.2).

Further reduction in reverberation can be achieved by the covering of the floor with carpet, cork, or rubberized squares. This will, in addition, cut down much of the internally generated sound of footsteps and scraping chairs. If adequate floor covering is not possible, an attempt should be made to use furniture that has rubber caps on the chair and table legs. In quite a lot of kindergarten classes in normal schools, children are required to wear sneakers to cut down noise levels. This example might be followed in special schools and classes for the hard-of-hearing. Remember that we are concerned with the role that noise plays in the amplified signal-to-noise ratio for people for whom the redundancy in speech is already at a minimal level. Unless we constantly bear this in mind, such factors as we have just discussed may seem inconsequential to those of us who have normal hearing.

The problem of visual distraction to the hard-of-hearing person in training sessions also requires attention. It is a tenet of teaching that the learning situation should contain as few distracting stimuli as possible to facilitate

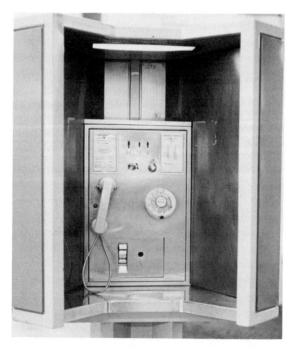

Fig. 7.2. Sound treatment of a small area is evident in this telephone booth.

concentration of attention on the subject matter. The hard-of-hearing person's increased dependency on vision for information may lead to increased sensitivity to visual distraction. Ultimately we must train him to tolerate the visual noise, but in the early stages we need to eliminate this as far as possible. If the room in which the auditory training is to take place overlooks a playground or hallway in which there is frequent movement of people, one should either seat the subject in such a position as to eliminate these activities from his visual field or use shades on the windows and doors. The use of a fairly small room for individual or small-group training, or the isolation of a training area with screens in a larger room, permits one to more easily control the visual distraction provided by books on bookshelves, pictures on walls, or activities seen through windows. At more advanced stages in the program these restrictive measures gradually can be eliminated as a means of building tolerance for the levels of auditory and visual distraction that will be encountered in everyday situations.

The physical equipment needed for providing a wide range of auditory and visual communication training activities in situations other than the ideal sound-proofed acoustic suite includes a separate work table and chair for the therapist and for the student. The use of two tables and chairs facilitates activities in which the student is asked to match sound-making objects by the acoustic stimulus. When written responses are used, this eliminates the need for either person to attempt to hold materials on his lap. For adults, chairs with a writing ledge may replace one of the two tables. When working with small children, the therapist should be able to sit at the same level as the child, making it easier for the child to observe the visual cues that he will be encouraged to integrate with auditory cues. For the same reason, the therapist should be seated so that the light falls on his face.

Many of the lessons will involve the use of the written form as reenforcement for the spoken message. The availability of a blackboard provides for flexibility in lessons. The therapist is able to write up examples or test items as the need occurs. It also permits the lesson to be developed progressively instead of being given to the student complete in typewritten or dittoed form. The blackboard should be positioned so that the therapist can stand to one side of it and still be facing the light source.

An excellent material holder for use with children is available from Scott, Foresman and Company (Fig. 7.3). This small portable stand has recessed metal slots, each of which can be pushed out to hold visual aids. Because each row of slots is recessed, the number of rows and therefore, the size of the spaces between the rows can be varied.

Finally, if possible, the therapist should arrange to have a space in which materials may be placed so as to be readily accessible during the lesson, without providing a source of visual distraction. While this is not essential when working with adults, it is an important consideration where

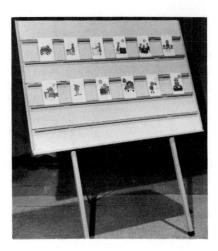

Fig. 7.3. A convenient materials stand, available from Scott, Foresman and Company. The sequential picture cards shown on the stand are available from Developmental Learning Materials.

children are concerned. Such storage space can easily be provided by a portable open-shelf bookstand, the back of which may be enclosed by a large sheet of cardboard or covered with a piece of material. The various toys and materials can then be stored on the shelves where they can be easily reached by the therapist, though they are not visible to the child.

Unfortunately a therapist or teacher, not completely aware of the implications of carrying out a program of aural rehabilitation under inadequate physical conditions, may fail to present a strong enough case to the administrators regarding the need for improvement of those conditions. The strength of the therapist's argument rests, not in the fact that she is dealing with a group of children who need exceptionally good listening conditions in order to be adequately trained, but in the fact that she is simply requesting a closer approximation to the minimal standards recommended for the education of children with normal hearing. She should point out that the improvement she is requesting will not benefit only the hard-of-hearing child, but all children taught in the room. For the speech and hearing therapist the point should be made that auditory training in a modified form comprises an important part in the rehabilitation of speech-impaired children, and that this large group of children alone constitutes sufficient justification for the request she is making.

The problems that the speech and hearing therapist in a school system encounters in obtaining the necessary funds to make some of the structural modifications that have been suggested in this section are not underestimated. Nevertheless, let us remember that, generally speaking, support of all kinds goes to the person who is able to make the strongest case. It is my personal belief that in a great many situations a tenacious teacher or therapist, well

214

equipped with appropriate information, will meet with more success than might be anticipated.

Assessing Auditory Perception

Before beginning the auditory training program, the therapist will need to carefully evaluate the information she already has available. We should keep in mind, as we attempt to interpret the various test results, that our purpose is to obtain as full an understanding as possible of the nature of the total communication difficulty. Many of the factors that we shall consider may not in themselves be particularly useful; the examination of them, however, may throw more light upon the problem and cause us to see certain other information within a more meaningful framework.

Pure-tone Audiometric Results

The first source of data to which the therapist will turn will be the pure-tone audiogram. The value of a pure-tone audiogram rests in the information it provides about the intensity and frequency distortion that the hearing impairment imposes upon the incoming speech signal. From the audiogram we can assess the extent of the residual hearing, and we can estimate the dynamic range by comparing the pure-tone thresholds with the threshold of discomfort. We can gain some information of the nature of the frequency distortion that will be imposed upon the incoming signal by noting the over-all configuration of the audiogram and the frequencies for which hearing is most severely affected. We should not predict speech discrimination from the pure-tone results, as this involves too many variables.

The free-field audiograms, if available, will indicate the best results obtainable with binaural hearing. Comparison of unaided and aided free-field audiograms will show to what extent loss of sensitivity can be compensated for by amplification.

Speech Audiometric Results

Having examined the unaided and aided audiograms, we will next turn our attention to the speech audiometric data. Once again we will be interested in making a comparison between the unaided and aided speech reception thresholds and speech-discrimination scores. When we look at these results, we must remember that all speech audiometric findings represent a statement of the person's auditory discrimination for the type of speech sample used for the particular conditions under which the test was conducted. Since this information is usually obtained before any auditory training has been given, it represents a statement of present function, not a prognosis for future communicative ability.

Speech Reception

The unaided and aided speech reception threshold levels provide an indication of the minimal intensity level at which speech must be presented before the person is able to derive enough information from the acoustic signal to be able to predict the content of the message. By comparing the two free-field measures, we will be able to judge the contribution that amplification makes in combatting the loss of redundancy caused by the decrease in sensitivity of the ear. Table 7.2 provides us with free-field pure-tone and speech

TABLE 7.2. Pure-Tone and Speech Audiometric Data for Three Subjects Discussed in the Text

| | Pure-Tone Thresholds in Hertz | | | | | | Speech Audiometry | |
	250	500	1000	2000	4000	8000	SRT	Discrimination
Subject A								
Unaided	0	15	25	40	55	80	25 dB	92%
Aided	0	0	0	5	45	80	5 dB	90%
Subject B								
Unaided	25	35	40	35	35	25	35 dB	96%
Aided	15	10	10	5	20	20	5 dB	92%
Subject C								
Unaided	55	70	85	110+	110+	110+	90 dB	58%
Aided	40	30	45	95	110+	110+	50 dB	50%
Using auditory trainer							30 dB	46%

test results for the three subjects. You will observe in this table that the speech reception threshold for subject A without amplification was found to be 25 decibels. Since we normally listen to speech in a conversational situation at 60 to 65 decibels of intensity, a speech reception threshold of 25 decibels means that almost half the intensity redundancy has been removed. This considerably increases the effort that must be made by the listener to obtain a sum total of information adequate for comprehension. Although, in many situations, with an SRT of 25 decibels this person will probably be able to follow a conversation on the basis of supporting information obtained from the other sources we have discussed, he may be expected to experience difficulty when the listening conditions deteriorate. Furthermore, the amount of strain that is placed upon him may be anticipated to be quite great. Observe, however, the effect that amplification has in compensating for this loss of intensity. The speech reception threshold, when the subject was wearing a moderately powered behind-the-ear hearing aid, was found to be 5 decibels. This improvement of 20 decibels represents a 33 per cent gain in loudness redundancy. Thus, when this subject uses a hearing aid we can be sure that sound, at least within the important speech-frequency range of 500 to 2000 cycles, is reaching him at approximately the same loudness level as that at which we like to listen. We must be careful not to assume, however, that because speech is loud enough it is necessarily clear enough. Speech reception thresholds should not be taken as anything more than an indication of the intensity level at which, on the basis of normative data, we would predict a person to be able to follow the gist of a conversation.

For our second subject the speech reception threshold is 35 decibels without amplification. This constitutes a loss of 50 per cent of the loudness of normal conversational speech. It has reduced the intensity redundancy to the point at which, should the strength of the speech signal be further reduced by 10 or 15 decibels, this person will hear speech at a loudness level of only 15 to 20 decibels, insufficient intensity to permit normal comprehension. This degree of hearing impairment will obviously result in marked difficulty in following a conversation in all except the most favorable conditions. We would anticipate this person to be very dependent for comprehension upon his ability to extract sufficient information from sources other than the auditory signal. When he is in a poor acoustic environment, is in a group situation, is unable to see the speaker clearly, is placed at a distance from the speaker, or is listening to particularly difficult material, he will probably be unable to obtain enough information to be able to understand the message. Once again, however, the use of a moderately powered hearing aid raises his speech reception threshold to within normal limits. Thus, with this person, as with subject A, we can be confident that while the aid is worn the speech is being received at a desirable loudness level.

Subject C presents a considerably greater problem. It was necessary to raise the intensity level of the speech signal to 50 decibels before this person was able to score 50 per cent on the spondee word list. From the audiogram and the speech reception threshold we learned that, although some of the strong lower tones of the speech signal were faintly audible without amplification, the residual hearing was insufficient to permit meaning to be attributed to the unamplified acoustic signal. The provision of a high-powered body hearing aid with an average gain of 70 decibels still failed to bring the speech reception threshold to within normal limits. The score of 50 per cent on the spondee words was not achieved at intensity levels less than 45 decibels. The obtaining of the speech reception threshold in this instance was further complicated by the fact that a great number of words had to be run before it was possible to ascertain a 50 per cent level, since the person experienced quite marked difficulty in discriminating words that he described as loud enough. This is reflected in the speech-discrimination scores, which will be discussed next.

It has been repeatedly stressed that neither the audiogram nor the SRT alone provides enough information for the assessment of a child or adult's rehabilitation needs. It is nevertheless true that these needs become greater and require more extensive rehabilitative work as the hearing level for speech decreases. Experience with large groups of children has made it possible for several authors [19, 23] to provide us with information that helps to formulate a general idea of the relationship that exists between the degree of hearing impairment and the rehabilitative procedures that will be required. These recommendations vary from providing an appropriate seating position in a normal school classroom for a child with a mild loss to full-time special education in the school for the deaf or the severely hearing-impaired child. For the adult they range from recommending a concentrated course in visual communication training to an extensive program of aural rehabilitation involving training in the use of a hearing aid, visual and auditory communication training, vocational counseling, and social and psychological guidance. While we cannot automatically assume that these statements are valid for an individual case, they provide us with a better understanding of the difficulties that may be predicted for certain degrees of hearing impairment.

Speech Discrimination

The results of the speech-discrimination scores obtained on the phonetically balanced word lists indicate the extent to which the person is able to extract sufficient information from the acoustic signal to be able to identify the word it represents. When examining the speech-discrimination score it is necessary to remember that *this is not an indication of the percentage of speech that the person is receiving, but a statement of the amount he is capable of identifying when the sound is amplified to a level of loudness that, for subjects with normal hearing, is adequate to permit a discrimination score of between 90 and 100 per cent.* In other words, in measuring discrimination ability for monosyllabic words, we wish as far as possible to compensate for the effect that loss of loudness will have upon discrimination. If you refer back to Fig. 5.3 you will observe the loss in discrimination that occurs as a simple function of decrease of loudness of the speech signal even when the hearing loss is of a flat conductive nature. For this reason the unaided speech-discrimination scores represent discrimination ability at 40 decibels above the speech reception threshold. They represent the usefulness that the person is able to make of his residual hearing at the time of testing.

Examine now the percentage discrimination scores obtained by our three subjects. From Table 7.2 you will see that subjects A and B both obtained scores that fall within the normal limit of 90 to 100 per cent. The provision of amplification through a hearing aid appears in both cases to result in a slight decrease in the discrimination score. However, since such small variations within the range of 90 to 100 per cent are observed when conducting tests with subjects with normal hearing; they cannot be assumed to be a function of the increased noise that we have already stated is inevitably added to the auditory system by a hearing aid.

In subject C, however, we observe a drop in the discrimination score in spite of the fact that when wearing a hearing aid the speech reception threshold is raised by 45 decibels. Since this subject showed a similar response for several aids, the decrease in discrimination cannot be attributed simply to the effects of a poor amplifying system. Further examination of this person's test results indicates that, unlike the other two subjects, she shows a reduced tolerance for loudness and poor discrimination in noise. This information in a confirmed case of severe high-frequency sensori-neural deafness is indicative of recruitment. This was confirmed by subsequent testing.

When we compare these three sets of scores, we can predict that subject A and subject B given adequate training in the use of amplification, have the potential, by the process of amplifying the incoming speech signal, for being able to make up for the loss of information resulting from the hearing impairment.

Subject C, even with a concentrated program of training in auditory discrimination, was never able to derive sufficient information from the amplified speech signal to be able to correctly and reliably predict the message signal. This person was dependent upon the additional information that she was able to derive from the visible aspects of the speech signal and from linguistic and contextual cues. It should not be concluded that, because the provision of amplification resulted in a reduction in the discrimination score, the hearing aid was therefore unsuitable for this person. The aural rehabilitation program included training to increase tolerance for loudness, part of which is a psychological adaptive process on the part of the hearing-aid user. As a result, the person was able to wear the aid and, therefore, was able to make use of 52 per cent of the information embodied within the acoustic signal heard at an intensity level of 45 decibels. Without the hearing aid the person was able only to determine that there was an auditory signal. She was quite unable to isolate any of the information it carried.

Social Adequacy Index

The information that we obtained for subject C indicates that, when considering the benefit provided by amplification, one must take into consideration both the intensity level necessary for the person to be able to follow the gist of a conversation received through hearing only and the maximum discrimination that is obtained when the signal is presented with adequate loudness. What we need, therefore, is some means of assessing the auditory communication function that results from the interaction of loudness and intelligibility. It was in an attempt to provide a means for doing this that Hallowell Davis and a team of co-workers at the Central Institute for the Deaf derived an index of social adequacy [6] (Table 7.3). The chart of social adequacy index permits one to obtain a score that represents the interaction of the speech reception threshold level and the percentage of discrimination loss for phonetically balanced words. This integrative score provides us with a descriptive quantity that can be compared to values designated for normal function. These normal values have been termed the threshold of social adequacy, or the point below which the person is no longer able to manage in a social communication situation without assistance. As Hayes A. Newby points out [18, pp. 116–18], the original article by Davis [6] describing the manner in which the social adequacy index was derived, explains that three discrimination scores were obtained at intensity levels selected to represent average levels of faint, average, and loud conversational speech. A discrimination loss was then computed as an average of these three scores. Newby also emphasizes that since the current methods of assessing discrimination for phonetically balanced words involve the use of the auditory test W–22, which constitutes a modified form of the original test material, caution should be taken when computing the social adequacy index on the basis of a single PB-test percentage loss as measured on the auditory test W–22.

The horizontal axis of the chart represents the speech reception threshold level for the better ear, or the free-field SRT. Note that the vertical axis represents, not the percentage discrimination score, but the percentage of phonetically balanced words missed. To obtain this figure, we simply subtract the subject's percentage discrimination score from 100 and read the resultant figure on the vertical axis.

Let us examine the threshold of adequacy scores that we would obtain for the three subjects we have been discussing.

Without amplification subject A has a speech reception threshold of 25 decibels and a discrimination score of 92 per cent, an 8 per cent loss in discrimination. We first locate the speech reception threshold figure along the horizontal axis. Since these are plotted in 2-decibel steps rather than 5-decibel steps, for 25 dB we will read 26. We next locate the figure on the discrimination loss that is closest to the 8 per cent loss exhibited by our subject; in this case this will be the 10 per cent line. If you now run your finger along the 10 per cent line on the horizontal axis until it intersects with the vertical column under the figure 26, you will observe that the social adequacy index score for this subject is 65, a figure that falls approximately midway between the limits of normal hearing function and the threshold of social adequacy. You will recall that the discrimination loss on the chart originally represented an average of three conditions of speech intensity; it is not difficult to understand that, while subject A shows a social adequacy index that falls well above the threshold of social adequacy, this index figure might

TABLE 7.3. Social Adequacy Index: Hearing Loss for Speech in Decibels (After Davis [6])

Column header (Threshold, dB): LIMIT OF NORMAL (94) applies to the lowest columns; THRESHOLD OF SOCIAL ADEQUACY (33) applies to the middle columns; LIMIT OF PURE CONDUCTIVE LOSS applies to the highest columns.

Left axis: **Discrimination Loss (percent PB words missed at high intensity)**

Discr. Loss	0	2	4	6	8	10	12	14	16	18	20	22	24	26	28	30	32	34	36	38	40	42	44	46	48	50	52	54	56	58	60	62	64	66	68	70	72	74
0	99	98	97	96	96	94	93	92	90	88	85	82	79	75	69	64	61	57	52	48	44	41	37	33	28	24	20	17	15	12	10	7	4	2	1	0	0	0
5	94	93	92	91	90	89	89	88	87	85	82	79	76	72	67	63	59	55	51	47	43	40	37	32	28	24	20	17	15	12	9	7	4	2	1	0	0	0
10	89	89	88	87	86	85	84	83	81	78	76	73	70	65	61	57	53	49	46	42	40	37	31	27	23	19	16	14	11	9	7	4	2	1	0	0	0	0
15	84	84	83	82	81	80	79	77	75	72	70	67	63	59	55	51	47	44	41	39	36	30	27	23	19	16	14	11	9	7	4	2	1	0	0	0	0	0
20	79	79	78	78	77	76	75	73	71	69	67	65	63	61	58	55	52	48	44	40	38	36	33	29	26	22	19	16	13	11	9	7	4	2	1	0	0	0
25	75	75	74	74	73	72	71	70	69	67	66	65	63	62	60	58	55	52	48	44	41	38	36	33	28	25	21	18	16	13	10	8	6	4	2	1	0	0
30	70	70	69	68	68	67	66	65	63	62	61	60	58	56	54	52	49	45	42	39	36	34	31	27	24	21	18	15	12	10	8	6	4	2	1	0	0	0
35	65	65	64	64	63	62	61	60	58	56	54	53	51	48	46	43	40	37	34	32	29	26	23	20	18	15	12	10	8	6	4	2	1	0	0	0	0	0
40	60	60	59	59	58	57	56	55	54	53	52	51	50	49	47	45	43	41	39	37	34	32	30	28	25	22	19	17	14	12	10	8	6	4	2	1	0	0
45	55	55	55	54	54	53	53	52	51	50	49	48	47	46	45	44	43	41	40	37	34	32	29	27	24	22	20	17	15	13	11	9	6	4	2	1	0	0
50	50	50	50	49	49	48	47	46	45	44	43	42	41	40	39	38	36	35	34	32	30	28	26	24	22	20	17	15	12	10	9	8	6	4	2	1	0	0
55	45	45	45	44	44	43	43	42	41	40	39	38	37	36	35	34	33	32	31	30	29	27	25	24	22	21	19	17	14	12	9	8	7	5	4	2	1	0
60	40	40	40	40	39	38	37	36	35	34	33	32	31	30	29	27	25	23	22	21	20	18	17	15	13	11	10	9	8	7	6	5	4	2	1	0	0	0
65	35	35	35	34	34	33	32	31	30	29	28	27	26	25	23	22	21	20	18	17	15	14	13	11	10	9	8	7	6	5	4	3	2	1	0	0	0	0
70	30	30	30	30	29	29	29	28	28	27	26	25	24	23	22	21	20	19	18	16	15	14	12	11	10	9	8	7	6	5	4	3	2	1	0	0	0	0
75	25	25	25	25	24	24	24	23	23	22	21	20	19	19	18	17	16	15	14	13	12	11	10	9	8	7	6	5	4	4	3	2	1	0	0	0	0	0
80	20	20	20	20	19	19	19	18	17	17	16	15	14	13	12	11	11	10	9	8	7	6	5	4	3	2	1	0	0	0	0	0	0	0	0	0	0	0
85	15	15	15	15	14	14	14	13	13	12	12	11	10	9	9	8	7	6	6	5	4	3	2	1	0	0	0	0	0	0	0	0	0	0	0	0	0	0
90	10	10	10	10	10	10	10	10	9	9	9	8	8	7	7	7	6	6	5	4	3	2	1	0	0	0	0	0	0	0	0	0	0	0	0	0	0	0
95	*(see note below)*																																					
100	0	0	0	0	0	0	0	0	0	0	0	0	0	0	0	0	0	0	0	0	0	0	0	0	0	0	0	0	0	0	0	0	0	0	0	0	0	0

When the discrimination loss is greater than about 90 per cent ordinary speech is not understood at any intensity, and it becomes difficult or impossible to measure the hearing loss for speech.

221

be expected to drop under adverse listening conditions. If, for example, the speaker's voice drops by 10 decibels, even if the percentage-discrimination loss remains constant, this would be equivalent to an increase in the SRT from 26 to 36 decibels, lowering the social adequacy index (SAI) from 65 to 46 and bringing the subject considerably closer to the threshold of social adequacy.

Subject B has an unaided SRT of 35 decibels, with only a 4 per cent loss in discrimination. The horizontal and the vertical scales for these two figures intersect at a point that gives us a SAI reading of 47. Note how much closer this person is to the point at which we predict he would be unable to manage adequately in a communication situation. In other words, the cushion of redundancy is considerably less for this subject than for subject A.

For both subjects A and B, the provision of amplification raises the SAI score to within normal limits.

Subject C was found to have an unaided SRT of 90 decibels, with a discrimination loss of 58 per cent. You will observe that the SRT values listed on the horizontal axis of the chart do not exceed 74 and that for all SRT values of greater than 66 decibels the SAI is zero. Since scores are available for discrimination losses up to 90 per cent at lower speech reception threshold levels, we can see that for this subject the first and primary problem is one involving inadequate intensity. Note the change that occurs when we provide amplification that raises the SRT to 35 decibels, even though the discrimination loss increases by 16 per cent to a 50 per cent loss. Using a SRT reading of 36, we find that at the point at which it intersects the 50 per cent loss we obtain an SAI score of 20, which is only one column removed from the social adequacy index. From this we can conclude that amplification has brought the speech signal within the hearing limits of our patient, though even in average listening conditions we cannot expect her to be able to function adequately in a communication situation on the basis of her hearing alone.

With this particular subject, an evaluation was also made of the speech reception threshold and discrimination score that could be obtained using an auditory training unit in an attempt to provide more powerful amplification and greater amplification in the 2000 to 4000 range. The results indicated only a slight improvement in the SRT, but some improvement in the discrimination score. When we calculate the SAI score for the new figures of SRT equals 30 decibels, discrimination loss equals 34 per cent, we observe that the score now falls above the threshold of social adequacy, indicating that this particular subject, who happened to be in college, would experience a significant increase in the amount of information she could obtain from the auditory signal if she were to use a binaural auditory training unit rather than a personal hearing aid in situations in which it was essential that she should derive as much information from hearing as possible. After a period of auditory training, the parents of this girl purchased a binaural training unit, which she found to be of considerable help in the classroom situation where her ability to use visual cues to supplement the auditory information was severely reduced by her need to take notes as the lecturer was speaking.

These three illustrations may be helpful in indicating the way in which we may approach the purely auditory data provided by the audiologist who performed the hearing-aid evaluation. In this chapter we are going to confine ourselves to the completely unrealistic situation whereby we are concerned only with hearing function. In Chap. 9, we will compare test results for groups of students for whom we have information not only on auditory function, but also on visual communication ability and the ability to combine visual and auditory cues.

We have stated that our first and second aim will be to attempt to counsel the hearing-impaired adult or the parents of a child concerning the nature of the hearing loss and the type of aural rehabilitation program that will be pursued. Because of the complexity of such a task, we shall at this point presume that such counseling has already been given and will continue to be given, and that the hearing-impaired subject is ready to begin the auditory training aspects of the rehabilitation program. Consideration will be given to the question of counseling and guidance later in the text. When we have evaluated the information made available to us, we will be ready to work with the student both for further testing and for training. Since we will be using amplification, we will now consider the controls of the amplifiers in more detail.

Using the Table-Model Auditory Trainer

You will recall from our discussion of this type of auditory training unit that we are able to modify the signal with respect to (1) the maximum output, (2) the gain, (3) the frequency-response characteristic. Our aim is to set these controls to provide the best possible listening conditions for the student.

The Maximum Output Control

The purpose of the maximum output control, you will remember, is to insure that the output signal at no time exceeds the maximum intensity level that the subject is able to tolerate. The limit of any auditory training unit is determined by the maximum tolerance level of the normal ear. Except where a child or adult shows evidence of recruitment, which results in a lowered maximum tolerance level for loudness in spite of the hearing loss, we should use the maximum output setting. This will insure that the aid is sensitive to a wide range of intensities.

For students who give definite evidence of recruitment or who initially reject high levels of amplification because of the unfamiliarity of this perceptual experience it may be necessary to begin the auditory training session at a lower level of maximum output. The same is true when working with very young deaf children for whom the degree of residual hearing has not yet been clearly established or when the nature of the auditory disorder is not definitely known. In these instances we must be cautious in our use of amplification for fear that we might prejudice the child against amplified sound. We must rely heavily upon our own clinical observations of the child's responses and adopt a pragmatic approach to the problem.

The Gain Control

The gain control permits us to determine, within the limits of the maximum acoustic output, the intensity of the signal reaching the ear. In assessing the amount of gain that an individual person requires, we are essentially asking how much amplification is necessary to compensate for the difference between normal threshold and the threshold of hearing of our student. The maximum amount of gain that can be added to the input signal to produce an increase in the output level will be limited by the maximum output selected. Thus, if we select the maximum possible output of 135 decibels and use an input signal of 60 decibels, the maximum gain that we can add to the input signal in order to utilize the upper limit of 135 decibels of output would be 75 decibels (60 dB input + 75 dB gain = 135 dB output).

The audiogram, however, often does not give us information about the level of tolerance that the person has for loud sounds. In order to take this into account, it is suggested that when the person is old enough the technique that you use in determining the setting should call for a subjective evaluation by the subject. The person is asked to listen to the therapist speaking and to say when her voice becomes unpleasantly loud. The gain control is turned on at the lowest setting and, while continuing to talk to the student, the therapist gradually increases the gain until the student indicates that the therapist's voice is too loud. The gain setting is then reduced in discrete steps, stopping at intermediate points to inquire whether the speech is still too loud. As the amplification of the input signal is gradually decreased by reducing the amount of gain, a point will be reached at which the subject may be expected to state that the speaker's voice is no longer too loud. At this point an inquiry is made, "Does it sound just right or does this make it sound a little better." The gain setting is then reduced one further step in order to permit the subject to evaluate which of the two settings he prefers. The value in this method of assessing the gain level rests in the fact that the patient is not asked to state when the sound is loud enough, a decision that may be difficult for him to make since he has no yardstick by which to ascertain what is loud enough. On the other hand, his physiological and psychological defense mechanisms will tell him when an input sound is too loud. Because the threshold of tolerance for sound may, in many cases, be increased after listening training, it is necessary to repeat the procedure for each session until a fairly consistent setting is arrived at. Once this has been reached, then it is only necessary to repeat the procedure periodically as part of an overall reassessment of the hearing function.

This type of approach can be used with children at a much younger age level than one might predict. Sympathetic handling of a three-year-old, and in some instances a two-year-old, makes it possible for them to give quite meaningful responses. Below this level, however, and with some more-difficult older children, you may be forced to work on the basis of the audiogram and careful observation of the child's responses. It is strongly advised that you begin at levels of amplification below what you might predict will be necessary and that the initial sound stimuli be very carefully selected to be those that might be most meaningful and most favorably received by the child. The intensity of the signal then can be gradually increased until either the maximum level is reached without protest from the hearing-aid user or some indication of discomfort is evident at a lower level.

The Tone Control

We have explained that the tone control serves to modify the frequency sensitivity of the amplifier. The various settings permit one to alter the pattern of modification in a way that provides for a relative increase in amplification of those frequencies for which a hard-of-hearing person has the greatest degree of impairment. In the less expensive models this selection is limited to two or three frequency responses, generally labeled either "Flat" and "High," or "Flat–Middle–High," referring to the range of frequencies for which the relative sensitivity is increased.

When an instrument provides a choice of several settings we must determine which will be most appropriate to a particular person. The first step is to ascertain from the specification sheet the frequency at which a reduction in gain begins. The attenuation will probably begin at around 1000 cycles and will extend down to the lower frequency limits of the amplifier. What we must determine is how rapidly we wish it to occur. Remember that the purpose of decreasing the sensitivity of the amplifier to the lower frequencies is to permit the overall gain to be raised, without over-amplifying the energy in the low-frequency range where a person may have relatively good hearing. This procedure results in a relative emphasis of high-frequency components of speech. We therefore make our assessment on the basis of the pure-tone audiogram for each ear. If a monophonic system is being used, the calculation should be made from a free-field, unaided audiogram. This tells us how the person's hearing functions when a single input sound is fed to both ears, a situation that is duplicated when we use an amplifier that feeds a signal from a single input microphone to binaural phones.

When the choice of alternative settings is limited to two or three positions, then we simply predict that, because an audiogram indicates a relatively flat loss effecting all frequency ranges by approximately the same amount, this person will derive the greatest benefit from selecting the tone-control position in which the sensitivity curve of the system remains unmodified. You will recall we discussed the criteria for developing a relatively flat sensitivity curve in an amplifier when we talked about amplifiers and hearing aids. A word of caution, however, should be added at this point. We have seen that the identifying second formant of some speech sounds is situated in the higher-frequency range, and that this second formant is often relatively weaker than the first. Furthermore, some sounds that have most of their energy concentrated in the high frequencies are also the least intense sounds. For this reason, although the audiometric configuration may be flat, these sounds will be more affected by the attenuation than a stronger sound situated lower in the frequency scale would be. As a result, one should attempt to assess whether relative high-tone emphasis may provide a better discrimination score than the flat setting.

The middle emphasis position is helpful when the audiogram shows an inverted bell configuration. The high-frequency emphasis is necessary where the subject shows much better hearing for the low and middle tones than for the high frequencies.

Some auditory trainers permit the selection of one of a number of rates of fall off. Each of these is represented by a figure indicating the number of decibels that will be progressively attenuated at each octave level below the frequency at which the fall off begins. For example, a setting of 8 decibels on the tone control of a unit with a fall off beginning at 1000 Hz indicates that we are attenuating from the gain-control reading 8 decibels at 500 Hz, 16 decibels at 250 Hz, and 24 decibels at 125 Hz. Similarly a 14-decibel rate of attenuation would attenuate 14 decibels at 500 Hz and an additional 14 decibels from the gain level at each octave frequency below this. This attenuation of the lower frequencies represents an attempt to balance the loss in the high frequencies. If this is achieved to a satisfactory degree, then we will have produced a condition in which the audiometric configuration, when listening through the auditory trainer, has essentially been flattened.

The desired rate of fall off can therefore be assessed from calculating the rate of fall off of the unaided pure-tone thresholds above 1000 Hz. By subtracting the unaided pure-tone threshold reading obtained at 1000 Hz from that obtained at 500 Hz (one-octave band), we will obtain a figure that represents the rate of fall off that we must attempt to equalize in the low frequencies. For example, with thresholds of 10 decibels at 500 Hz and

20 decibels at 1000 Hz we would obtain a fall-off rate of -10 decibels per octave. That is to say, with the gain control set at 45 decibels, the gain at 1000 Hz and for frequencies above would be unmodified and could be read directly from the specification data for the frequency sensitivity curve. For frequencies below 1000 Hz we would subtract 10 decibels at 500 Hz, 20 decibels at 250 Hz, and 30 decibels at 125 Hz.

Once we have the modified gain levels we can then compare them to the unaided pure-tone audiogram in order to see to what degree amplification equalizes the loss at each frequency. We will then be in a position to know whether we should use a different rate of fall off or whether we should aim with training to persuade the person to tolerate a higher level of amplification.

The Relationship of the Auditory Training Unit to a Personal Hearing Aid

We need to provide some clarification of the relative role of the auditory training unit and the personal hearing aid in aural rehabilitation. We may wonder whether it is realistic to use a high-quality auditory training system for training a person to make use of the acoustic aspects of speech, when in normal communication situations he will have to make his predictions on the basis of the reduced information that he is able to obtain through his personal hearing aid. It may be suggested that perhaps we should train him on the instrument with which he will have to function in most communication situations.

We have already recognized that speech perception and speech comprehension are not achieved purely on the basis of the analysis of the acoustic stimulus. This complex process also involves making prediction on the basis of linguistic cues and, possibly, on the association of the incoming auditory pattern with the motor pattern we would use in order to produce such a sound wave. It has also been stressed that communication between individuals involves a great deal of built-in redundancy. It is not necessary to receive the complete message signal in order to perceive what has been said and to be able to attribute meaning. It would seem, however, that when we are attempting to learn a new activity we require a great deal more information in learning to discriminate between sounds and words than we do to perform the same act of discrimination once we have learned these sound patterns. This is not difficult to understand when we remember that speech discrimination is dependent upon our ability to make predictions and that, in order to be able to do this effectively, we must be familiar with the rules that make these predictions possible. The amount of information necessary to verify a reasonable prediction is considerably less than that needed to learn to make such a prediction. We are justified in using a high-quality training unit for auditory training purposes because our aim is to provide the hard-of-hearing person with an acoustic signal that contains the greatest amount of information. During the process of learning to discriminate be-tween acoustic signals that may be completely or relatively unfamiliar, the hearing-impaired person will need as much information as possible to guide him in his predictions. His increasing familiarity with the acoustic patterns will be augmented by an unconscious, but nevertheless important, awareness of the linguistic rules that determine the ways in which we may sequence these patterns. In a good program of auditory training the student will also be encouraged to reproduce what he hears in spoken and, when possible, in written form. In this way the acoustic signal will be associated with its tactile-kinesthetic and visual-motor aspects. An efficient aural rehabilitation program that integrates sensory information through several channels through a program of listening, watching, saying, and writing will build up sufficient message-signal redundancy to permit the person to be able to tolerate the reduction in the information available through the auditory channel that may be expected when the performance of the high-fidelity auditory trainer is replaced by that of the wearable hearing aid.

This rationalization of the use of high-fidelity amplification in training situations can only be supported if we accept the concept of the information pool and the associated threshold of comprehension, which were discussed in Chap. 5. Some writers have cautioned therapists about the apparent waste of money represented by using wide-frequency, high-fidelity amplification with subjects for whom no thresholds have been determinable at frequencies above 1000 Hz. This is an acceptable criticism providing one recognizes that, unless modifications of an individual audiometer have been made, the pure-tone audiogram seldom represents the maximum limits of hearing, since it is not usually possible to test at sensation levels of greater than 100 deci-bels re: audiometric zero. Thus, before we rule out the value of high-intensity amplification of high frequencies, we must be quite sure that we have demon-strated, beyond reasonable doubt, that the hearing-impaired person is incapa-ble of detecting sound at these frequencies.

We are, however, justified in showing concern if our auditory training program is carried out exclusively with an auditory training unit without any comparative training in the use of the personal hearing aid. In addition to aiming to provide the subject with the best possible acoustic conditions for learning, we must teach him the relationship between the acoustic patterns he receives through the auditory trainer, and those he receives through his personal hearing aid. Thus, part of our training program will involve using speech materials with which the subject is familiar through his training on the auditory training unit to train him to perform the same task of discrimina-tion using his personal hearing aid. Similarly our early training lessons con-ducted under good listening conditions will be modified to provide experience in auditory discrimination under listening conditions of increased difficulty.

In summary, we may say that wherever possible we should provide our subject with the experience of listening to amplified speech through the best available system. We should design our training program to permit him to use his residual hearing to the maximum possible extent in the process of learning to represent internally the acoustic patterns of speech. Once this has been achieved, we must then teach him to associate a signal containing less information with the internal speech patterns that he has learned. In order to do this we must also conduct auditory training with the personal hearing aid. Once again, the concept of a pool of information is strongly stressed. The learning of auditory discrimination using a high-fidelity amplifying system involves the learning of the linguistic and contextual probabilities that are essential to the process of attributing meaning to speech. Furthermore, since the learning of the identifiable characteristics of speech sounds normally occurs simultaneously with the learning of the visual characteristics, teaching the person to correlate the visual and acoustic aspects of speech will enhance the total amount of information available to him.

TESTING AUDITORY DISCRIMINATION

The information that the therapist or teacher will have available concerning the subject's auditory-discrimination ability will probably be confined to the scores obtained by the audiologist who administered the phonetically balanced word-discrimination test. Unfortunately, the subject's performance on this test is reported simply as a percentage discrimination score. Each response is usually scored either correct or incorrect. Frequently no record is made to indicate how closely the subject approximates the test word. The omission of the final "s" sound is penalized in the same way as a word that evokes no response at all. In this case, the discrimination score represents little more than a quantative statement. We cannot tell from it which sounds the person is experiencing difficulty in hearing, nor can we predict with any degree of reliability how well he will comprehend connected speech. It is true that data are available that indicate the relationship between discrimination scores obtained on monosyllabic PB words and those obtained for sentences. However, these data were obtained on subjects with normal hearing and cannot, therefore, be generalized justifiably to people with impaired hearing. Furthermore, standard tests of auditory discrimination deliberately reduce the redundancy of the message signal to a minimum. It is purely a statement of the amount of information that the listener derives from the acoustic signal itself. In instances where a hearing-aid evaluation has not been made, no information will be available to indicate how well a person is able to make use of the amplified sound that the aid provides.

Our early sessions in auditory training should therefore seek to provide a more definitive statement of the listener's ability to extract information from the acoustic message signal. This information will provide us with a yard-stick against which we are able to measure subsequent improvement in performance. It should also indicate which sounds are presenting a problem to the student and thus make it possible for us to design our auditory training lessons to meet specific needs.

Assessing Speech Discrimination

The usefulness of hearing in communication can be roughly assessed by standing behind the subject and asking him questions about something with which he is well familiar. The degree of difficulty of the material can be progressively increased to see how well he functions with more complex information. Such an initial subjective evaluation can be very helpful in orientating the therapist to the degree of communication difficulty that the person is experiencing as a result of impaired hearing. Of course, such an evaluation should only be made after insuring that the hearing aid is in good functioning order and appropriately set. We may begin the questioning by setting up such a simple communication situation as will be illustrated by the following questions.

1. What is your name?
2. How old are you?
3. Where do you live?
4. Are you married?
5. What is your wife's name?
6. Do you have any children?
7. What are their names?
8. How old are your children?
9. What sort of work do you do?
10. Do you have any hobbies?

Note that the above questions are all confined to a particular topic and that there is thought progression contained within them. Each question is made easier to understand because one might logically predict it on the basis of the previous questions. Although the topic begins to expand as the questions progress, this widening of the scope of the questions is compensated for by the increased predictability that comes from the contextual constraints. In other words, although the relationship between the first and each subsequent question decreases, the relationship between each adjacent question remains relatively constant.

At a more advanced level the task can be made more difficult by increasing the complexity of the ideas that are being discussed. Note, however, that, while the basic structure of the task remains approximately the same, it demands a higher level of performance in both cognitive and communicative areas.

1. What was the name of the man who discovered America?
2. From where did Columbus set sail?
3. Who paid for his trip?
4. How many ships did Columbus have?
5. Do you know the names of his ships?
6. How many ships actually reached the continent of North America?
7. Where did Columbus think he was when he first sighted land?
8. In the days of the sailing ship, how did sailors preserve their food?
9. What problem arose from using salt as a preservative?
10. How did sailors counteract this problem?

For a child with a mild-to-moderate loss, one might, for example, ask such questions as the following:

1. Does Christmas come in the summer or the winter?
2. In what month do we celebrate Christmas?
3. What is it we decorate at Christmas time?
4. What is the name of the man who wears a red coat and hat and has a white beard?
5. What does Santa Claus ride in?
6. What makes his sled go?
7. Where do you find all your Christmas presents?
8. What would you like to have next Christmas?
9. Why is it the mailman is always so busy at Christmas?
10. What kind of pictures do you find on Christmas cards?

Whenever we are considering a person's ability to discriminate speech, we must remember that comprehension of speech requires a more complex process than the recognition of gross sounds. In selecting speech material for evaluation and training, the age and educational level of a person are obvious factors that need to be taken into account. Other less apparent factors, such as unfamiliarity with what may be presumed to be a common experience, may play a role. Careful attention must also be paid to insure that the topic falls within the person's experience. For example, the questions pertaining to Christmas might well place a Jewish child at a disadvantage. His apparent difficulty in responding to what one might consider to be easy questions might mistakenly be attributed to his impaired hearing rather than to his unfamiliarity with the topic. The questions asked should be at an appropriate level of complexity and must avoid the use of unfamiliar names or vocabulary unless these have previously been reviewed. The relationship between aural rehabilitative procedures and language training for the child has already been emphasized. Failure to respond to a spoken direction may indicate insufficient auditory discrimination of the message signal, but it may equally indicate unfamiliarity with linguistic structure or with the content of the message.

Having obtained a general measure of the person's ability to follow progressively developed ideas presented through the auditory channel, we next assess the effect on his performance of presenting ideas that are not related. This requires the person to depend more on the acoustic information, since the contextual cues will be significantly reduced. Such questions may be illustrated by the following:

1. How many days are there in a week?
2. What is your favorite flower?
3. Who is the president of the United States?
4. What time do you generally go to bed?
5. What is the capital of France?
6. What color are the shoes you are wearing today?
7. For what sport are the New York Yankees famous?
8. At what time of the year do we traditionally eat pumpkin pie?
9. For what was Abraham Lincoln famous?
10. How much would two dimes and a nickel be?

Similar questions for children could be as follows:

1. What color are the shoes you have on?
2. What do we use a toothbrush for?
3. How many eyes do you have?
4. When do we eat turkey?
5. What is your favorite color?
6. What is the name of your school teacher?
7. What do you like to eat best of all?
8. Who said "I'll huff and I'll puff and I'll blow the house down"?
9. What does mommy say if you do something very naughty?
10. Hold up two fingers.

We cautioned earlier against presuming that failure to respond to a question necessarily indicates that the person has not heard it adequately. However, it will often be noticed that as redundancy is reduced, the hearing-impaired person experiences increasing difficulty in responding. The decrease in the amount of the information he normally obtains from situational and contextual cues will often be perceived as a deterioration in his ability to hear. He experiences a sense of frustration as he is forced more and more to make predictions on fewer cues. When the stimulus material has been appropriately selected, such a reaction to a decrease in redundancy provides a helpful indication of the contribution that hearing is making to speech comprehension. If no such difficulties are encountered, we may presume that amplified speech provides sufficient information for adequate communication under favorable listening conditions.

The information obtained from several informal evaluations of this type cannot be quantified exactly. Nevertheless, a written summary of these observations will prove valuable in permitting us to formulate an idea of the extent of the communication handicap that the person experiences when listening conditions are optimum.

Discrimination of Individual Speech Sounds

Once we know how well the person can follow related and unrelated messages, we seek more specific information about the nature of his discrimination problems. For the adult student our first clues to this may be obtained by repeating the phonetically balanced word lists. These should be presented with the auditory trainer set at a comfortable level of loudness. The student should be asked to write his responses, if this is possible.

When several tests have been presented, they can be analyzed according to the nature of the errors made. This will indicate how many errors showed a close approximation of the sound pattern of the test word, and how many were incorrect simply because one phoneme was wrongly identified. In this way we obtain our first information concerning the specific speech sounds that present difficulty. Obtaining similar information for young children is more difficult, particularly when vocabulary is limited. In order to compensate for the linguistic deficiency, it is necessary to limit the range of test words to include only those with which the child is familiar. Testing the auditory discrimination of small children frequently necessitates the use of multiple-choice picture tests such as those developed by A. Simm [22], F. L. Nasca [17], and most recently by B. M. Siegenthaler and G. S. Haspiel [21]. The authors of the latter test have demonstrated that it not only produces "reliable and satisfactory estimates of hearing ability of children, but also includes the strong clinical impressions that the obtained scores are meaningful to the child's audiological status." It must, however, be recognized that the reduction of the number of possible choices from which the child must identify the word, generally to four or five pictures, greatly increases redundancy. We must therefore be cautious in generalizing the percentage discrimination scores obtained on these tests to the discrimination performance we might expect to occur when the demands on auditory perception are greater, as occurs when the number of alternative choices is increased.

Vowel-Sound Discrimination

We are now ready to carry out specific tests of the accuracy with which the listener is able to distinguish between phonemes, particularly those that are rather similar in acoustic structure. For the person with a moderately severe or severe hearing impairment, we may not even be sure of the degree to which he is able to recognize the vowel sounds. If we consider it necessary, we will conduct auditory-discrimination tests in order to assess this. Once again, when working with children we will need to do this by the selection of appropriate pictures; for adults it is possible to use the written forms of the words and to select the stimulus materials from a much wider range of choice.

In testing vowel-sound discrimination, as far as possible, we shall attempt to keep the consonants surrounding the vowels constant. This makes it essential for the listener to correctly identify the vowel in order to discriminate between the items' names. The following list, which is read across columns, illustrates the way in which multiple-choice lists can be constructed to test most of the vowels and diphthongs. The test item is in the first column.

well	wall	wool
bat	beat	boat
pin	pen	pan
moon	main	man
bud	bead	board
boy	bow	bean
bear	bar	beer
pain	pine	pin
man	mine	mean
been	burn	born
cat	cut	caught
like	look	lick
low	lie	lay
tea	to	tie
rat	rot	rut

By repeating several such lists with variations of the test word used within each group, it is possible to demonstrate whether the listener consistently identifies a particular vowel sound. If his responses are inconsistent, then we would predict that certain vowel-consonant combinations provide more information in the transients than others. From these findings we should be able to decide whether auditory training for vowel-sound discrimination is indicated or if it is possible to begin working with consonant-sound discrimination.

Consonant-Sound Discrimination

A number of tests have been constructed to provide information about the particular consonant sounds that present discrimination difficulty to the listener. Each of these lists attempts, to some extent, to control the vowels or diphthongs used while varying the consonant combinations. In this way, a limitation is placed upon the linguistic redundancy that occurs when the vowels, as well as the consonants, differ. In the following list only one phoneme is varied in each item; thus, the acoustic information carried by that particular consonant is high.

pan	man	fan	ban	can	ran
will	fill	wing	wit	wig	whim
wall	fall	ball	tall	hall	call

The test of consonant discrimination may be presented in one of several ways, the easiest of these is the forced word choice. The student is asked to listen to the test word and then to identify it from one of two alternate choices. This is the approach used in the recorded consonant-discrimination test developed by Laila Larson [14]. This test (Table 7.4) comprises 34 sets of five or more paired words. The words in each pair differ by only one phoneme. The lists have been prepared so as to require the student to make discriminations between phonemes that might be easily confused. Where appropriate, the lists represent an attempt to present the phoneme in the initial, medial, and final position of a word. In administering the test, one word of each pair within each set is presented to the student, who is asked to identify the spoken word by drawing a line through it on the response sheet. Analysis of the results will indicate the specific sounds with which the student is experiencing difficulty. Within the test, a given phoneme is matched with several other phonemes with which it might possibly be confused; therefore, the results will provide some idea of the types of confusions that the student is experiencing.

The Multiple-Choice Word Intelligibility Test, developed by John W. Black [2], increases the difficulty of the auditory task by increasing the selection from which the choice must be made. The list shown in Table 7.5 is one of 24 such lists. The student is given a copy of the test list to be used and asked to identify a test word from each group of four. The 27 test items are preselected by the tester. While this test provides a measure of percentage intelligibility, the words in each group are not sufficiently strictly controlled to permit the determination of the particular consonants that are presenting difficulty for the listener. For this reason it provides less information than the Larson test.

TABLE 7.4. Larsen Recorded Test (After Larsen [14])

Score: (Errors) _____ /165

Name: _____

With Aid _____ (_____)

Date: _____

Without Aid _____

Directions to be Given the Listener: Draw a line through the words that are pronounced to you from each box.

Box 1	f and ch	Box 2	l and z	Box 3	l and n	Box 4	d and n	Box 5	m and l
few	chew	lip	zip	lame	name	dot	not	mine	line
fin	chin	loan	zone	light	night	die	nigh	mast	last
filed	child	dale	daze	loan	known	deed	need	moan	loan
calf	catch	mail	maze	pail	pain	ode	own	name	nail
four	chore	hail	haze	rail	rain	did	din	home	hole

Box 6	b and m	Box 7	l and v	Box 8	k and g	Box 9	p and b	Box 10	m and v
bill	mill	lane	vane	coal	goal	pin	bin	mice	vice
boast	most	lie	vie	came	game	pie	by	ham	have
bake	make	lace	vase	coat	goat	pole	bowl	glum	glove
robe	roam	lull	love	luck	lug	cap	cap	mine	vine
tab	tam	rail	rave	rack	rag	rope	robe	mile	vile

Box 11	n and v	Box 12	sh and f	Box 13	f and k	Box 14	f and b	Box 15	s and sh
nice	vice	show	foe	fit	kit	fun	bun	lease	leash
nurse	verse	shore	fore	four	core	fig	big	sew	show
nine	vine	shade	fade	find	kind	cuff	cub	sigh	shy
loans	loaves	cash	calf	cliff	click	calf	cab	sip	ship
lean	leave	leash	leaf	laugh	lack	graph	grab	save	shave

236

TABLE 7.4. (Continued.)

Box 16	p and f	Box 17	s and z	Box 18	v and f	Box 19	ch and sh	Box 20	b and d
pour	four	ice	eyes	five	fife	chop	shop	bid	did
pile	file	seal	zeal	vase	face	chair	share	big	dig
par	far	bus	buzz	leave	leaf	watch	wash	buy	die
cap	calf	lice	lies	view	few	catch	cash	rob	rod
cup	cuff	juice	Jews	loaves	loafs	cheap	sheep	robe	rode

Box 21	d and g	Box 22	t and p	Box 23	f and s	Box 24	b and v	Box 25	v and z
doe	go	tail	pail	fine	sign	bet	vet	live	lies
date	gate	cat	cap	flat	slat	dub	dove	have	has
drove	grove	cut	cup	cuff	cuss	base	vase	rave	raise
bud	bug	tar	par	knife	nice	bigger	vigor	view	zoo
dad	gag	toll	pole	lift	list	robe	rove	wives	wise

Box 26	th and f	Box 27	t and th	Box 28	k and t	Box 29	k and p	Box 30	m and n
thin	fin	tie	thigh	kick	tick	pike	pipe	mine	nine
thirst	first	tin	thin	kite	tight	car	par	new	knew
three	free	trill	thrill	code	toad	crock	crop	time	tine
thought	fought	mit	myth	shirk	shirt	cry	pry	dime	dine
thrill	frill	pat	path	park	part	coal	pole	dumb	done

Box 31	Word endings	Box 32	th and s	Box 33	th and v
store	stores	thumb	sum	than	van
will	wills	truth	truce	thy	vie
start	starts	path	pass	that	vat
cough	coughs	thing	sing	thine	vine
cap	caps	thank	sank	loathes	loaves

237

TABLE 7.5. Multiple-Choice Word Intelligibility Test—Sample List (After Black [2])

1	deed	protrude	train
	weed	conclude	crane
	seed	construed	strain
	feed	include	terrain

2	virtual	hide	pack
	curfew	five	patch
	virtue	hire	catch
	virgin	fire	cat

3	dimmer	envy	rumor
	dinner	empty	roamer
	thinner	entry	rubber
	tinner	ending	rover

4	sphere	gull	petal
	fear	gall	mettle
	spear	gold	meadow
	beer	goal	settle

5	fault	burst	trade
	vault	hurt	trace
	dog	first	praise
	fog	birch	pray

6	black	kernel	graft
	track	curdle	draft
	slack	turtle	drab
	flak	hurdle	grab

7	glow	late	break
	go	laden	rake
	grow	lazy	great
	goat	lady	grape

8	change	pen	hard
	chain	pin	part
	stain	tent	harsh
	shame	ten	heart

It may be considered helpful with some adults to conduct a highly detailed analysis of auditory-discrimination ability for specific phonemes. This should be carried out over a period of sessions. It was explained in Chap. 2 how the structural cues within a language greatly influence our ability to identify words. For this reason, nonsense syllables are used instead of words as the test items. The use of nonsense syllables in a test situation provides as accurate a measure as it is possible to obtain of the amount of information that is derived from the acoustic message signal itself, since the linguistic clues have been all but eliminated. Nonsense syllables do, however, present certain difficulties as test items, since some combinations are difficult to record in writing. On the other hand, if the responses are given verbally by the student, we are in essence testing not only his ability to recognize, but also his ability to reproduce the nonsense syllable, and we are also involving the auditory-discrimination ability of the tester who is scoring the responses. Nevertheless, if these limitations are borne in mind and allowed for, valuable information can be obtained from such a detailed analysis. Table 7.6 shows the results obtained on such a test by a hearing-impaired young adult. A section of the test was presented at the beginning of each of five sessions. This was considered necessary in order to avoid any learning influence and to counteract the rather rapid growth of boredom that arises from having to repeat a series of nonsense syllables.

You will notice that the first test items are comprised of various consonant sounds combined with the vowel /a/. In each instance the consonant sound is placed in the initial position. Three patterns of responses can be observed on the record sheet. The first type of response is that which indicates a correct recognition of the sound on all of the five tests. This suggests that the person has no difficulty in identifying this consonant by its acoustic pattern alone. The second type of response is that in which the sound was on no occasion correctly recognized, indicating that the acoustic message signal provides insufficient information for the correct recognition of the sound in any of the test items presented. The third pattern is that in which the response was not consistent, as indicated by the correct recognition of the sound on some presentations and the incorrect identification on others. It is reasonable to expect that a subject with normal hearing might also incorrectly identify a particular sound on one of the five occasions. One false identification was therefore not considered to be significant.

Let us examine a little more closely the results that were obtained for this subject. We observe that the phonemes /θ/, /ð/, /j/, /ʒ/, /ʃ/, /v/ all fall under the category of total failure to be recognized. This allows for the fact that two of these sounds were correctly identified on one of the five presentations; however, this might have been a fortuitous recognition rather than a definite discrimination and, therefore, was not considered significant. When we examine the substitutions that were made for the sounds we find there is a degree of consistency in that on four of the five occasions the voiced "th" sound /ð/ was recognized as an /f/, the /j/ sound was identified as an /r/, and the /v/ was identified as its unvoiced counterpart /f/. Within the other sounds there was not such a high degree of consistency. The unvoiced "th" /θ/, for example, was confused with both /s/ and /f/, while the /dʒ/ sound was confused with /w/, /r/, and /j/.

When we turn to the second category, those sounds that are identified part of the time but not consistently, we find that the /k/ and /t/ sounds

TABLE 7.6. Test Results for Phoneme Discrimination Test

Stimulus	Response 1	Response 2	Response 3	Response 4	Response 5
pɑ					
kɑ	t (incorrect)			t (incorrect)	t (incorrect)
tɑ	χ (incorrect)				
bɑ					
gɑ					
dɑ		g (incorrect)	g (incorrect)		g (incorrect)
sɑ					
zɑ					
ʃɑ					
tʃɑ				ʃ (incorrect)	ʃ (incorrect)
θɑ	s (incorrect)	s (incorrect)	f (incorrect)	s (incorrect)	f (incorrect)
dʒɑ		r (incorrect)			
ðɑ	f (incorrect)	f (incorrect)	f (incorrect)	r (incorrect)	f (incorrect)
jɑ	r (incorrect)	r (incorrect)	r (incorrect)		r (incorrect)
ʒɑ	w (incorrect)	r (incorrect)	r (incorrect)	j (incorrect)	dʒ (incorrect)
fɑ	ʃ (incorrect)		ʃ (incorrect)	ʃ (incorrect)	ʃ (incorrect)
vɑ	f (incorrect)	f (incorrect)		f (incorrect)	f (incorrect)
lɑ					
rɑ					
mɑ	l (incorrect)				
nɑ		m (incorrect)			
wɑ					
hɑ					

Key

☐ Correct response

■ Incorrect response

240

show a natural confusion, though the /k/ appears to be more difficult to identify than the /t/. Note that although the /d/ sound is often mistaken for a /g/ sound the reverse is not true.

Table 7.7 shows what happens when we isolate the phonemes that the first test indicated to be presenting discrimination difficulties and test them in combination with other vowels. The first two phonemes, the voiced and unvoiced "th" sound /ð/ /θ/ were not made more discriminable by changing the vowel. Essentially, the same confusion pattern existed with /s/, /f/, /v/, and /z/, which constitute the sounds that were predicted on the basis of

TABLE 7.7. Test Results Illustrating the Effect Upon Consonant Discrimination When the Vowel Is Changed

Pair	Col 1	Col 2	Col 3	Col 4	Col 5
θi / ði	t / v	f / v	s / z	f / z	s / z
ji					
ʒi	g	j	j	j	g
fi / vi	s / z	s / z	s / z	s / z	s / —
ki					
ti	—	k	—	k	k

Pair	Col 1	Col 2	Col 3	Col 4	Col 5
θou / ðou	s / z	s / z	s / z	f / —	s / —
jou	—	—	r	—	—
ʒou	r	r	r	j	j
fou					
vou	—	—	z	—	ð
kou					
tou					

the distorted acoustic signal received by the subject. Note, however, the difference that occurs in the recognition of the /j/ sound when the vowel is changed. When /j/ was combined with the /a/ sound, it was recognized only once in five trials. When the same consonant is combined with the diphthong /ou/, it is missed on only one occasion, while when it is combined with the short vowel /ɪ/, it is correctly identified on each occasion. The consonant /f/, which was recognized only once when in combination with the /a/ sound, was not recognized at all in combination with the /i/ sound, when it was consistently confused with the /s/ consonant. Surprisingly, one finds that when the /f/ sound is combined with the diphthong /ou/ it is recognized 100 per cent of the time. Similarly, the voiced sound /v/, recognized only once in five presentations when combined with the vowel /a/ and only once when combined with /e/, was recognized on three of the five occasions when combined with the diphthong /ou/. The consonant /k/, which presented significant difficulty when combined with the vowel sound /a/, with a resultant confusion between /k/ and /t/, presented no difficulty for discrimination when combined with either the long vowel /i/ or the diphthong /ou/.

These results provide us with some insight into the complexity of the process of auditory discrimination. The essential problem that faces us is in reaching some conclusion concerning the relative importance of the information actually conveyed within the acoustic message signal itself relative to the amount of information that one needs in order to correctly predict a phoneme. Yet it is important that we should give careful consideration to this question, since it is fundamental to the way in which we set up our auditory training program. Should we ignore the fact that a person experiences auditory-discrimination confusions between certain phonemes when they are presented in the form of nonsense syllables? We might justify doing so by saying that speech perception never requires the individual to make discriminations between meaningless sound units. Since he will always have access to structural and contextual cues, we need not be concerned with the confusions that he is likely to make when these are absent. Our lesson plans, we might claim, should concern themselves only with meaningful materials. The drill-type approach, involving the careful comparison of sounds that may be confused, might be considered to be meaningless to the student and a waste of his and the therapist's time.

On the other hand, we have subscribed to the concept of verbal communication as involving the utilization of "bits" of information, derived from a variety of internal and external sources, that together must exceed a given amount in order that the threshold of comprehension may be crossed. Therefore, we are not justified in jettisoning a limited amount of acoustic information that, with training, the subject may be able to use to augment the amount in the pool. It is not true to claim that the listener will never need to utilize the maximum informational context that can be wrung out of the acoustic signal. Since the cushion of redundancy that we have built into our communication system is severely reduced in the case of a person with a significant hearing impairment, the amount of information that can be derived from all available sources becomes critical. For this reason, with the adult client we may well wish to investigate whether some intensive training in the auditory discrimination of phonemes might not result in an improvement in the phonemic discrimination that would be reflected in an overall increase in communication ability.

Testing Auditory Discrimination Under Conditions of Noise

The final evaluation is designed to indicate how well the person functions when the listening conditions are poor. Noise, in the sense that we are using it in the subheading above, refers to the various kinds of noise that we discussed in Chap. 2. For training purposes this noise can be divided into two major types: acoustic noise, which reduces the signal-to-noise ratio and therefore makes discrimination more difficult, and acoustic and nonacoustic noise, which constitutes distracting stimuli. We shall first consider the noise as it relates to signal-to-noise ratio. Since a normal environment contains varying types and levels of acoustic noise, it is unrealistic to assume that because a person functions adequately with amplification in the clinic he will necessarily manage well outside. Our testing and training should therefore include materials that require the listener to function under acoustic conditions similar to those he might expect to encounter in his everyday activities. This can be achieved in two ways: the sound can be duplicated within the clinic situation by the use of tape recordings, or the therapy situation can be set up in an actual environment in which the acoustics are poor. Bringing the sound into the therapy situation is best achieved by pre-recording the test items in the presence of the noise against which one might encounter them. Ideally one would like to be able to use a stereophonic recording played back through a stereophonic output system. In this way we should be sure that the person was provided with as faithful a reproduction of the auditory environment as possible. On the other hand, since most hard-of-hearing people depend upon a single monophonic personal-hearing-aid system for their amplification, the use of a monophonic tape recording should not result in too serious a deviation from what the person would have heard through his hearing aid. Test materials for the evaluation and training of a person's ability to discriminate in noise can conveniently be made in the house. Using a battery-operated tape recorder, recordings may be made on a busy street, in a restaurant or store, or in an office environment. By constructing recordings in this way, one obtains a message signal recorded against the actual environmental noises that would be encountered. Development of materials appropriate to the background against which they are recorded increases the nonverbal situational cues; this permits the person to develop an appropriate auditory set. The recordings should be made first with the microphone held at a favorable distance of about 6 inches from the speaker and then at a normal conversational distance of 3 to 4 feet, so that the relationship between the speech and the noise is similar to that encountered by a person with normal hearing. If the microphone is held further away, the intensity level of the speech items is reduced in relationship to the noise, and the task becomes increasingly difficult.

If it is not possible to actually record the test material against its appropriate noise environment, environmental noise may either be recorded alone and played separately as a background to the speech material presented by the instructor, or professionally available recordings of noise may be used. Personal experience suggests that this second, more artificial way of providing a noise background is less satisfactory than when the recording is actually made within the environment.

The white noise available on clinical speech audiometers may also be used. It is helpful in determining how well a person is able to function against a background of this type of noise, compared to what we would expect for a person with normal hearing. The advantage gained in using white noise is that the signal-to-noise ratio can actually be controlled by the attenuator dials of the audiometer, since the input intensity can be held constant. However, this broad-spectrum noise is not representative of the type of noise that the person experiences in normal environmental situations. White noise is a continuous noise of constant intensity; environmental noise, on the other hand, fluctuates rapidly both in its intensity level and in its spectral composition, producing a different pattern of speech interference.

If we wish to assess the person's ability to function in white noise, we will make a comparison of his performance versus what we would expect of the person with normal hearing. It takes approximately 12 decibels more noise than signal before a person with normal hearing is unable to correctly discriminate a list of monosyllabic words. The hard-of-hearing person, because of the reduction in acoustic redundancy that his hearing impairment has already placed upon the acoustic message signal, will frequently be able to tolerate far less than this amount of noise.

If we wish to obtain a subjective evaluation of how the person will manage in a noisy environment, we may utilize the recordings that we have discussed above.

The second type of noise is that which serves as a distraction without necessarily seriously interfering with the signal-to-noise ratio. The person may be able to manage perfectly easily in a situation involving only himself and one other person. On the other hand, he may exhibit a low tolerance for the interference that occurs when a conversation is simultaneously being carried out by two other people in the environment. For this reason, the hard-of-hearing person may often experience difficulty in situations involving groups of people in which there may be more than one person speaking at the same time.

In the testing and therapy situation it is not difficult to reproduce such conditions through the use of tape recordings. Recordings of the test or training materials that we have already discussed may be made against a background of conversation being carried on by members of one's own family in the living room at home or a conversation being carried on by three people, or they may be made against the noise of the radio or television being played at a comfortable loudness level. As was recommended in our discussion of recording test items against environmental noise, care should be taken to insure that the recording level represents a realistic signal-to-noise ratio. The test words should be recorded at conversational loudness, with the microphone held at distances from six inches to four feet from the speaker. When recording group conversations, the microphone should be set in a position equal to that which the recorder would assume if he were to enter into the group conversation.

The materials and procedures outlined above, systematically administered over a number of visits, will provide the therapist with both a subjective and objective measure of the individual's auditory performance. With patience, it will be possible to obtain the data necessary for a comparison to be made between the subject's performance wearing his own personal hearing aid and that achieved using a true binaural auditory training unit.

Once again it is necessary to stress that the results, which will be obtained before an exacting program of auditory training is begun, represent the subject's performance at the time of testing. Although one will be able to obtain an indication of the prognosis for communication through the auditory channel, care should be taken not to permit these results to prejudice one's attitude negatively toward the value of providing intensive training. If our attempt to improve the communication of the hard-of-hearing person is to be successful, then we must be unrelenting in our efforts to train the person to extract the last bit of information from the incoming signal.

THE AUDITORY TRAINING PROGRAM

We stated our first aim in the training program as being to familiarize the person with a hearing loss (or in the case of a child to advise his parents) with the nature of his auditory and communication problem. The first stage of auditory training involves, therefore, the presentation of a simple explanation of how the normal ear functions and the reason why the hard-of-hearing person is having difficulty in understanding speech. It is often wise, at this point, to emphasize to the student with a sensory-neural loss that, although his hopes may be raised when he hears of people whose hearing has been restored through medical treatment, such cases are always those in which the person has suffered from conductive hearing problems. No such hope can be held for a person with a medically diagnosed sensori-neural hearing loss. For these people, all one's aspirations must be pinned upon an improvement in communication achieved through the diligent pursuit of the aims of a rehabilitation program. Although such information will undoubtedly have been provided to the student or his parents by the otologist who made the diagnosis, hopes for a cure frequently linger on and often detract from the determination with which the person approaches the aural rehabilitation program.

When the type of hearing problem has been explained, it is helpful to show the person the pattern of his hearing loss as represented by the audiogram. It is quite simple to explain that each speech sound is made up of a variety of different frequencies or pitches, each having a different intensity or loudness. It may be pointed out that the audiogram indicates how sensitive the subject's ear is to sample frequencies or pitches within the range of those that are found in conversational speech. By looking at the chart we are not only able to gain information concerning which pitches are proving difficult for him to hear, but we are also able to obtain a measure of how much sensitivity loss is present. We measure this loss, we explain, using a unit known as a decibel. The level at which a person with normal hearing is able to first detect a tone we designate as zero decibels. When a person requires 20 decibels more than this amount of sound before he is able to detect the tone, we consider that his hearing is no longer normal. Some indication of the relative intensity of sound can be given by explaining that speech that is barely above a whisper is produced at an intensity of 40 decibels, normal conversation at 65 decibels, and a loud shout at 90 decibels. If we speak at a normal conversational loudness level but move our mouth to approximately one inch from a person's ear, we put back the 30 decibels of sound that is lost as the voice travels from the mouth to the listener's ear; for this reason, conversational speech at a distance of one inch from the ear produces a loudness level of 95 decibels. This piece of information is valuable to a mother who is encouraged to speak with her mouth very close to the ear of her hard-of-hearing infant when he is sitting on her lap.

After a simple explanation of the audiogram, the therapist should discuss with the student or the parent the types of speech-discrimination difficulties he is experiencing under the various listening conditions that were tested.

If a hearing aid is being used for the first time, the components of the aid and the basic steps that are necessary for its maintenance should be explained in the simplest manner to the wearer or his parents. It can be explained that a hearing aid is essentially a small amplifying unit designed to pick up the sound created by people and things in the environment and to make it louder. It should be pointed out that the aid does relatively little to make the sound clearer to the person. The sound is picked up by an internal microphone, which turns the movements of the sound wave into electrical impulses that are then amplified or made stronger by the internal components of the aid, using power drawn from the batteries. The amplified electrical current representing the sound waves is then carried by means of a connecting cord to the earpiece or receiver, which serves to change the electrical impulses back into sound waves and to feed these sound waves into the earmold. The purpose of the earmold is to hold the receiver in the ear and to convey the sound into the ear canal. The on-off switch, which is either a separate switch or one that is incorporated in the volume control, should be pointed out and its use demonstrated. It is helpful to use the method of setting the loudness level of the hearing aid that was explained earlier. A person should also be told which tone-control setting is appropriate to his type of hearing problem. Instructions in the care of the hearing aid should include mention of the sensitivity of the aid and the need to avoid knocking it or dropping it. The student should be told how to put the batteries in correctly and should be advised to use two or three batteries in rotation. It is advisable that the batteries be removed from the aid each night to prolong their life and to permit the wearer to check to be sure that they are not leaking.

The fit of the earmold should be such that it is tight, yet comfortable. The wearer should be told that he should mention any soreness or irritation that might be caused by the earmold. The connection between the earmold and the earpiece, or receiver, should also be firm. If necessary, a small plastic washer can be used to tighten the fit. Similarly, the two- or three-pronged plugs on the cord, which connect it at one end to the amplifying unit and at the other end to the receiver, should fit snugly. It can be explained that the concern for the correct fitting of these various parts is an attempt to eliminate the effect of feedback, in which the leaking of sound between the receiver and the earmold or the effect of a poor fitting plug may give rise to a high-pitched squeal that is both unpleasant and acts as an important source of noise in the system.

The need to keep the earmold clean should be stressed. This can be achieved by running warm water through the hard plastic mold to clear out wax and by use of a pipe cleaner to keep the channel open. If water is used in the mold, great care must be taken to check that the passage is completely dry before reusing the mold. If this is not done, it is possible for an air bubble to be trapped in the earmold canal, resulting in an attenuation of sound. The mold should therefore be banged hard against the palm of the hand or blown through if a pipe cleaner is not available for the purpose.

It is wise to separate the earmold and the receiver each night, placing the receiver faced down on a pad of facial tissue in order to allow any moisture to dry out.

The therapist should also explain to the hearing-aid user any special accessories that the aid has built into it. This will include pointing out and demonstrating the use of the telephone switch (Fig. 7.4) and instruction on how to set the level of the automatic volume control, if one is included. Too frequently this advice is never given by the therapist because she, herself, is unfamiliar with the components of the aid—often as unfamiliar with them as the beginning user. She may be further handicapped by a feeling of inadequacy resulting from lack of knowledge of an essential topic with which she feels she should be familiar. Such inadequacies are easily overcome by seeking the advice of one of the hearing-aid representatives in the area. These representatives are flattered by being asked to advise on these matters, and they prove to be very careful in explaining to the therapist the procedures with which they, themselves, are extremely familiar. Such a contact

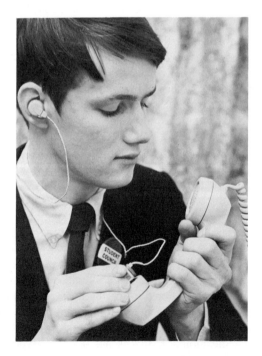

Fig. 7.4.   The hearing-impaired person should be instructed in the use of special features of the hearing aid. (Courtesy of St. Mary's School for the Deaf, Buffalo, New York.)

also proves invaluable when the time arises to seek assistance in the further care and maintenance of the hearing aid.

After the nature and the use of the basic controls of the aid have been explained, the therapist should discuss with the student some of the experiences that he might be expected to encounter until he is thoroughly accustomed to the aid. It should be explained that the aid is not particularly selective in the sounds that it amplifies, and for this reason the person will suddenly be exposed to many environmental noises that in the past have either not been audible to him or have been sufficiently soft not to attract his attention. It can also be explained that whether or not we pay attention to sounds is, to a great extent, determined by our familiarity with them. Initially, many of the sounds the student hears will seem new to him, and his mind will constantly draw his attention to them. However, after he has worn the aid for a while and has received auditory training in gross-sound discrimination, these sounds will no longer be unfamiliar to him, and his mind will be able to accept them and fit them into a background without making him particularly conscious of them. We should point out, however, that some of the noises that he hears will prove to be very meaningful to him in helping him to assess the environmental situation at any given moment. Furthermore, they will frequently provide him with additional cues that will be helpful in evaluating the spoken message.

When a hearing-aid user uses an aid for the first time or changes his own aid for a new one, he may be disturbed by the quality of the sound that the amplifier provides. It is not uncommon for a person who has worn an aid for several years to object to the quality of a new aid, even when it can be clearly demonstrated that the new aid provides a clearer pattern of amplification. This is a function of the auditory-perceptual pattern that the user has developed; the incoming sounds no longer exactly match that pattern and, as such, they have a degree of unfamiliarity to them. This perceptual phenomenon should be explained to the user, who should be encouraged to be patient in the knowledge that it takes a little time for the mind to modify the internal auditory pattern so that the new sounds become acceptable.

Two booklets that are helpful in familiarizing the child and his parents with the use and maintenance of the hearing aid are *Tim and His Hearing Aid*, revised edition by Eleanor C. Ronnei and Joan Porter [20], and *Caring for a Child's Hearing Aid,* by Charlotte Dempsey (Fig. 7.5). The first of the two booklets uses an illustrated story to familiarize the child with the aid—why he wears it and how to look after it. The Dempsey booklet, written for parents, provides all the essential information for care and maintenance of the child's aid, with a detailed chart to aid in the diagnosis of minor hearing-aid problems and their causes.

We specified as our second goal in auditory training the development of an understanding by the student of the approach to aural rehabilitation

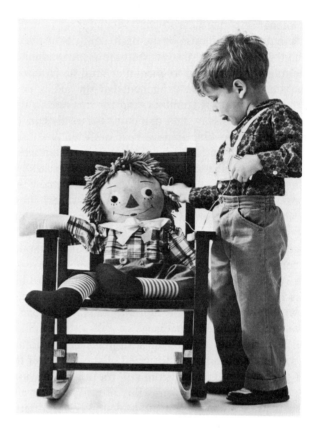

Fig. 7.5. *Caring for a Child's Hearing Aid,* a helpful publication by Charlotte Dempsey, published by Zenith Hearing Aid Sales Corporation. (Courtesy of Zenith Hearing Aid Sales Corporation.)

that will be used. In the case of the younger children such an explanation should be provided to the parents. It is important to convey the concept of communication as involving the use of a pool of information. Parents or students often find it difficult to understand why one spends a considerable amount of time in listening training when they know that their hearing is not sufficiently good to permit them to be able to understand the spoken message under certain listening conditions. Parents not infrequently express the opinion that, since the hearing cannot be improved, one's efforts would be perhaps better spent in training the person to use his eyes instead of his ears. It is important for motivation in auditory training that the people involved clearly understand that, although the hearing itself cannot be improved, the use that is made of the information in the auditory channel generally can be enhanced. They should be told that in an integrated approach the auditory information will be combined with the visual and that when this happens the total amount of information is greater than that represented by the sum of the two parts.

It should be explained to the student why the auditory training program begins with practicing gross-sound discrimination, why we work not only with whole sentences but also with individual sounds in controlled words, and the way the lessons are sequenced to move from situations in which speech discrimination is relatively easy to those that are likely to present the greatest amount of difficulty.

For the teenager or adult, an effective auditory training program should serve not as a series of drill sessions in listening, but rather as an ongoing course designed to familiarize the student with the auditory communication. It must necessarily involve a discussion on a simplified level of many of the concepts that we considered in the first half of this text. In this way, one is developing a mode of behavior in the student. It is well to reflect frequently upon the thought that the only part of any rehabilitation program that is of any value at all is that which the student internalizes and takes with him in the form of an adaptive change in behavior.

Our third and fourth aims we designated as being the development of an awareness of sound and its referential function, and the development of a mobilization toward auditory stimuli. For the young deaf child we shall need to devote the initial stages of training to the development or improvement of gross-sound discrimination. We shall aim to develop in the child an interest in listening to sound and an awareness of its usefulness as a source of information about what is going on in the environment. Our aim for the older child or adult who may be listening to amplified sound for the first time will be to help them to reorientate themselves to sounds that were previously either too soft or too distorted to be of value to them.

Finally, we shall seek to achieve our fifth aim of teaching the person to discriminate sounds under conditions of decreasing redundancy by structuring our lessons in speech-sound discrimination so that he moves from listening under the most favorable conditions to extracting information from the speech signal when the listening conditions are poor.

Types of Lesson Activities

Although the type of materials and activities that will be used with adults and children will obviously be quite different, the progressive stages of auditory training will be essentially the same. Our rationale for these stages is based upon our understanding of the progressive steps that an infant with normal hearing goes through in learning to attribute meaning to auditory stimuli. He first learns to discriminate between highly dissimilar sounds that, by virtue of their nature, contain a high degree of acoustic redundancy. He learns to identify these sound sources in their environmental context, receiving information about them simultaneously through several sensory pathways. Later, after learning has taken place, he is able to recognize them on the basis of reduced cues represented by their acoustic characteristics alone.

Our rationale leads us to attempt to reconstruct for a person first provided with amplification the same progressive experiences that, by virtue of a congenital impairment, may have been missed, or that, because of a subsequent deterioration in hearing and the consequent necessity for the use of a hearing aid, need to be repeated in order that the process may be applied to the modified auditory impressions that the person is now receiving. The following stages of the auditory training program represent, therefore, the progression of normal auditory-perceptual development.

It must be strongly emphasized that the sample lessons presented in this chapter and in Chap. 8 should be treated only as examples. It is essential, when developing similar lessons for a particular child or adult or a particular group of students, that the language level and content material be very carefully controlled.

Training Discrimination of Gross Sounds

Techniques with Young Children

When working with young deaf children, one should begin this training stage using actual sound-making objects (Fig. 7.6). Small bells, toy animals that make noises when squeezed, music boxes, or xylophones are some of the many types of sound-generating toys to which the child will be able to relate. The child's motivation to learn to recognize them by their sounds will arise from his interest in them as toys (Fig. 7.7). He will initially relate to them holistically, not differentiating between the various sensory impressions he receives from them. We wish to incorporate into this gestalt the acoustic characteristics of the toys. Thus, he is presented with the same initial learning experiences as occurs with an infant with normal hearing.

We first permit the child to become familiar with the training objects. He is allowed to examine them and to play with them. It may be found helpful to use some of his own noise-making toys brought from home. This initial familiarization stage can be carried out in an unstructured play situation. The teacher draws the child's attention to the sound of the toy by holding it first to her own ear and indicating, through speech and appropriate facial expressions, that she hears and enjoys the sound. This is an illustration of the value of the visual message signal in communication, which we discussed in Chap. 4. The therapist will then hold the toy close to the microphone of

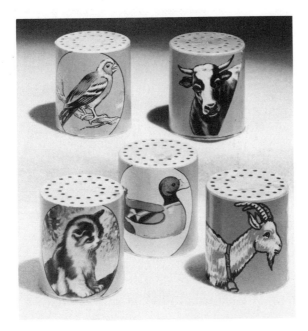

Fig. 7.6. Noise-makers are helpful in early auditory training activities. (Courtesy of Foster and Gallagher, Inc., Peoria, Illinois.)

the auditory training unit or to the child's own hearing aid, encouraging him to handle it and to cause it, in the same way as she used it, to make a noise and indicating her pleasure when he does so.

For small children, who will almost inevitably be wearing a body-type aid, it may be found helpful to have the parent obtain the longer 18-inch cord connecting the microphone and amplifier to the receiver. With this longer cord, it is possible for the mother to hold the aid close to the noise-making toy that the therapist is showing to the child.

You will remember that in our discussion of auditory development it was explained that the young child at first does not respond to mother's voice, except when she is actually catering to his physical needs. Later he learns to use the sound of her voice to predict the other characteristics that together constitute his concept of mother. The next step in gross-sound-discrimination training, therefore, is to encourage the child to learn to predict the presence of an object when he can neither see it nor feel it. We do this by playing games in which a sound-making object is held behind the therapist or, perhaps, under the table. She gains the child's attention through her facial expressions and through holding her finger toward her ear while fixating her glance as an indication of listening. When the child's attention has been obtained, she will make the sound with the toy several times and then

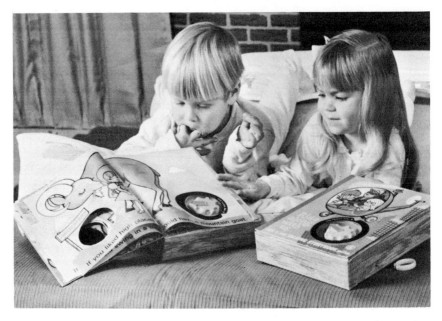

Fig. 7.7. See 'n Say Talking Storybooks, by Mattel, Inc., can be useful in stim-
ulating the hearing-impaired child. (Photo courtesy of Mattel, Inc.,
Hawthorne, California and Harshe-Rotman and Druck, Inc., New
York.)

bring it into his view, make the sound again while he can see the object, and
then finally hand the object to the child and encourage him to make the sound
himself. This step is the first in the process of separating the auditory aspects
from the visual and tactile aspects of the toy. The child is being asked to
identify it by its sound when the other characteristics are absent. He will not,
however, experience frustration, since the amount of information available
to him in this task is increased by adding vision to hearing and then, finally,
by adding touch to the other two pathways. After a while, with patience, we
will observe that the young child will begin to anticipate the object he hears.
He will begin to respond to the auditory clues in a more and more positive
manner, indicating a growing ability to identify objects by the sounds they
make (Fig. 7.8).

    Although at this early stage we are not directly concerned with the
teaching of speech, we must not neglect the fact that the newborn child with
normal hearing is generally spoken to by his mother from birth onward.
The fact that the infant apparently shows no comprehension of what is being
said does not disturb her; she's talking as much to herself as she is to her
child. Unfortunately, parents tend to react negatively if they fail to observe
evidence of comprehension by the child before the second birthday. At the

University of Manchester, England, where the principles of the early training of very young deaf children and their parents have been studied extensively, both from a clinical and research point of view, we found that the number of times the parents spoke to the child decreased rapidly once they became fairly certain that he was not hearing what was said to him. Some parents of deaf children, prior to receiving guidance, had ceased entirely to talk to their babies on the assumption that, since the child obviously could not understand what they were saying, there was no value in talking to him. The idea that he might be receiving at least part of the acoustic signal and that this part might contain information that would be valuable to him quite understandably did not occur to them. We are dominated by the concept that either you hear enough to understand or the auditory signal is of no value to you. You can imagine how serious such a misconception is when the parents are made aware that their child is deaf when he is no more than a few months old. Unless the parents are given guidance in how to provide the child with maximum learning opportunities, they may talk very little to him. He will therefore be deprived of the auditory information that he might be able to glean through his residual hearing, patricularly if he has been fitted with a hearing aid. He will also be deprived of the visual cues to speech.

We have pointed out that during the first one or two years of life the child is as much concerned with developing the concept of speech as a means of communication as he is with the learning of the actual vocabulary and grammar. Before a child can learn to speak he must be exposed to the experiences that will convince him that by listening to these noises and by learning to make them himself he will be able to exert considerable control over his environment. Therefore, while we are working on gross-sound discrimina-

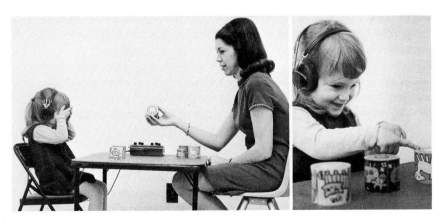

Fig. 7.8. As the child begins to utilize the auditory cues more efficiently, his confidence in his predictions grows. (Courtesy of Speech Communication, State University of New York at Buffalo.

tion, we should always make quite sure that we expose the child to speech that is appropriate to the toys we are using and the ways in which we are using them. When we are working with the hearing-impaired child, we will certainly insure that we are more deliberate in our behavior—we will be more conscious of why we are doing things. We will need to insure that those experiences that the child is deprived of by virtue of his hearing impairment are deliberately repeated more frequently than would be necessary with the child with normal hearing. Thus, when we are playing gross-sound-discrimination games, we should not forget to talk about what we are doing.

"There's the teddy bear; listen to teddy bear squeak. Squeak, squeak, teddy bear. Here, you hold teddy bear; you squeeze him; there. Squeak, squeak, squeak." Then, hiding teddy bear behind your back, "Where's teddy bear gone? Where's teddy bear? Squeak teddy bear." And then, when teddy bear is squeaked, "I hear him. Listen. Do you hear teddy bear squeak? There he is. Hi teddy bear. You squeak teddy bear."

This constant patter during the play activities is extremely important to young children. We have seen how a great deal of learning occurs through identification and imitation. We are encouraging the child now to identify with his mother, with his other immediate-family members, and with the teacher or therapist as speaking beings. We want him to recognize that we too are sound-generating objects and, eventually, that he can discriminate between the sounds that we make in the same way as he is already beginning to be able to discriminate between the sounds that his toys make. Furthermore, by doing this we are causing him to associate speech communication with pleasurable experiences, further motivating him to adopt the same pattern of behavior.

When we have carried out this form of activity with several sound-making toys, the next step is to make the process of prediction harder for him by increasing the probabilities from which he must make his choice. We will now move to a game in which he has to choose between the sounds made by two objects, both of which are familiar to him. We first demonstrate to him how the game is played. To do this we need the cooperation of mother. Holding the child on her lap or, if he is somewhat older, crouching beside his chair, she tells the therapist, "Cover your eyes." While the therapist has her hands covering her eyes, the mother causes one of the objects to make a noise. Having done so, she then, very deliberately so that the child can grasp what is going on, asks the therapist to choose which toy made the sound. For the first one or two occasions, the therapist should experience failure. However, she should be encouraged by the mother to try again. The therapist now begins to show that she is able to choose the toy correctly on the basis of the sound it makes alone. It is important while doing this to give the child a large amount of visual information concerning what is happening.

Small deaf children must depend upon what they see occurring in order to be able to analyze the situation. When the therapist makes a correct selection, the mother should therefore clap her hands and nod approval. When she fails to make a correct selection, the mother should simply shake her head without showing any other negative reaction, saying, "Try again." The procedure can then be repeated, with the child choosing the toy and causing it to make its noise. This involves him in the activity.

Once the child is able to participate well, he is asked to cover his eyes, or mother places her hand over his eyes, while the therapist causes one of the toys to make a noise. Having done this, she then encourages the child to make a selection. His successes should be strongly reinforced, his failures should not be reacted to negatively. When the child fails to identify correctly the source of the sound, he should be shown which toy was used, permitted to listen to it while he is watching it, and allowed to make the sound himself. The activity is then repeated, selecting the toy that he just previously failed to identify. One expects him to predict that you will squeeze the same toy; this is, in fact, a positive step, since it is his ability to predict that we are attempting to train. Whether or not he has learned to recognize the toy can only be determined on a subsequent presentation when he does not have the justification for making such an assumption and must make his choice on the basis of the acoustic cues he receives. Various modifications of this type of activity can be used (Fig. 7.9).

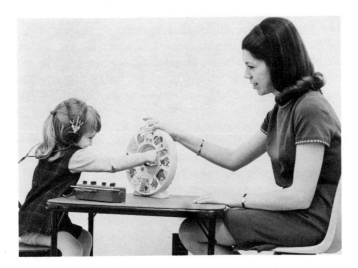

Fig. 7.9. For the child with considerable residual hearing, one anticipates a noticeable growth in the ability to identify by auditory cues. Shown here is an example, using the Mattel See 'N' Say toy. (Courtesy of Department of Speech Communication, State University of New York at Buffalo.)

It is quite helpful to duplicate the sound-making objects so that the child is able to sit at a small table with a set of noise makers in front of him. The therapist, with a similar set on a small table behind the child, is able to present the sound without any fear that the child will be able to use visual cues, such as the particular position of the object, as clues to which one had been touched. In this way, matching games can be played. The therapist, seated behind the child, opens the music box. The child, listening to the sound, identifies it correctly and proceeds to open the music box before him. The therapist then may squeeze a small toy horn, and the child attempts to match the sound from his own selection of objects.

The sound-making objects that are selected should not be confined to toys. There are many everyday sounds around us that can be duplicated in a therapy situation. For example, some of the sounds that might be used would include a spoon stirring in a cup, a banging together of a knife and fork, the shaking of coins in one's hand, the jangling of keys, or an alarm clock ringing. When one moves to these types of sounds, it is possible to narrow the differences between them by selecting objects that would fall into the same category of sound makers, yet for which the actual sounds are not identical. For example, the noise of a spoon being stirred in a cup will vary, depending upon the cup that is used. In this way, providing he can hear the differences, we can teach the child to group and classify sounds into the same category, even though they differ somewhat in acoustic structure.

When the child is able to perform this activity fairly successfully, we can decrease the redundancy of the situation by increasing the number of noise makers from which he must make his choice. Initially we do this simply by placing more noise makers in front of him, permitting him to see the group from which the sounds will be selected. The task can be made more difficult by increasing the number of noise-making objects on a small table behind the child. The therapist then makes a sound and the child is asked to come to the table and make the same sound. Since the child can be prevented from knowing exactly which selection of sound makers are on the table from time to time, the difficulty of the task is increased quite considerably, and he is therefore forced to depend more and more on his ability to identify the acoustic characteristics of the sound and to remember them (Fig. 7.10).

Once the child is old enough to be interested in pictures, the scope of possible activities is considerably increased. By using pictures we are able to extend the range of gross sounds that we can use in training sessions. We will be able to depict many environmental sounds for which the sound maker itself cannot be brought to the classroom. We may use carefully selected pictures together with either commercially or personally pre-recorded materials to present sound within the limits of situational constraints. This use of sounds that are appropriate to a particular situation is illustrated by the recording *Sounds Around Us,* available from Scott, Foresman and Company. In this

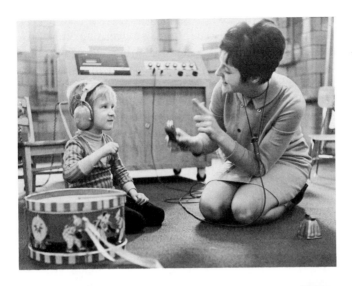

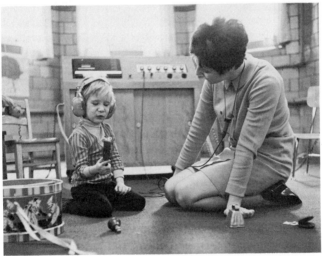

Fig. 7.10. The discrimination task becomes more difficult when the number of alternatives is increased. (Courtesy of St. Mary's School for the Deaf, Buffalo, New York.)

record, the child is presented with sounds around the house, town, and farm. The household sounds, for example, include the telephone ringing, the door-bell buzzing, the vacuum cleaner humming, water running in the sink, and a dog barking. The grouping of the sounds within a context permits the listener to develop a perceptual set, which improves his ability to predict. This ability may be further enhanced by the presentation of pictures representing the sound-making objects and then, later, by depicting situations in which such sounds might be expected to occur. In this way, we encourage the listener to make use of contextual and situational cues to limit the possibilities from which he must make his identifying choice. Other such sound groupings may include animals, musical instruments, and forms of transportation. Using the same technique, it is relatively simple to make a tape-recorded story in sound in which, for example, the activities of a child's day may be characterized by the sounds he hears and makes.

Gross-Sound Discrimination for Older Children and Adults

The activities we have discussed constitute the beginnings of auditory training for the very young hearing-impaired child. It should not be thought, however, that training in gross-sound discrimination plays no role in the auditory training of the older child or adult who is wearing a hearing aid for the first time. The acoustic differences between familiar gross sounds are much greater than those that exist between speech sounds. They are therefore much easier to discriminate between, and they provide an excellent introduction to the process of auditory discrimination. This is true regardless of the age of the student or the degree of hearing loss. The amount of gross-sound discrimination that adults will require is, however, much less than that required by small children. The hard-of-hearing adolescent or adult is familiar with environmental sounds; his problem is that they have become fainter and fainter as his hearing loss has progressed, and their quality has deteriorated. When these sounds are amplified, he may find them relatively unfamiliar. Gross-sound-discrimination training is therefore helpful when a hearing aid has been provided, since it offers an opportunity to orientate the person to his new acoustic environment. For this reason, even when we predict that the student will be able to correctly identify all of the familiar sounds presented to him, we may still choose to devote one or two lessons to gross-sound-discrimination training as an enjoyable and entertaining introduction to the type of activities that will be undertaken with more difficult speech materials.

Discrimination Training for Speech Under Conditions of High Redundancy

The type of material included in this second stage of sound discrimination is often referred to in other texts as "discrimination of simple speech materials." We have explained how the ease with which a person is able to attribute meaning to the acoustic signal is not simply a function of the acoustic message signal itself. While it is true that syntactical redundancy contributes to the ease of recognition of speech, contextual and situational constraints also play an important role in increasing redundancy. Furthermore, we have seen how that same redundancy can be reduced by the introduction of competing stimuli through any of the input channels. The simplicity of the speech material, if one interprets this to mean the ease with which it may be perceived, must therefore be considered to result from several interacting factors.

The aim of this second stage of auditory training is to introduce the student to the task of ascribing meaning to speech in situations in which the amount of noise in the total system is kept at a minimum. The value of this is that it provides the student using amplification with initial success in speech communication activities. It will also permit him to become familiar with the sounds of speech in a situation in which failure to comprehend the message does not carry a penalty. It should permit learning without anxiety.

The factors that we can manipulate in order to provide this high degree of message redundancy are as follows:

1. Simplicity of the message. The statements made should be simply worded. They should not contain vocabulary that might be difficult for the student to comprehend even if he had no difficulty in receiving the message. Insuring simplicity of material is less difficult with older children and adults than it is with young children. It is also easier to achieve when the child has a considerable amount of usable residual hearing. The reason for this is that the young deaf child is almost invariably handicapped by his limited language development. Auditory training for these children must be an integral part of a continuous language development program.
2. Familiarity of the listener with the topic to which all of the messages will be related. By insuring familiarity, the listener can adopt an anticipatory set for information relative to a particular situation. The progressive development of the ideas that are being communicated will permit contextual structure to be built. This further increases message redundancy by limiting the choices from which the speaker may select and, therefore, those from which the listener will predict. In this way, we increase both situational and contextual redundancy.
3. The number of acoustic and nonacoustic distractions.
4. The presence of visual cues to further limit the selection of possible messages. Such cues include the physical items that may be talked about, pictures of items or situations, key words or sentences written on the blackboard, and of course, the visual cues obtained by watching the speaker.

By manipulating these four factors, we are able to control the amount of redundancy in the communication and, therefore, the ease with which the person may correctly interpret the message signal. The approach to training in speech discrimination that we advocate follows our philosophy of providing maximum opportunity for prediction and then gradually reducing the amount of redundancy. In this way we increase the listener's dependency upon the information contained in the acoustic message signal.

Activities for Children

When you decide upon the type of activity you plan for a lesson, bear in mind the following requirements.

1. Be certain about what you wish to achieve and then make sure that the activity you choose provides for this.
2. Be as creative as possible in insuring that the activities are fun for the child. If you structure them wisely, they will motivate active participation and a desire to succeed. Whenever you find it necessary to place pressure on the child to participate, the value of the lesson is at best highly questionable. We must create enjoyable learning situations rather than impose teaching upon the child.
3. Insure that the materials are appropriate to the child's language level. Any new vocabulary must be taught before it is included in auditory training lessons. Familiarity with a new word requires recognition and an understanding of the various meanings that the word may convey. The student should be able to use the word in sample sentences.
4. Choose for activities attractive and interesting pictures such as those found in glossy magazines. Avoid using poorly drawn and uninteresting ditto sheets.

One of the most valuable tools for a hearing therapist is a collection of everyday objects or their toy representatives and a complete set of commercially available pictures of objects, people, and activities. A set of such unrelated items as illustrated by the list below will prove extremely useful.

doll's shoe	comb	shell
sock	hammer	bar of soap
airplane	dolls' tea cup	paintbrush
car	and saucer	can opener
boat	pencil	toy clock or watch
ball	safety pin	toothbrush
	fir cone	

Using such objects or pictures the therapist can begin by asking the child to select the items she names. If he experiences difficulty in choosing familiar objects, the therapist begins to provide additional cues. For example, if he fails to recognize the word "shell" she might say:

I found a beautiful shell on the seashore.
Shell.
We find the shells by the ocean.
Inside the shell is a fish.
We call it a shellfish.
An egg also has a shell.
It is called an eggshell.
A baby chick grows in an eggshell.

Where necessary, we should take time to teach the language concepts represented by unfamiliar words. When the problem is one of difficulty in discrimination rather than one of vocabulary we can enhance auditory awareness of the sound of these words by limiting the number of items from which the student must make his choice. We might, in this instance, place the shell with the comb and the boat. The child is now helped in choosing the shell by the constraints placed upon his selection by limited choice and by the auditory patterns of the words *boat* and *comb*. When the sound he hears is neither of these, he will predict the word *shell*. In this way, we provide him with an experience of success in selecting the shell when the item is named. We then increase the number of items from which he must choose until we are back with the original group with which he first experienced difficulty.

A student who can easily select the object named can be asked to select, from a wider collection, groups of two or three objects. This requires the storage and recall of sequenced auditory information. In a group situation, each child is told what to choose, but he must wait until all the children have been given their instructions before carrying them out. Sequenced commands can be used in place of object selection.

For the next step, a limited number of items are placed before a child. This time, instead of naming the item, you tell the child something about it. He must try to recognize the object about which you are speaking (Fig. 7.11). For example, the objects may be:

A fir cone
A toothbrush
A ball

The information might be:

This is something that grows on a tree.
The tree stays green all winter.
At Christmas we decorate this kind of tree.
This is the seed of the fir tree.

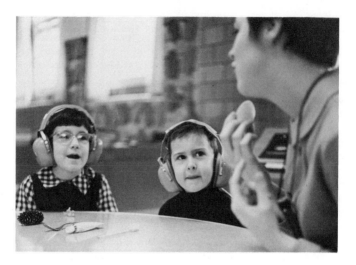

Fig. 7.11. The child must learn to predict the object from the content of the spoken message. (Courtesy of St. Mary's School for the Deaf, Buffalo, New York.)

Or:
    We use this after we have eaten a meal.
    We put paste on it.
    If we forget to use it, we may not have good teeth.

Using this technique, we are training the child to identify an object on the basis of information about it. In this way we are improving the usefulness of hearing. By using a relatively simple situation containing a high degree of redundancy, the child may experience success in the listening situation. It is an enjoyable activity, it presents a challenge, and it permits the student to handle his failures in a positive way.

The same activity can be presented at a more advanced level through the re-creation of everyday situations. Playing grocery shopping with empty cartons and containers of foods and household commodities can be enjoyable and useful. The items are placed on a table and the child is given a verbal list of things to buy. Duplicate items permit variation of the quantities to be bought.

In a group situation, each child can be responsible for shopping for three or four things. The children are told what to buy, but no one goes shopping until everyone in the group knows what to get. This requires the child to remember the items named. The activity can be made a little more difficult by describing rather than naming the items.

Older children can participate in a similar task by using labels or pictures of items on a larger master card. The student then indicates which item is being discussed. Picture-lotto games can be modified for the same purpose. The classification of stimulus items is practically unlimited. They include domestic and wild animals, fruits and vegetables, musical instruments, gardening tools, household appliances, etc. Mail-order catalogues provide an excellent source of illustrative materials for building master cards.

Active participation in play stories is always appealing to young children. A set of farmyard figures can be used to describe what is happening on the farm, while the child manipulates the figures to conform to the story. For example:

It is early morning. The farmer goes down to the cow shed to milk the cows. Now the farmer's wife is coming out of the farm house. She is going to feed the chickens. The farmer brings the cows out of the shed and drives them into the fields. Now he is going to feed the pigs (Fig. 7.12).

The story continues, and the child follows the directions. Similar action stories can be set up with a doll's house and furniture, with miniatures for a doll's tea party, or with a set of toy vehicles such as cars, buses, fire engines, ambulances, and police cars. Buildings can catch fire, traffic accidents can occur, and robberies can take place.

Pictures and stories can be used as a means of conveying information to the student who is then asked to answer a series of questions about them.

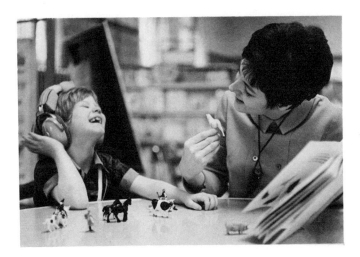

Fig. 7.12. Children enjoy auditory training activities centered around play stories. (Courtesy of St. Mary's School for the Deaf, Buffalo, New York.)

The questions should be presented in a sequential order. If a question is not understood, the information related to its answer should be presented verbally and the question repeated. The most helpful method of doing this is to use what might be termed a constructive or developmental technique. Presume, for example, that a question about a picture is, "What did the little boy's dog do?" Since the student failed to understand the question, we may develop the information necessary for the answer in the following manner:

> Can you show me the little boy in the picture? That's right. Now show me his dog. You see the dog has a leash. The dog pulled at the leash and the boy let go. Then the dog ran into the road. He was almost hit by the car, but the car swerved and hit a lamp post. The little boy's dog *caused an accident.*

At this point we would repeat the initial question. The same procedures can be used in discussing a story that has been read to the child. Although there are a number of stories and games for use in auditory and visual communication training of children, the greatest source of materials will be found in the school or public library. Picture storybooks designed to be read to preschool through first- or second-grade children, if chosen carefully, provide excellent source materials. One should look for simple, but interesting, stories with good illustrations. The illustrations are particularly important as visual aids and should therefore depict the text clearly. The more unusual type of creative drawings to be found in some books tend not to lend themselves to this type of activity. Should you wish to build an inexpensive library of materials for this purpose, many of the 29-cent books in the Golden Book series [15] lend themselves extremely well to auditory and visual communication training. These should be selected carefully, since by no means all of them are suitable. When you look at a book as a possible source of a lesson plan, remember that you will almost invariably have to rephrase the story for the child. Ask yourself how easy this will be, and then look at the pictures to see whether they clearly illustrate the main concepts of the story. With such inexpensive books as these, you may wish to buy two copies in order to cut the pictures out and mount them on separate cards to facilitate story development.

You may also wish to vary the story-telling approach by using the commercially available records. Those that combine sound effects with the stories are particularly useful for this purpose. Remember, however, that the nature of recorded materials is such that it makes it difficult to allow for flexibility. Most of the stories that are recorded for children with normal hearing are rather too long and too complex to provide appropriate training material. Too much must be heard before feedback, in the form of questions and answers, can be obtained.

As the student begins to progress, we can increase the difficulty of the discrimination task by eliminating all cues other than the auditory stimulus. A number of activities can be used for this purpose. One of the most popular is that in which objects are placed in a paper bag and information about them provided to the student in the developmental pattern that we spoke of before, until the child is able to guess what the object is. This task is most difficult when the children have no idea in advance of what the objects might be. It is, of course, simplified by letting the child know in advance which objects are in the bag and thus constraining his choices. Multisensory techniques can be used by letting the child feel, though not see, the objects. Such games as "I Spy" or "Guess What I Bought at the Store" fulfill the same purpose. Question-and-answer activities around a particular topic, such as a visit to the seashore, winter sports, a birthday party, or a trip to the zoo, can be progressively developed using appropriate pictures, film-strips, color slides, and sound recordings. Well-known children's stories can be used in auditory training by asking the child to identify the story depicted on the basis of progressively developed cues.

This is a story of a little girl. One day she went for a walk in the forest. She discovered a little house. No one was at home. She went inside. She was very hungry. Someone's breakfast was already on the table, etc.

For younger children, nursery rhymes may be substituted for stories. Duplicate cards are given to the child for matching games. The test items may consist of naming the rhymes, reading the first line, or telling about the story. The activity may be made more difficult by reading the last line of the rhyme or one of the intermediate lines; two lines drawn from different rhymes may be presented and the child asked to identify the two nursery rhymes involved. Other activities may include packing a suitcase for a trip, using doll's clothes and a doll's suitcase, and identifying the verbal cues to such categories as games we play, people's occupations, or national holidays.

The same approach to auditory discrimination of speech under favorable listening conditions is appropriate for adults. In many cases, the only difference between the activity for children and grown-ups is the actual contextual material that is used. Working with the older student permits one to make much heavier use of the written word as the test item. The student can be asked to identify the test word from among a group of words. These words can be selected to be progressively more similar in acoustic structure to the test item, thus making the task more difficult. As we suggested in the training outline for children, it is then possible to feed the listener information about the test item rather than actually naming it.

The topics around which lesson activities can be planned may include many of those we used for children. For example, an adult activity equivalent to the grocery-shopping game for children might include identifying at which type of store one would obtain the items named. A list of items is compiled, and the subject listens to the list until he is able to identify the type of shopping that is being done. It may be that some of the items on the list are not recognized by him; therefore, once he has identified the store, the therapist then reads the list again, asking the student to repeat the names of the items. Those he has difficulty with may then be worked on individually.

In order that we establish a communication situation and avoid a too-persistent use of simple repetition, we can modify this activity by requiring the student to respond to the item named by specifying the manner in which it is purchased.

bread	eggs	flowers
loaf	carton or dozen	bunch
lettuce	milk	cauliflower
head	pint, quart,	head
flour	gallon, or carton	cereals
pound or bag	pears	box
soap	pound or can	tea bags
box, tablet, or	celery	box
cake	bunch	paper towel
jelly or jam	toothpaste	roll
jar	tube	cigarettes
matches	tomato sauce	package or carton
box, book, or	can or jar	
package		

Key lists can be compiled that use as their topics states of the union, famous people, famous places, the names of well-known movies or plays, the titles of well-known books or current magazines. Once again, either these lists may be read to the subject who is asked to repeat them or interest can be stimulated by feeding progressive clues about the person or film that constitutes the test item.

Adults often enjoy an activity in which the therapist presents on a master board a series of cartoons for which he has deleted the caption. A typed list of captions is given to the student who is asked to identify them through hearing and place them with the appropriate picture. The task can be made more difficult by including in the list of captions given to the student a number that are not appropriate for any of the cartoons depicted. To provide a real challenge, one should ask the student to carry out the task without knowing in advance the list of captions from which he must make his selection. The latter activity requires very careful listening on the part of the student. Advertising slogans from well-known products can be used in the same way, with the student being required to identify the product by its slogan. The task can be facilitated greatly by limiting the choice of the student to a group of products for which either the actual items or a label or advertisement is visible to him. The labels or advertisements clipped from magazines can be conveniently placed on large master cards.

Auditory training lessons can also be structured around specific activities in which the adult is likely to experience some difficulty. Topics such as "The Car" can be used to require auditory discrimination of phrases appropriate to purchasing gasoline, having repairs carried out, buying tires, as well as comments that might be made by a driver with regard to the amount of distance that has been traveled, the wearing of seat belts, the fatigue of a trip, the driving conditions, etc. One should insure that the phrases one uses are as natural sounding as possible; try to bear in mind what one would actually say. For example:

"Oh Lord, I just went through a stop sign. Is that a police car behind us? I can't see a damn thing through this windshield. Make sure your door's shut, will you?"

Other topics of this nature could include statements made with reference to the home, the garden, a visit to a play, things that one's husband or wife does that prove aggravating, problems one has with one's children, comments made when visiting a dentist. For a man, several lessons may be devoted to the vocabulary and topics appropriate to his type of employment.

The number of topics that might be used is unlimited. They should be chosen so that they are relevant to the interest and needs of the students with whom one is working. It is often quite helpful to ask the students to suggest topics around which questions may be developed and then, later, to have them work them up themselves for presentation to the class.

The third stage of auditory training involves helping the subject to improve his ability to discriminate between words or phrases that may be confused easily on the basis of their auditory pattern. For young children it is necessary to provide visual cues in the form of pictures illustrating the test words or sentences (Fig. 7.13). Such sets of paired pictures are commercially available for illustrating paired words; paired sentences are also visibly depicted in some of the pre-reading workbooks.

For those students who are able to read, the paired words that comprise the *Larson Consonant Discrimination Test* [14] and the extensive lists that can be found in *The Clinician's Handbook for Auditory Training*, by J. C. Kelly [12], constitute excellent sources of test materials. The usual technique of administering these is to provide the student with a dittoed answer sheet, requesting him to underline the word in the series that he

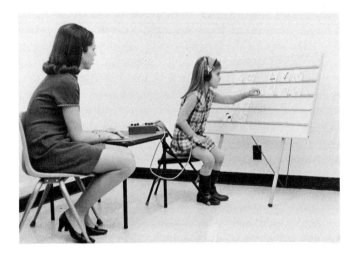

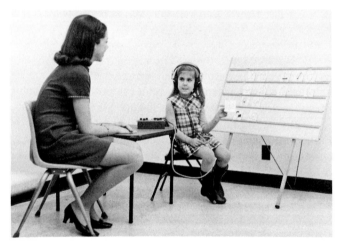

Fig. 7.13. Auditory discrimination between word pairs with similar phonetic patterns is facilitated by use of pictures. (Courtesy of Department of Speech Communication, State University of New York at Buffalo.)

heard. Sometimes more than one test item is presented at a time, and he is asked to underline each of these. Another technique is to request the student to place a number over each word in the list in the order in which it is heard.

The therapist can also construct her own items without a great deal of effort. Such comparative sentences as those listed below may be taken as examples of those that may be confused.

I hope this is all right.	I hope this is all white.
How much did it cost?	How much have you lost?
I need some brown thread.	I need some brown bread.
This way, please.	Just wait, please.
Do you think you'll have	Do you think you'll be
to wait?	that late?

It is true that it is unlikely that the listener would confuse the sentences above were they presented with the appropriate situational and contextual constraints. However, the purpose of the exercise is to eliminate these clues, thus forcing the listener to make better use of the auditory signal. If we can improve the subject's ability to discriminate speech sounds under conditions of low redundancy, then we may be sure that he will function much better when the additional cues are added.

Individual sounds that present difficulty in discrimination can be incorporated into practice material that combines these consonants with different vowels and places them in contrast with other consonants, most particularly those with which they are most frequently confused. Drill sessions of this nature can serve to train the listener in becoming familiar with characteristics of speech sounds presenting difficulty. These may be sounds that he is able to hear but of which he has not been made sufficiently aware to be able to use. Remember that identifying cues may also be derived from the transients of speech, so that it is possible for a person to learn to recognize the sound on the basis of the influence it exerts upon adjacent sounds.

Carhart has stated precisely the goal to which we are aspiring:

Skill in discrimination cannot be considered properly restored until sounds are recognized accurately and quickly on the first presentation. This level of mastery is required if hearing is to be adequate for everyday life, where most remarks are made only once. Consequently, the training program must develop precise and rapid recognition of phonetic elements. [4, p. 382]

Training Discrimination for Speech Under Conditions of Low Redundancy

The everyday situations that a person encounters require that he be capable of understanding speech under adverse listening conditions. A reference to Table 2.3 of Chap. 2 will remind you of some of the sources of noise, both acoustic and nonacoustic, that contribute to reducing the redundancy in a communication situation. Our training program must aim to increase the student's ability to function under these conditions. From the factors listed in the table under the heading "Noise Sources within the Listener," you will see that some of the factors that we must take into account involve an attempt to increase the listener's vocabulary and general linguistic ability where this is inadequate, to develop an ability to listen for general content rather than to worry about individual words, and to be able to disregard distracting environmental stimuli.

We must train him to tolerate the effect of environmental noise that may result in a reduction in the signal-to-noise ratio or of a distortion of the acoustic patterns due to reverberation. Finally, he must be able to handle the problem of poor message encoding, which is a function of speakers, by increasing his ability to make predictions on limited cues.

The materials and activities that may be used to provide training in speech discrimination under conditions of low redundancy are essentially those that we outlined in our discussion of the evaluation of speech-discrimination ability under poor listening conditions. There are two major ways of providing the training: we may present the speech items by live voice against a background of pre-recorded random noise or a competing speech stimulus, or we may record the speech samples against actual background noise. Research findings [5] have shown that speech discrimination is easiest when the speech and noise are separated by an angle of 90°. In other words, we are best able to tolerate environmental noise or a second competing stimulus when our mind perceives them to be spatially separated. We can achieve this by placing the tape recorder with the recorded environmental noise or competing speech stimulus at right angles to the student. We begin our training sessions by setting the noise at a very low level, providing a highly favorable signal-to-noise ratio. The training exercises are then carried out in the same way as was suggested for speech discrimination under good listening conditions. The ability to concentrate on the training materials while ignoring the distraction provided by the tape recording is to a great extent psychological. It is a function of attention, and it has been demonstrated that a subject can learn to improve speech discrimination under these conditions. As his performance increases, the level of the noise is gradually increased, thus reducing the signal-to-noise ratio and making it necessary for the subject to pay greater and greater attention to the acoustic stimulus.

The nature of the distracting speech stimulus can be varied from recordings of a series of numbers or monosyllabic words to conversational speech presented by one or several people. The distraction materials may either be recorded by the therapist or by another adult. Various combinations of male and female voices should also be used for the recorded test items. It is possible, for example, for a female therapist to have a list of test words or sentences recorded by a male while she reads distracting materials to the student. This technique obviates the need for two tape recorders to perform this type of activity.

The advantage that the normal person obtains through the ability to spatially separate signal and noise is lost when the subject is using his own hearing aid or a monophonic auditory training system. In these situations it is perfectly possible to use a single tape recorder in which the test items have been recorded against various levels of environmental noise. These recordings are easily made at home, using the television, radio, or record player as a means of adjusting the intensity level of the background noise.

The therapist should also attempt to carry out this activity using test items that vary in difficulty. While a student may be perfectly able to resist a competing stimulus when the test items consist only of simple sentences, he may experience considerable difficulty in obtaining information of a more complex nature. Test activities should therefore include those that require the student to listen to anecdotes or messages. Comprehension may be evaluated by asking specific questions about the material he has just heard. This activity can be modified to provide training in the ability to shift attention rapidly from one speaker to another. To achieve this training, we tell the student that he is going to be asked to repeat or to record in writing a set of words or sentences. We tell him that test items will be read by the therapist at the same time as lists are played on a tape recorder. The therapist will indicate to him from time to time that he should attend to the materials that she is reading, or that he should shift his attention to concentrate on what he hears from the tape recorder. She may do this simply by preceding the list of sentences by saying, "Listen to me," and then a few sentences later, "Listen to the tape recorder." In this way, the student must learn to be flexible in the figure-ground relationship that he develops.

Some individuals wearing their hearing aid for the first time, or even those who have had amplification for a while, may need training designed to increase their tolerance for sound. We have already stated that some types of hearing losses are associated with a decrease in the physiological thresholds of pain and discomfort. Nevertheless, a perception of loudness and the discomfort that occurs when a sound becomes too loud is at least in part, if not to a considerable degree, a psychological or perceptual function. Inasmuch as there exists a perceptual aspect, we can hope to increase a person's tolerance. If a person has a relatively small dynamic range of residual hearing—that is to say, that the distance between the threshold of detection and the threshold of discomfort represents only a small range of decibels—then it is important that we should attempt to broaden this range. Frequently, the listening habits have been developed so that the individual likes to wear the hearing aid at a relatively low level of amplification. He has developed a perceptual concept of the loudness of sound and may be psychologically resistant to increasing this. Therefore, over a period of training sessions we present test materials first at the level of loudness that the subject identifies as comfortable, and then at each session we present materials at an intensity level slightly above this. Over a period of time it is often found that the person ceases to object to hearing sound at the slightly higher level and the intensity can then once again be slightly increased. Care should be taken, however, that the increments are only small increments, represented by the individual's comment that it is a little bit too loud. The aim of this training is not to permit the individual to listen to unusually loud speech. It is an attempt to overcome the difficulty experienced by a person who has a decreased tolerance for loudness. As a result, he may wear the hearing aid at an amplification level that reduces the strongest peak signals to below tolerance level but in doing so reduces the overall intensity of speech to a point where less information is obtained. We are hoping that, as a result of the training, the individual will be able to wear the hearing aid on a slightly higher setting, thus increasing the dynamic range of the usable residual hearing.

In summary, we might say that the purpose of auditory training is to modify the various aspects of listening behavior in such a way as to increase the total amount of information that the listener can derive from the auditory stimulus. We aim to modify the pattern of listening that the adult has established in such a way as to increase the usefulness of residual hearing or, in the young child, to train him to develop habits that are most appropriate to the perception of speech.

REFERENCES

1. Acoustic Materials Association. "Performance Data." *Architectural Acoustical Materials Bulletin,* AIA no. 39–B (1965).

2. Black, John W. *Multiple Choice Intelligibility Test.* Danville, Ill.: The Interstate Printers and Publishers, Inc., 1963.

3. Beranek, Leo L. *Acoustics.* New York: McGraw-Hill Book Company, 1954.

4. Carhart, R. "Auditory Training." *Hearing and Deafness,* ed. Hallowell Davis. New York: Holt, Rinehart, & Winston, Inc., 1961.

5. Davis, Hallowell. "The Articulation Area and the Social Adequacy Index for Hearing." *The Laryngoscope* 50 (1948): 761–78.

6. Dempsey, Charlotte. *Caring for a Child's Hearing Aid.* Zenith Hearing Aid Sales Corporation.

7. General Radio Company. *Handbook of Noise Measurement.* 5th ed. West Concord, Mass.: 1963.

8. Goldstein, Max. *The Acoustic Method for the Training of the Deaf and Hard-of-Hearing Child.* St. Louis, Mo.: The Laryngoscope Press, 1939.

9. Hirsh, Ira J. *The Measurement of Hearing.* New York: McGraw-Hill Book Company, 1952.

10. Hudgins, C. V. "Auditory Training: Its Possibilities and Limitations." *Volta Review* 56 (1954): 1.

11. John, J. E. "Acoustics in the Use of Hearing Aids." *Educational Guidance for the Deaf Child*, ed. A. W. G. Ewing. Manchester, England: Manchester University Press, 1957.

12. Kelly, J. C. *Clinician's Handbook for Auditory Training*. Dubuque, Iowa: William C. Brown Company, 1953.

13. Knudsen, V. C., and C. M. Harris. *Acoustical Design in Architecture*. New York: John Wiley & Sons, Inc., 1950.

14. Larson, Laila L. *Consonant Sound Discrimination*. Bloomington, Ind.: Indiana University Press, 1950.

15. Little Golden Books. New York: Golden Press, n.d.

16. Miller, B. A., G. Heise, and W. Lichten. "The Intelligibility of Speech as a Function of the Context of the Test Materials." *Journal of Experimental Psychology* 41 (1951): 329–35.

17. Nasca, F. L. "An Investigation of the Picture Identification Test for Children of Standard Index." Ph.D. thesis, Indiana University, 1964.

18. Newby, Hayes A. *Audiology*. New York: Appleton-Century-Crofts, 1964.

19. O'Neill, John J. *The Hard of Hearing*. Englewood Cliffs, N.J.: Prentice-Hall, Inc., 1964.

20. Ronnei, Eleanor C., and Joan Porter. *Tim and His Hearing Aid*. Rev. ed. Washington, D. C.: Alexander Graham Bell Association for the Deaf, The Volta Bureau, 1965.

21. Sanders, D. A. "Noise Conditions in Normal School Classrooms." *Exceptional Children* 31 (1965): 344–53.

22. Siegenthaler, B. M., and G. S. Haspiel. "Development of Two Standardized Measures of Hearing for Speech by Children." University Park, Pa.: Speech and Hearing Clinic, Dept of Special Education, Pennsylvania State University, 1966. Available from HEW, Project no. 2372, Contract no. OE-5-10-003.

23. Simms, A. "Word List Picture Identification Test for Speech-Hearing in Preschool Children." Master's thesis, Louisiana State University, 1961.

24. Streng, Alice, et al. *Hearing Therapy for Children*. New York: Grune & Stratton, Inc., 1958.

25. Thomas, H. "Architectural Acoustics as a Fundamental Factor in the Design of Schools for the Deaf." *The Modern Educational Treatment of Deafness*, ed. Sir Alexander Ewing. Manchester, England: Manchester University Press, 1960.

26. Watson, T. J. *The Use of Residual Hearing in the Education of Deaf Children*, Reprint no. 770. Washington, D.C.: The Volta Bureau, 1961.

27. Wedenberg, E. "Auditory Training of Deaf and Hard-of-Hearing Children." *Acta Otolaryngologica Supplement* 94 (1951): 1–129.

28. Whetnall, E., and D. B. Fry. *The Deaf Child*. London: William Heinemann, 1961.

CHAPTER EIGHT

Visual Communication Training

It is important at this point in our study of aural rehabilitation that we again remind ourselves that the division between auditory and visual communication training represented by these two chapters is a completely artificial one. To separate these channels would be contrary to our basic philosophy of a holistic approach to rehabilitation. Such a separation, made for convenience in the study of communication, carries with it the real danger that the reader may come to think of each channel as an independent system and may consequently establish separate therapy sessions for work with each modality. We must constantly bear in mind that, although we may devote parts of a rehabilitation program to the emphasis of either visual or auditory characteristics of speech, we should never do so without reintegrating the information thus derived with the complementary characteristics of the other channel. Having made this point, we will now continue with our theoretical separation in order that we may study the nature and methods of visual communication training more specifically.

IMPLICATIONS OF THE HISTORICAL BACKGROUND

It is not our purpose to present a detailed account of the evolution of visual communication as a method of rehabilitating the hearing impaired; such a presentation has already been made by Fred DeLand [3]. However, some knowledge of the historical background from which it arose is helpful in understanding the role that visual communication training has played, and still plays, in aural rehabilitation. To study the growth of the use of the visual pathway as a means of receiving the information contained within a speech signal is to a great extent to study the development of oralism as a method of educating the deaf. The word "deaf" in the term "deaf mute," which was for so long the label used to identify individuals who suffered from severe congenital or early-acquired hearing impairment, did not imply, as we might now think, that these individuals were deaf and consequently mute. It signified, rather, that the deafness and mutism represented symptoms in a syndrome of mental deficiency. The causal relationship between the deafness and the failure to speak was not recognized. It was not until the skepticism of such early pioneers as Jerome Cardan [3, p. 19] and Ponce de Leon, in the early sixteenth century, led them to challenge the prevalent concept of the nature of deaf mutism, that the education of the child with defective hearing began to be considered.

Without electrical amplification any person with a hearing loss in excess of 40 or 50 decibels SPL was denied the possibility of utilizing hearing in communication. Thus, by current standards, most hearing-impaired people were deaf rather than hard of hearing. The impracticality of using residual hearing for purposes of speech communication caused the early teachers to depend almost entirely upon the visual channel. However, it was not the visual aspects of speech that were exploited for purposes of communication with the deaf child, but a system of manual symbols representing either whole concepts or individual letters of the alphabet. Remember that the whole purpose for the development of this system of manual communication was to educate the deaf child. It was essential to be able to feed information into and extract information from the student with the relative ease necessary for the communicative interaction between human beings. The manual method was therefore not concerned with providing the deaf individual with a system of communication that would permit him to integrate with the hearing society. Contact between deaf people and those with normal hearing was only established by a relatively few hearing people who had a personal interest in learning the system. This rapidly led to the development of a separate society of deaf people. Nevertheless, it would be grossly unfair to ignore the fact that the manual system was remarkably successful in achieving its aim of the education of a section of society that had previously been considered ineducable. However, because the major goal of manualism was education rather than communication, no consideration was given by the method to the possibility of teaching the deaf child to extract enough information from the visual characteristics of speech to be able to predict what the speaker wished to communicate. It is logical, therefore, that the child was not taught to speak.

Although manualism developed and flourished as a successful formal system of education of the deaf, there continued to exist a small nucleus of people scattered across Europe who were committed to the idea that the visual aspects of speech might be used to convey information to the deaf child. It was not, however, until John Bulwer [3, p. 41] wrote *The Deafe and Dumbe Man's Friend* that it was suggested that visual communication might also be used as a means of teaching the deaf to speak. This idea, and subsequent demonstration of its feasibility, greatly enhanced the value of what was to become known as the oral system. Visible speech communication was from this time destined to become an integral part of the teaching of speech, the expansion of language, and consequently the enhancement of the overall possibilities for learning.

The late birth of oralism proved to be a handicap to its development, since it faced the established and accepted system of manual education. Even in the latter part of the nineteenth century it was still not widely accepted that the deaf were capable of speech. The growth of oralism, first in Europe and the United Kingdom and later in the United States, was erratic. The application of its principles was dependent upon a few dedicated teachers such as Samuel Heinicke in Germany [7], and Thomas Braidwood in Britain [8]. It was, however, the pupils of such teachers as these who began to turn the tide in favor of the oral education of the deaf based primarily on the use of the visual aspects of speech communication. The success of the system, as demonstrated by its students, encouraged the development of a number of small private oral schools in the United States. The commitment of Alexander Graham Bell to a system of education using visible speech symbols, developed by his father, added impetus to the acceptance of oralism. The method was gradually adopted by an increasing number of major schools for the deaf. This focused attention upon the need for formalizing the methods of teaching visible speech communication.

The specific methods that were evolved are sometimes classified as either analytical or synthetic. Careful study of the various methods suggests that such a distinction is misleading, since each method at some point combines elements of both analytical and synthetic techniques. It is not our intention to present a detailed account of the various schools; the reader is urged to examine the original texts for himself. What we shall try to do is to examine the salient concepts and techniques contributed by the best-known systems.

We have already mentioned that the two basic approaches to visual communication training are generally classified as analytical and synthetic. For the moment, let us assume that there is some value in such classification; we will consider the advantages embodied in each technique.

THE ANALYTICAL APPROACH

This technique is based upon the assumption that development of the ability to recognize individual speech components with accuracy and at speed carries over into the recognition of those same characteristics when they are encountered in connected speech. The value of the analysis of the nature of the visible speech signal in visual communication training lies in the principle that speech is comprised of a number of differentiated articulatory movements, each of which has varying degrees of identifiable characteristics. It may, therefore, reasonably be assumed that one's comprehension of speech is dependent upon the ability to identify component phonemes rapidly enough to be able to predict what the speaker is saying. To this end, the analytical aspects of visual communication training emphasize a careful study of the nature of individual speech sounds and stress syllable recognition rather than the recognition of words or sentences.

The methods that are most usually classified as analytical are the Mueller-Waller method, as expounded by Martha Bruhn [1], and the Jena method, explained by Anna Bunger in her description of Karl Braukman's original techniques [2]. Both methods utilize practice materials that emphasize the characteristics of individual phonemes. The student is trained through a series of drill lessons to increase the rapidity with which he is able to recognize rhythmically presented groups of syllables. Like most schools of visual communication training, the Mueller-Waller method and the Jena method both emphasize eye training. They are committed to the concept that the interpretation of speech by way of the visual channel must be based upon the ability to distinguish between and relate the characteristic visible movements of the speech organs during articulation.

The argument advanced by Bruhn in support of the use of syllable drill, rather than drill with single meaningful words, is that the absence of the semantic constraint present in words causes the student to concentrate his whole attention upon recognition of movements, rather than upon attempting to attribute meaning. The separation of what are considered the two most mental processes of reception and perception is claimed by Bruhn to permit the development of the essential movement-recognition skill to a level not attainable when linguistic redundancy is added. Both methods make use of rhythmic exercises to develop in the student a feeling of the movements of speech and a recognition of the information conveyed by the fundamental rhythms of normal speaking. The Jena method even uses simple bodily movements, such as clapping hands or bouncing a ball, to aid in the associative recall of rhythmical patterns.

The Jena method approaches the definition of visual characteristics of speech sounds by considering the vowels as representing variations in the shape and extent of the opening of the mouth cavity, which is modified by the lips, tongue, and jaw. The consonants are considered as brief closures of the vocal channel occurring at three distinct positions: (1) the lips; (2) the tongue, the hard palate, and the teeth; and (3) the back of the tongue and the velum. All consonants are classified according to these three positions, or closures, which are referred to as "ports." The student is first trained to classify the speech movement according to one of these three ports. The Jena method also defines consonants in terms of movement. Bunger explains that they perform two functions in syllables: firstly, to close the vocal channel partially or completely at the beginning of the syllable and then to release the syllable pulse and, secondly, to close the vocal channel at the end of a syllable, thus arresting the syllable pulse.* Consonants are defined as either simple or compound. For example, the consonant in the words *on* and *no* is simple. On the other hand, in the words *three* and *inked* the consonants are compound. Recognition is made of the fact that the transitions of speech also exert an influence on the appearance of the syllable production. The releasing consonant invariably overlaps the vowel and doesn't link the syllable; on the other hand, the arresting consonant does increase the syllable length. When syllables come together in connected speech, the arresting consonant, if followed by a vowel, will move over to a releasing position as occur in the words *bad apple* or *ten eggs*.

Of the two systems, the Jena method provides an even more analytical introduction than that suggested by the Mueller-Waller school. The Jena technique places a great deal of stress in the beginning on the recognition of consonants and vowels as individual units. A student is even required to memorize the basic vowel series. The Mueller-Waller method, however, is more immediately concerned with syllable recognition without a careful analysis of the nature of the consonant and vowel structure.

THE SYNTHETIC APPROACH

The synthetic approach, perhaps best represented by the method advocated by Edward Bartlett Nitchie [9], who himself became deaf at the age of 14, approaches visual communication training from the opposite view of the basis of speech reading. The advocate of the use of synthetic techniques is dedicated to the concept that the ability to predict meaning, rather than identifying individual speech components, should be the paramount aim in visual communication training. The exponents of this approach recognize the value inherent in linguistic and situational constraints. They claim, quite correctly, that it is not necessary to be able to identify each and every articulatory movement, but only some of them, in order to be able to identify the idea being communicated. Unlike the analyst, who considers the syllable to constitute the basis of speech, the synthesist considers the complete thought or sentence to be the essential unit.

---

*It is interesting to note how these concepts later played such an important role in R. H. Stetson's work on motor phonetics.

Like the analyst, Nitchie is also concerned with training visual recognition of articulatory movements; he achieves this, however, through the use of syllable drills. A student studies pairs of movement words that illustrate a particular articulatory movement in an initiating and releasing position. Each new movement is developed in contrast and in connection with previously studied movements, providing a progressive approach to training. Nitchie's lessons begin with a description of the observable characteristics of the groups of sounds to be studied. Awareness of these visual characteristics is emphasized through mirror practice. The student is then presented with a series of movement and contrast words. For example:

pay	way	fay
pea	we	fee
pie	why	fie

may	lay	day
my	lie	die
me	lee	dee

In this way a new movement is contrasted with movements that have already been learned. The ultimate aim is to develop instant recognition of speech movements. Key words, presented first in isolation then in context, are used to provide practice in recognition of groups of speech movements.

Another school that is generally classified as synthetic is the Kinzie school of lipreading. The method set forth by the Kinzie sisters in their books, *Lip Reading for Children* [5] and *Lip Reading for the Deafened Adult* [6], places heavy emphasis upon the recognition of meaning. They teach vowel and consonant recognition through the use of carefully selected words and sentences. Nevertheless, because of Cora Kinzie's personal experiences, the method is more eclectic in nature than the other schools. Cora Kinzie, who developed a hearing impairment while at medical school, took leave of absence from her studies and set out simply to improve her own communication skills. She became so inspired by her teacher, Martha Bruhn, that she decided to work in the field of training deaf students rather than return to medicine. She studied the Mueller-Waller method under Bruhn and opened her own school in Philadelphia in the spring of 1914. Not completely satisfied with the method she had learned, Kinzie decided to study Nitchie's approach. Nitchie suggested to her that she should develop an eclectic system of her own, incorporating the best of the two schools with which she was acquainted. Thus, the fundamental principles of the analytical approach of the Mueller-Waller method and the synthetic approach of Nitchie were combined to make the Kinzie method of lipreading.

The trend toward eclecticism, which was established by Kinzie, has continued. Most teaching institutions today utilize systems of visual communication training, the framework of which can clearly be seen as representing the integration of what, perhaps, might be considered to have been no more than a theoretical division between analysis and synthesis. It is clear that the so-called analytical schools, like the so-called synthetic schools, utlimately seek to encourage the students to apply skills learned in the recognition of speech sounds to the identification of meaningful speech units. Neither the Mueller-Waller method nor the Jena method neglect or underestimate the importance of synthesis. In the 40 lessons in her book, Bruhn moves quickly from rapid syllable drill to practice material involving the recognition of sentences. She makes a serious attempt throughout her lesson plans to encourage the student to see and grasp the whole. She lists as her second important goal the training of the mind to grasp the meaning as a whole and to be able to substitute the sounds that are not recognized in rapid speech, suggesting that such synthesizing power is overridingly important to the good lip-reader. She recognizes that homophenous phonemes and words are indistinguishable and must be predicted on the basis of linguistic and semantic rules. Bruhn also points out that a great deal of information is to be derived from the natural tendency of a speaker to model sentences upon a predetermined linguistic pattern—patterns that aid in prediction. Furthermore, many phrases and sentences occur so frequently in normal conversational speech that they become highly redundant. She suggests that we respond to them as a "memory whole" and that only a slight glimpse is necessary in order to start an automatic train of recognition. A key word or sentence may serve as a compass to a hard-of-hearing person who has lost his way in the ever-changing terrain of conversation. From a familiar key phrase or sentence, it may be possible to obtain a bearing on the whole topic of conversation, permitting one to piece together the information that one has already received.

The Jena method, which is even more truly analytical than the Mueller-Waller approach, also uses the concept of the sense group as a unit of understanding. Furthermore, this method also evidences a realization of the role that predictability plays in the interpretation of the visual attributes of spoken language.

Perhaps the separation of the various traditional schools of visual communication training into analytical and synthetic groups is yet another piece of conventional wisdom that doesn't really hold up under scrutiny. Rather than distinct and unrelated approaches, we are looking at a shift of emphasis. Each of the schools start out to achieve the same end; it is really only a question of the starting point that is different. Like Cora Kinzie, we should surely seek to develop an individual approach to auditory and visual communication training that incorporates both analysis and synthesis in training the person to utilize the information in both sensory pathways. Our justification for isolating a particular phoneme, articulatory movement, or word from the thought unit is, as Martha Bruhn suggested, the only way in which we can insure that the student is forced to pay careful attention to the revealing movements of the speech sound in order for him to be able to identify it. By eliminating linguistic and contextual constraints in this way, we are driving up the information value of the visible signal. If, by this approach, we can teach the preconscious recognition of specific speech sounds, or at least groups of sounds, under conditions of minimal redundancy, then the student will be better equipped to continue to function adequately when the conditions of speech communication deteriorate. Through the use of analytical techniques in both visual and auditory communication training, we attempt to insure that the student is capable of extracting the maximum amount of information from each of the input channels whenever the communication situation reduces the redundancy to a minimum.

The synthetic approach probably has more immediate appeal than the analytical. From all that we have already said concerning the role of constraints in increasing the listener's ability to predict the components of an incoming signal, it follows quite logically that we should make every attempt to train the hearing-impaired person to look for whole ideas or concepts, without worrying about the individual components from which they were constructed. Certainly, the training of the mind to impose an appropriate figure-ground structure upon incoming stimuli (perceptual set) and to provide for the filling of gaps in information (perceptual closure) must play an important role in successful communication. It is to this ability of synthesis that Nitchie devotes much of his discussion. On the other hand, one cannot fail to recognize that synthesis is only possible when one receives information. Although it is true that a person may respond to a gestalt without a conscious awareness of the individual components from which he has constructed that gestalt, its ingredients must nevertheless have been received. We might therefore reasonably hypothesize that, by concentrating attention upon the individual components, we will be able to improve the person's ability to recognize the gestalt. Although the synthesists do not advocate the use of nonsense drills for improving recognition of individual sounds, they do include the use of practice and contrast words designed to increase the awareness of the differences between the visible identifying characteristics of specific speech sounds.

On the basis of what has been said, it seems that the division of the approaches to the visual communication training into analytical and synthetic is purely an artificial one. None of the schools that are traditionally classified under these two headings can be considered to be devoted exclusively to one or the other technique. It is, therefore, not only difficult to support these classifications, but it proves confusing to a student teacher or therapist.

What is important is that you should recognize that in the teaching of visual and auditory communication skills the ultimate goal is the improvement of total perception. This final perceptual gestalt occurs as the result of the interaction of numerous stimuli organized according to an internal schemata or set. In attempting to improve this process, we should direct our efforts both toward increasing the subject's conscious awareness of the specific characteristics by which component parts may be identified (analytical) and toward the enhancement of his ability to grasp the relationship that these parts have to each other, filling in the gaps in the information when necessary (synthetic).

DEFINITION AND AIMS

We said, with reference to auditory training, that our ultimate goal was to increase the amount of information that the hard-of-hearing person could extract from the stimuli reaching him through the auditory channel. Likewise, the goal of visual communication training is *to increase the person's awareness of the constraints represented by the visible aspects of speech communication.* We seek to increase the amount of information that visual cues will contribute to the pool.

Our definition of visual communication training is essentially the same as that which we adopted for auditory training. Throughout our discussion we have maintained a concern that we seek an improvement in overall communication ability. The total system will function with varying degrees of efficiency at all times; what changes is the relative emphasis placed upon each of the sensory input channels. Our definition is, therefore, that *visual communication training is a systematic procedure designed to increase the amount of information that a person's vision contributes to his total perception.*

Our general aims will also be similar to those suggested for auditory training. We include among these the following:

First, *to familiarize the person with the nature of the role that vision plays in communication.* It should be explained that we are not seeking to replace hearing by vision, nor even simply to add vision to hearing as J. O'Neill and H. Oyer have suggested [10, p. 71]. We are seeking to blend visual and auditory information so that the resultant perception is more complete than a simple additive process would permit. The value of the auditory information is enhanced by the visual cues, which themselves became more useful when interpreted together with the auditory sensations. It is important to stress this effect that each channel has upon the value that is given to information coming in through other channels.

Second, *to develop, as far as possible, a mobilization or perceptual set toward visual stimuli.* We shall aim to make the student more aware of visual cues, which may be both directly or indirectly related to the spoken message signal, and to develop his ability to unconsciously incorporate this information into the total pool. What we are attempting to develop is a pattern of communicative behavior that places a greater emphasis upon the use of the visual cues that, under favorable listening conditions, constitute redundancy for the person with normal hearing.

Third, *to teach the person to discriminate between samples of speech in which the visual redundancy progressively decreases.* This trend toward the use of more difficult materials is characterized by lesson plans that progress from training in visual discrimination between highly visible and dissimilar groups of speech sounds, such as the /p//b//m/ group and the /ʃ/ /tʃ/ /dʒ/ group* to those that are highly similar in appearance, for instance, the /t/ /d/ /n/ group and the /l/ sound or /w/, which is visually hard to distinguish from /r/. This also includes the training of the person to make better use of visual cues in the presence of competing auditory stimuli.

PREPARING FOR THE TRAINING SESSION

The environmental factors that are important to satisfactory viewing conditions are primarily those of the lighting and the distance of the student from the speaker. In Chap. 3 the importance of adequate light for good visual acuity was emphasized. In a teaching situation, if there is a major light source, such as sunlight passing through the windows, the teacher should position herself so that the light falls upon her face. She should avoid standing with her back to the windows, since this places her face in shadow and makes it hard to observe facial expressions and articulatory movements. The glare from sunlight will also bother the viewer as he turns to be able to see the speaker.

Distance plays a role in the efficiency with which information can be obtained from the visible characteristics of speech. The optimum distance between the speaker and student is approximately ten feet. In a group situation the chairs should be set up in a semicircle around the teacher, so that by varying the student's position he is given experience in observing facial cues from different angles.

When setting up the aural rehabilitation program, the therapist may wish to consider the relative value of individual versus group therapy ses-

*The phonetic symbols /ʃ/ /t/ /dʒ/ refer to the written sounds /sh/, /ch/, and the sound /j/ as in jam or judge.

sions. In the public school system it may be very difficult to find enough hard-of-hearing children to establish a group program; on the other hand, the needs of pupils in a school for the deaf may outstrip the amount of the teacher's time available to them, making it difficult to justify an extensive training program for individual children, which would be achieved at the expense of the class as a whole. The possibility of choice between the two systems is more likely to occur with adults. However, whether it arises with children or adults, when the opportunity does present itself, the therapist should be familiar with the advantages of each system.

Clearly, the value of individual training rests in the flexibility it provides for meeting the needs of an individual child or adult. Such flexibility is considerably more limited in a group situation. The materials that are used in individual training sessions can be highly relevant to the person's interests and needs. It is possible to provide the businessman with experience in listening and discriminating between phrases appropriate to his communication with his business associates, secretarial staff, and clients. The recognition of specialized vocabulary and expressions can be given concentrated practice. Similarly, the difficulties that a child may be experiencing with vocabulary and terminology of a particular subject area in school may more easily be alleviated through personally tailored lessons than in a group situation. When providing individual training, the therapist will probably find it necessary to shorten considerably the duration of the session compared to the amount of time spent with the group. However, the attention that the student receives is highly concentrated and permits the development of a more intense relationship with the teacher. She becomes more aware of the student's communication strengths and weaknesses and is better able to provide for his specific needs. The disadvantages of individual rehabilitation sessions constitute the advantages of the group system.

There are several reasons why a therapist may decide to put a group of hard-of-hearing people together in a rehabilitation program or to include an individual student in an existing group. We should, perhaps, be honest and recognize that the most common motivation for group work is generally one of economics. It is quite frequently the only way in which a therapist can train a number of hard-of-hearing persons for whom he is unable to justify the amount of time taken out by individual sessions. The reason adult groups are formed is often to make it financially possible to offer services at a reasonable fee. Let us not, however, be cynical about these motives. We are not all fortunate enough to work in a university or community clinic, where individual therapy sessions are made possible by student training needs or by a subsidy from the United Fund. The therapist, faced with the reality of the economics of financing services for the hearing-handicapped, can be reassured by the fact that there are a number of excellent reasons for using group therapy.

Although the individual training session permits a great deal of personal attention from the teacher, it nevertheless represents a communication situation in which the hard-of-hearing person is least likely to experience difficulty. The hearing-handicapped person almost invariably complains that he experiences his greatest frustration in a group situation. He finds that he is required to understand a variety of speakers with different patterns of speech and varying degrees of visibility of articulatory movements. He must be able to adapt to the constant change in speakers and the rapid progressions and shifts in conversational topics. The group situation makes it possible for him to become more familiar with the reasons for the failures that he experiences in such social situations and to learn the techniques by which he can handle these. This listening is facilitated by the fact that the type of activities that can be undertaken in a group situation are considerably broader in scope than is possible when working with an individual student. Real-life situations can be more easily structured and activities can be set upon a partner basis, so that each individual derives a great deal of feedback concerning his performance. The student also has available to him the comments and reactions of a group of people who share many of the same problems that he experiences. Furthermore, group activities stimulate a degree of competitiveness, which serves as an excellent motivation to the student members to strive more persistently to reach the communication goals of the group as a whole.

The effect of being together with people with similar problems constitutes another important advantage to be gained from the group structure. Because the problems experienced by each member will be different, the chances are that no one will experience either success or failure all the time; thus, the student is less likely to feel embarrassed by his own handicap. Instead of being the one person at a disadvantage in a communication situation, he may even find himself on occasions having understood something that the other members of the group have failed to comprehend. The mutual sympathy and cooperation that a competent therapist should be able to engender in a well-selected group does much to help the individual to reassess his problem and his reactions to it in a more realistic way. The increase in security that he is likely to experience as a result of shared difficulties can lead to a more positive approach in communication situations in the outside world.

If the teacher or therapist permits it, the group situation tends to encourage the discussion of social experiences that for the hard-of-hearing person may evoke quite intense feelings. This is a frequent occurrence when any group of people with a particular problem come together to exchange and discuss common experiences and their reactions to them. The therapeutic value that is to be found in this aspect of group activities is very important. For this reason we will defer our discussion of it until the final chapter, when we will consider it in more detail with reference to the broader aspects of rehabilitation.

The success or failure of any kind of group is heavily dependent upon the compatibility of its members. In setting up a group for aural rehabilitation, the therapist must insure that those chosen demonstrate a similar level of communication ability and share sufficient interests to make appropriate lesson activities relatively easy to structure. I recall as a student, the frustration of trying to develop some form of cohesion in a group that consisted of the elderly wives of senior faculty and three young hard-of-hearing college students. The problems arising from the incompatibility of such grouping proved to be insurmountable.

Equally difficult situations can arise if the degree of communication difficulty that the members of the group experience is markedly different. In such situations it frequently occurs that a particular student will have more difficulty in performing a task than the other class members. Although the therapist may divert her attention to helping the student to overcome his difficulty, the amount of time that she can devote to him is relatively short. She diverts her attention at the risk of losing both the continuity of the lesson and the attention of the rest of the members of the group. Thus, it becomes necessary for the lesson to continue, leaving the one member of the class disheartened by his public failure in an activity in which the other members of the class have experienced success. The effect that this can have upon his morale may be quite serious.

Therefore, whenever possible the therapist should seek to provide the student with the experience of both learning situations. Concentrated individual attention should be given whenever it is clear that the student is not yet ready for placement in a group or when he is already experiencing difficulty in group situations. However, the aim of the individual training sessions should be to equip the person to move into, or to maintain his place in, the group training session. The degree of continued individual attention that will be necessary to retain him within the group should be carefully assessed; it should be progressively decreased as the student's communication performance improves.

In this discussion we have done little more than summarize some of the major advantages and disadvantages to individual and group therapy approaches. For a more detailed consideration of these topics, the student is referred to Chaps. 9 and 10 of Oyer's book, *Auditory Communication for the Hard of Hearing* [11]. Although these chapters are directed specifically to auditory training, the evidence that they present is equally valid for any type of individual or group training session. The same comment must be made about our own discussion of this topic. Although it is included in this chapter on visual communication training, the statements made are equally applicable to the training of the student in processing auditory information. The actual placement in this chapter is simply another artifact of the unnatural dichotomy of visual and auditory processes.

ASSESSING VISUAL COMMUNICATION SKILLS

It is unlikely that the therapist or teacher will find an assessment of visual communication skills in the audiological report. This is generally concerned with the evaluation of auditory function and with the evidence upon which a diagnosis of etiology and appropriate recommendations will be made. The assessment of total communication function is generally deferred until medical attention has been provided and, where necessary, a hearing aid has been fitted. The audiologist then makes an assessment of communication ability as part of his planning of rehabilitation.

In many instances, the person receives rehabilitation training somewhere other than at the clinic where the audiological work-up was carried out. Probably one of the first tasks of the therapist will be to make an assessment of both auditory and visual communication performance. The information that is obtained by tests of visual communication skills will provide the basis for determining the amount of emphasis that needs to be placed in training the visual pathway to contribute to the total process of communication. It will also help the therapist to determine at what level of difficulty the visual communication training might begin and will serve as a yardstick against which progress may be measured.

When we discussed the assessment of auditory communication skills, we mentioned that informal evaluations, although they cannot be quantified, do provide the therapist with a general impression of the extent of the handicap in auditory communication. The same holds true for the visual aspects of communication. The first question that arises is how this assessment should be conducted. Should the tester present the material while the student is wearing his hearing aid? Should a normal voice be used, or should the therapist simply mouth the test words? In order to answer these questions we need, once again, to take a careful look at what it is that we are trying to assess. Although, on various occasions, the hard-of-hearing person may be called upon to depend entirely upon the auditory cues to speech for his comprehension of the message signal, it is highly unlikely that he will be faced with a situation in which he is deprived completely of whatever residual hearing he has and made entirely dependent upon vision as his channel of information. Thus, while we can justify isolating hearing from vision in a testing situation, it is harder to justify evaluating vision without hearing. We may ask what value would rest in a score obtained when the material was presented visually in the absence of audition? Actually, visual presentation alone provides relatively little information; however, as we have said several times previously, we must take advantage of any information available to us. Even though by itself it may not have a great deal of significance, it may contribute to the enhancement of our overall understanding of the problem. The data that we obtain when we test visual communication in isolation is important if we are to assess the effect that vision and audition have upon each other in the communication process. We shall be discussing this more fully in the next chapter; however, an example would seem relevant at this point. Presume that a student obtains a score of 60 per cent discrimination on a given test item when using the auditory channel alone and that his score, when the input is confined to the visual channel, is only 12 per cent. From these figures one might presume that the visual contribution is very small and that it does not play an important part in the student's communication function. We might expect that the score that he would obtain when vision and audition are presented simultaneously would probably be around 72 per cent; however, when we test the two channels simultaneously we may well find that the person obtains almost normal comprehension. This would indicate to us that, although the visual channel alone does not convey sufficient information to bring the material above the level of comprehension, it has a marked affect on the way in which the person is able to utilize the information coming in through the auditory channel. In another case, it might well occur that the discrimination score by the auditory channel alone is inferior to that achieved by vision. As a result of certain learning patterns or in some types of deafness involving an auditory-perceptual problem, it is possible that the integration of the two channels might result in a reduction in performance. In such instances, as John Gaeth has suggested, the addition of the acoustic stimuli may constitute a distracting factor (see Chap. 9 bibliography).

Our first measure of auditory communication performance might therefore be made in the absence of auditory cues. If one is testing in a facility that provides an acoustic suite that permits sound isolation between the tester and the student while permitting visual contact to be maintained through a window, then it is perfectly possible for the material to be read at normal conversational loudness without the student being able to hear what is being said. However, when such a facility is not available, the therapist is faced with the problem of eliminating the auditory cues. It is a well-accepted fact that the process of devoicing tends to lead to a change in the speech pattern of the tester. In particular, there is a tendency to overexaggeration of articulatory movements, which in fact serves as a distortion factor. It is therefore advisable for the therapist to avoid mouthing the words and to attempt only to reduce the amount of auditory information to a minimum. This can be achieved by asking the student to remove his hearing aid and then by presenting the material at minimal voice level. The use of minimal voice insures the retention of normal speech patterns, though the loudness is reduced to a level that forces most hard-of-hearing persons to depend almost entirely upon visual cues. Furthermore, this situation approximates the least favorable situation in which the student may find himself. For a person who has a minimal hearing loss, relatively little value is obtained from a measure of his ability to follow speech through vision alone, since a comparable situation does not normally arise in real life. With this type of case, unless sound isolation is possible, it is best to confine testing to a comparison of speech-discrimination ability through audition alone, and then through audition and vision combined.

The types of test materials used for testing and teaching visual communication skills will, for the most part, be the same as those used in auditory training; only the mode of presentation need differ. Test items should progress from evaluation of visual communication of highly redundant material to more advanced tasks requiring a much greater dependence upon visual cues. The student's ability to follow related ideas should be tested first, then if he performs well, unrelated test items can be presented. The use of objects, pictures of objects and events, or pictures of situations permits the therapist to vary the degree of complexity of the task. Visual discrimination for individual speech-sound groups can be tested by constructing test items that place heavy emphasis upon a particular group of sounds.

Formal Tests

The formal testing of visual communication ability involves the use of a standardized tool administered under controlled environmental conditions. The only way in which this can be achieved is through the use of filmed test material. The scores obtained by different subjects, or by the same subject on different occasions, can in this way be compared. O'Neill and Oyer, in Chap. 3 of their text *Visual Communication for the Hard of Hearing*, review the various filmed lipreading tests and the research data pertinent to their use [10, p. 71]. The reader is referred to this source for a detailed discussion of the available filmed tests and teaching materials. In general, it may be stated that the use of standardized test materials, as represented by these films, is essential for research into the variables involved in visible speech communication. It is also important where comparative information about the performance of groups of subjects is necessary. However, the use of filmed test materials may not be practical for the teacher or therapist responsible for only a few students, nor may she consider it necessary to obtain an exact measure of visual-perceptual ability. She may therefore need the flexibility inherent within the informal test materials but absent from the predetermined test items of the film. The therapist using a film is much more restricted in the allowances she is able to make for the language abilities of each child.

Certainly, the use of standardized film materials would seem to provide a controlled approach to the problem of evaluating visual communication ability. However, like so many other aspects of aural rehabilitation there is still an absence of conclusive research evidence to indicate the superiority of the evaluation and teaching of visual communication skills by means of film as compared to the use of informal test materials. The therapist is therefore forced to rely, more heavily than we would like to think necessary, upon empiricism. All one can do is encourage you, as a teacher or therapist, to maintain an open mind on these matters. It is important that you keep up with current research into the variables involved and that you select a method or technique that, after careful consideration, seems to you to be the most appropriate in meeting the particular needs that arise from the situation in which you are working.

METHODS AND TECHNIQUES OF VISUAL COMMUNICATION TRAINING

In Chap. 4 we said that the visible stimuli pertaining to communication may be considered conveniently under three categories:

1. Stimuli arising from the environment
2. Stimuli associated directly with the message but not part of the speech production
3. Stimuli directly related to speech sounds

Training In the Use of Stimuli Arising From the Environment

In the first category, cues arising from the environmental stimuli, we are attempting to train the person to be able to adopt an appropriate set for the communication on the basis of the constraints that one predicts the environment imposes upon the speaker. We have seen how the adoption of a particular set is closely related to the establishment of a specific figure-ground relationship. This involves concentrating attention on what are considered to be related stimuli, while permitting the remainder to constitute the ground. The resultant set should not be considered stable, since during communication the figure-ground relationship is constantly subject to trial and check, both within and between channels. The nature of visual perceptions may be markedly modified by information reaching the receiver through audition. Each sensory set is, in fact, more truly a subset of the total perceptual gestalt. The subsets must fit together in a meaningful pattern, or they will be subject to reassessment. We must consistently consider visual cues in relation to the affect that they will have upon the interpretation of oher sensory cues, and we must remember that they, in turn, will be modified by the constraints imposed by the other sensory data.

Unfortunately, there is virtually no experimental evidence available to prove that systematic training to improve awareness of situational cues improves communication performance. We still lack conclusive findings concerning what exactly goes into the successful use of visual information. We do, however, know that the amount of information that the trained eye or ear of a detective, espionage agent, or orchestra conductor is able to extract from a situation is greater than that obtained by the lay person. Most of us are well aware how much more we derive from an experience when we are oriented toward it. We benefit from the guidebook when we visit a foreign city, an art gallery, or a museum. We see more clearly the shapes of people and objects in a Picasso painting or collage when we have read about the painting beforehand, just as a course in music appreciation helps us to perceive more about a symphony or concerto. This increase in the quantity of information extracted is due to our preparedness, which permits us to adopt an appropriate set of expectancies. Thus, the reliability of our predictions is increased. Once again, therefore, we justify what we do on the basis of such empirical evidence, drawn from various similar situations and supported by a logical theoretical model.

The overlap of activities and materials used for training visual communication ability must obviously be great, since we are not dealing with different methods of communication, but only with different sets of cues—visual instead of auditory. The emphasis shifts either to the ear or the eye, depending upon the aspects of the message signal that we emphasize. A few aspects are peculiar to a particular channel, such as gross-sound-discrimination training and visual observation training; yet even these are related at all except the simplest level. Every gross sound originates from an object that can be apprehended through other senses, vision generally included, while visual observation will be influenced by what we hear. One simply cannot escape the holistic nature of the act of total perception.

Visual Awareness

A number of techniques can be used to develop visual awareness. The basic nature of these activities is illustrated by an old Boy-Scout game known as "Kim's Game." For this activity, a number of objects are placed on a tray and covered with a handkerchief or scarf. These are then placed before the viewer who is told that when the cover is removed he will have 20 seconds to observe the objects on the tray, after which they will be covered and he will be asked to recall the objects present. The task can be made progressively more difficult by increasing the number of objects that the person is to observe. As the number of items is increased, it is helpful to present them in concept groups. For example, to a pencil and pen might be added an eraser, a paper clip, an elastic band, and a small pencil sharpener, all of which might be found in a desk drawer. In this way we encourage the student to see the relationship that might exist between particular objects.

The same game can be slightly modified by permitting the student to observe the objects as before, after which, while his eyes are covered, one or two are removed. The student is then asked to observe the tray again to determine the missing objects. This makes an interesting activity for both adults and children. It can be made increasingly challenging by constituting the items from less and less familiar objects.

With very young children it helps to duplicate the objects. The child is presented with a particular selection, which he is then asked to match by memory from larger selections that he has before him. Memory for visual sequencing can be given practice by requiring that the objects not only be remembered, but that they also be placed in a line in the same order as they were shown to the child. If this is done behind a card placed between the child and the therapist's line of objects, the matching can be visually checked by the child on completion of the task (Fig. 8.1). A second brief exposure to the therapist's model may then be used to encourage the child to think again and to make necessary corrections in either the objects selected or the

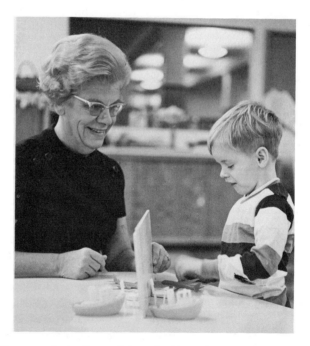

Fig. 8.1.   The use of visual matching of objects by memory seeks to improve visual retention span. (Courtesy of St. Mary's School for the Deaf, Buffalo, New York.)

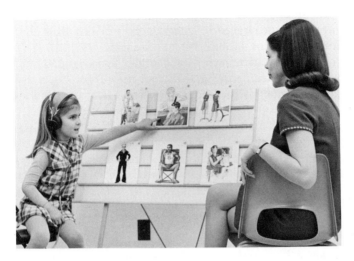

Fig. 8.2. The message to be speech read is easier if constrained by the contextual material. Here, the pictures taken from the Peabody Language Kit help the child to predict the probable nature of the message. (Photo courtesy of Department of Speech Communication, State University of New York at Buffalo.)

order of alignment. The variety of items or item groups can be greatly increased by using pictures instead of actual objects.

Another activity to stimulate observation in visual memory is to present the student with a picture of an object, person, or activity of varying complexity. The stimulus is then removed, and the student is asked either to give a detailed description of what he has observed or to answer specific questions. The technique of questioning may be used to show the student how to observe in a systematic manner. When observing, he should be taught to ask himself such questions as: "Where? How many? Who? What are they doing?" etc. The number of possible sources of pictures is almost unlimited. You should try this activity yourself in order to experience how little detail we normally record consciously. For the most part, these details constitute redundancy for which we have little need. The hard-of-hearing person, however, needs to be trained to make use of this additional source of information, which is available to him as a result of attention and the adoption of an appropriate perceptual set.

Other activities might include the use of a series of unrelated pictures to which statements obtained through watching or listening, or both, are to be related. The situational cues provided by the picture are, in this way, related to the verbal message signal. Pictures of people in various roles may be used in place of environmental pictures (Fig. 8.2). Statements are presented to the student, who attempts to relate them to the people shown. In this way, he is encouraged to integrate cues arising from the situation with those reaching him through the speech signal.

Training in the adoption of appropriate figure-ground relationships can be provided by telling the student that he will be shown a picture in which a lot of activities are occurring. He is told to ignore everything in the picture (ground) except a particular category of objects (figure). He is to attempt to identify as many as possible of the objects that fall into the category named. For example, in a picture of a man working in a garden shed, the task may be to identify all the tools that are visible, or all those tools that are used for certain purposes. Another example would be a picture of a mother in the kitchen preparing a meal. The amount of time allowed for observation can be varied. This can also be presented as a modified form of "Kim's Game," requiring the child to look for and remember only certain types of objects from the total group.

A similar activity is illustrated by the pictures in children's magazines that have embedded within them outlines of objects to be located. Such tasks appropriate to young children will be found in prereading books. Although these may be too simple for older children, the ideas they provide can be exploited by the therapist. One such activity is that of identifying incongruities in a picture. Such an activity can be modified by using groups of toy items of pictures, grouped according to concepts of varying complexity, with inclusion of an item incongruous to the idea represented.

Such activities can also be carried out using words. The subject is given a limited exposure to a group of words from which he is asked to identify specific types, such as the names of fruits, places, or professions. These words are embedded among a background of unrelated words. He may be presented with a list of words with the instructions to identify a meaningful grouping. Anagrams or sentences in which the word order has been scrambled will also help to develop an ability to organize visual information in a meaningful manner. This involves the process of closure. Activities for training this ability also appear in children's prereading books and children's magazines. They generally present a series of pictures, the last of which is omitted in order that the child can make closure himself by telling what he thinks what has occurred. The activities that were mentioned in the section on auditory training, involving the matching of captions to appropriate cartoons or of watching or listening to the reenactment of a situation and then predicting what might next have been said, are similarly involved with the process of closure. With older children and adults, incomplete sentences may be used, where the student is asked to fill in the missing words or to complete the sentence.

Jigsaw puzzles encourage the growth of visual-perceptual closure, since when a child begins to seek a particular missing piece on the basis of visual cues predicted from the completed section, the closure has already been made in the child's mind. He is simply seeking to realize this in the pattern before him. He has assessed the cues available to him, has made a predicted perception, will choose the missing piece, and will subject the piece to trial and check before being satisfied that it is appropriate to the goal before him.

Nonverbal Cues Related to the Message

It is much more difficult to provide training in the category of nonverbal cues related to the environment because of the variety of personal gestures that people use. The constraints placed upon the nonverbal communicative behavior are considerably fewer than upon verbal behavior, which makes it less predictable. Nevertheless, it does add to the total amount of information. Therefore, the student's attention should be drawn to the fact that there frequently exists a close relationship between what a person is doing and what he is saying. One can help bring these cues to the awareness of the student by planning sections of lessons to include activities that require him to predict which comments might be associated with certain roles, actions, or facial expressions. It is fairly easy to depict a series of situations to which the student can respond. The following are examples of some of the actions that may be demonstrated.

1. The therapist is writing on a pad when his pencil point breaks; he looks up to say something.
2. He reaches into his pocket, pulls out a handkerchief, and sneezes.
3. He looks at his watch.
4. He holds his watch to his ear and shakes it.
5. He loosens his tie and wipes his forehead with his handkerchief.
6. He tries to thread a needle and fails, then holds out the needle and thread to the student.
7. He tries to make marks on a piece of paper with an empty ballpoint pen.
8. He places a stamp on an envelope and hands it to the student.
9. He goes to the door, which he either opens or closes.
10. He hands the student a magazine open at a particular page and points to a paragraph.

Some therapists may find it relatively easy to imitate facial expressions appropriate to certain emotions. The student may be asked to identify these emotions and to predict statements that might be made in association with them. Most therapists, however, will find that pictures from magazines and newspapers provide a more reliable source for depicting facial expressions

(Fig. 8.3). The student is given a list of remarks, not all of which will be appropriate to the picture he will be shown. He is given a picture and asked to determine which of the comments on the list might be associated with it.

The intentional gesture is a deliberate constraint placed by the sender upon the interpretations of the message signal that the receiver might logically make. For this reason it is more highly predictable and contributes more information than do implemental activities. The role of the intentional gesture can be illustrated in the following examples.

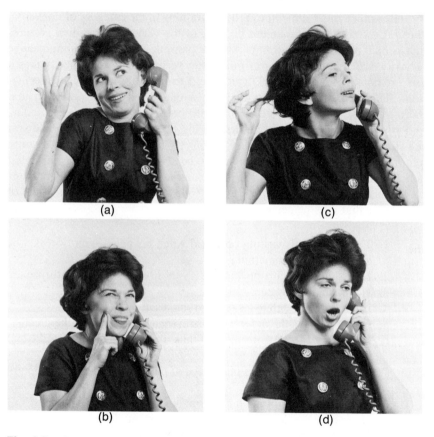

(a)   (c)

(b)   (d)

Fig. 8.3. Practice may be given in interpretation of facial expression by matching appropriate remarks to pictures. (a) recruit a den mother; (b) find a home for the last of the puppies; (c) make an appointment for a smashing new hairdo; and (d) lay down the law to the repair man. These photographs appeared as a magazine advertisement for American Telephone and Telegraph Company. (Courtesy of Ormond Gigli, Inc., New York City.)

1. The therapist says, "Would you please close the _____?" omitting the all-important final clue; however, at the same time she points to the window.
2. The therapist beckons to the student.
3. The therapist places a collection of metal screws in front of the student who is asked, "Could you give me one about this size?" The approximate size is depicted by the distance between the forefinger and thumb.
4. The student is told to ask the therapist three simple questions. To the first, the therapist shrugs her shoulders; to the second, she nods her head in the affirmative; to the third, she shakes her head quite emphatically in the negative.
5. The therapist asks the student to read from a book, pointing with a pencil where she wishes him to begin and end. He is then asked to say how much he is to read.

The scope of this activity is limited. One hopes to do little more than make the student more conscious of the value of intentional gestures. In therapy sessions, the student's attention should be drawn to these whenever they occur naturally. He may be given an assignment to keep a written record of intentional gestures that he observes being used by his family or friends in everyday communication situations.

Cues Arising from the Spoken Message Signal

The visual cues that we have considered up to this point have all been concerned with providing a framework within which the spoken message signal will be interpreted. If they have given rise to a selection of an appropriate set of expectancies by the listener, the amount of remaining information that he will need in order to correctly reproduce the spoken message signal transmitted by the speaker should be considerably less than would have been needed without the nonverbal cues. The specific information associated with the verbalized thought will be derived from the visual articulatory movements of speech. This we have seen involves the following:

Observation: the act of noticing
Discrimination: the process of elimination and choice
Integration: the combining of data into a meaningful pattern
Verification: intrasensory and intersensory trial and check
Association: the relating of previous experiences
Total perception: involving the final evaluation of the significance of the restructured message signal

Let us think about the various steps that we will need to take if we are to improve the student's ability to perform the rather difficult task of what might appropriately be referred to in this connection as "speech reading."

Motivation

Motivating a student to concentrate upon his visual communication ability can sometimes be much more difficult than achieving the same concentration in the improvement of auditory skills. Most hard-of-hearing persons, particularly adults, tend initially to refute the idea that they are able to speech read, though in most instances it is possible to varying degrees to demonstrate this to be a fact. They are unaware of the extent to which they have come to rely upon the additional information that they derive from watching the speaker. When you mention speech reading or lipreading to them, their immediate reaction is to consider this to be a difficult task that they feel doubtful about being able to perform. There is a tendency to feel that what they have come for is training to improve their hearing. They are frequently of the opinion that if they can learn to use a hearing aid well they will not need any other kind of training. For this reason, it is wise to begin by demonstrating to them the role that you will have explained vision plays in communication. This can be done by asking them to repeat a list of monosyllabic words or sentences, depending upon the amount of residual hearing the person has, read at minimal voice level without amplification or vision. A written record is kept of his performance. The same test is then repeated with the student watching the teacher, and a comparison of the scores is made. For students with severe or profound losses, the auditory stimulus alone may be presented with amplification, then vision is combined with hearing. The reaction to the observed differences between the scores obtained under the two conditions very often comes as a surprise to the person convinced that he does not lip-read.

Perhaps the most important factor in motivation is the experience of success. Early exercises in visual communication training should therefore be selected to contain high levels of visual, linguistic, and contextual redundancy. The initial aim is to demonstrate to the student that he is able to speech read, and that improvement of this skill will enhance his overall communication ability.

The Development of the Ability to Make Closure

We have already discussed the role of closure in general perception and with reference to the interpretation of the auditory signal and the nonverbal aspects of visual communication. In Chap. 3 we examined the factors that limit the amount of information inherent within the visible speech signal. We listed these as the low degree of visibility of many articulatory movements, the rapidity of movements, the similarity in their appearances, and the variations in intersubject patterns of speech-sounds production. These factors affect various sounds to different degrees, though even the easiest sentences still do not contain 100 per cent information. Our aim is to train the students to become so familiar with word or phrase gestalts that he will be capable of making closure on the basis of limited visual cues. In order for him to do this, we must train the speech reader's mind to store visual impressions in individual articulatory movements even before he has enough information to attribute meaning to them. This is one of the valuable aspects of the use of analytical procedures. We frequently find that a person who initially fails to grasp what is being said will later identify the message. This demonstrates that he has stored the visual impressions and has achieved closure on the basis of using the total visual cues within the constraints imposed by linguistic and contextual rules. It stresses the importance of training visual memory span.

The Development of Accuracy and Speed in Speech Reading

The two factors of accuracy and speed are essential to the effective use of speech reading in everyday situations. Accuracy can only be achieved by persistently working in exercises selected to train discrimination between the visual speech patterns that present the student with difficulty. There is no shortcut; material that has been learned in earlier lessons must be reviewed frequently, while discrimination of problem sounds must be repeatedly attempted.

Accuracy alone, however, it not sufficient unless it can be achieved at speed. It is rather like the typist who is able to type with 100 per cent accuracy, but who takes hours to complete a letter. Her accuracy is of no more value than the speed of another typist who types rapidly but makes numerous errors. Efficient performance only occurs when the two assets are combined. We must therefore work toward building up the rate at which the speech reader is able to process the visual information accurately. This is achieved through overlearning, which results in the whole process being so automatic that the person is aware only of the comprehension of speech. In the words of Edward Nitchie:

> The conscious effort to see the movements, to associate them with the sounds and words, seriously interferes with the understanding of the thought. It is an analytic process, whereas effort to understand the thought is a synthetic process. The brain cannot carry on two such opposite conscious processes at the same time. How difficult it would be to grasp the thought of this printed page if you stopped to think consciously of each letter or even of each word! Everyone has some sub-conscious knowledge of the movements. No one can know them perfectly, but as far their obscurity, rapidity, and

variability will allow them to be known, the knowledge should be without the consciousness of efforts. To illustrate in my own case I know them so well that in my dreams I always read the lips and cannot understand if the lips be covered or the face turned away any more than I can in my waking hours [9].

This state is achieved when the person is completely relaxed in processing visual information, confident that his mind has assumed an appropriate mental set, and is storing the information he will need to interpret the message. This only comes through training and practice. The initial apprehension, frustration, and failure, which the beginning speech reader may be expected to experience, are no different from those encountered by the beginning motorist, swimmer, pianist, or artist.

Planning Speech-Reading Lessons

Before we examine particular lesson outlines, we will do well to take note of several underlying principles discussed by Nitchie. He stresses the importance of naturalness in the presentation of all materials, cautioning against mouthing or exaggerating words and against speaking unusually slowly. These practices distort the natural speech pattern and do not provide experience in the type of speech reading that the student will need for normal encounters. He reminds us that the temporary improvement in performance that may initially result from such behavior is only obtained at the expense of making the ultimate success in speech reading more difficult.

The second principle that Nitchie stresses is thoroughness. By this, he refers to the persistence and tenacity that both student and teacher must show in repeatedly returning to the difficult task. Repetition of exercises must occur both within the training sessions and from session to session, until those reasonable goals that have been set are obtained. Since we are seeking to train the student to use the incoming visual stimuli to improve his ability to respond appropriately to speech communication, it is necessary to guard against the tendency that he will have to simply repeat what is said to him rather than to respond to it. This reaction is understandable, since it is something we all tend to do when we are uncertain that we have understood what has been said. Just as you are about to leave the house, a member of your family calls downstairs.

> Pick up two cartons of cigarettes while you're at the drugstore.
> Two cartons of cigarettes?

With this response to the request, you are seeking verification that you have received the message signal correctly. We have already referred to the lack of self-confidence that a person experiences in performing a new task. The beginning speech reader will often manifest this by repeating what he thinks a speaker has said. Unfortunately, the teacher may use this repetition as a means of verifying that the student has understood, thus reinforcing an undesirable pattern of communicative behavior. Furthermore, as Nitchie points out, it tends to develop an analytical rather than a synthetic pattern of thinking, in which the student is more concerned with accuracy of word recognition than he is in grasping the concept as a whole. The student, therefore, should be encouraged in most activities to give an appropriate response to what is said to him. If he is asked a question, he should give the answer. If he is truly in doubt about what has been said, he should be trained to tell the speaker that this is the case: "I'm sorry I didn't understand." The wisdom in rejecting the repetition form of feedback lies in the fact that it forces the student to decide either that he has enough information to respond appropriately, or that he must respond in a manner that will give rise to further information being provided by the other party.

Finally, Nitchie advocates that the teacher should insure a varied approach to the development of communicative skills. He, too, argues for a holistic approach to communication training rather than one that concentrates upon a particular aspect (lipreading) with a single purpose in view. He suggests that with a little thought almost all activities can be used to achieve several different beneficial results. Throughout a lesson, every possible opportunity should be taken to exploit each aspect of the process of communication as it arises. The flexibility that permits such vital digression from a lesson plan should be fundamental to rehabilitation.

We shall now examine some of the approaches to lesson planning that are commonly used by teachers. However, remember that the approach that you decide to use should be based on your own theoretical model, derived from what you have read about communication and what you will learn from the experience of working with the hearing-handicapped.

There are three major ways in which visual and auditory communication training can be approached. These are the informal approach, the formal approach, and the correlated approach.

Although it is possible to structure a lesson or a whole series of lessons exclusively within one of these frameworks, where appropriate it proves more interesting and more valuable to the student to be exposed to two or three approaches.

The Informal Approach

The informal approach involves the least structure and, therefore, accords the greatest flexibility. This does not mean that there is an absence of structure but that it applies only to the activity as a whole, not to the individual components. For this reason it is particularly appropriate for use with children. The method involves teaching the basic principles of visual and auditory communication, or both, in a nondirective manner. This is achieved through setting up situations and, through the use of games and stories, training the children to watch, to notice visible differences between words and phrases, to make guesses based upon synthesis, to remember, and to concentrate. Many of the activities that were suggested for auditory training of young children lend themselves equally well to visual communication training. We simply let the children watch instead of listen. The intriguing object that we placed in the bag for the children to identify must now be recognized on the basis of visual rather than auditory speech cues. The teacher encourages the habit of watching by gaining the child's visual attention before she speaks. In this way she insures the reception of the visible cues from the beginning of the message. In teaching very young children to recognize the spoken names of objects, holding the object up to the face will make sure that both the object and the articulatory movements associated with its name fall within the child's visual field.

In the early stages of visual communication training you must make sure that the child's attention is not distracted from your face by something else that you are doing, even though this may be related to what you are talking about. For example, when you are showing a picture, the book should be held almost at face level so that both can be seen at the same time. When this is not possible, the picture should be shown first, then the spoken message should be given, and finally the picture should be shown again. If you talk about something that necessitates the child looking away while you are speaking, you deprive him of the added information available in the visible speech cues. For the same reason, when you are referring to something you have written on the blackboard or have placed in a card holder, you should not begin talking until you have completed what you are doing and have turned toward the student. Teachers who have the unfortunate habit of talking while they are actually writing on the board—a bad teaching technique under any circumstances—place the hard-of-hearing child at a serious disadvantage.

There are many informal situations that a teacher might utilize for the teaching of auditory and visual communication. For example, a play situation might be introduced in which a toy doll is bathed and dressed. Verbalization of what is happening is provided by the teacher who, each time, makes sure that the child is watching before she speaks. Simple instructions and requests are given at minimal voice levels.

> We'll need some soap. Can you find the soap for me?
> The wash cloth is too wet; squeeze out some of the water.
> Don't forget to wash her ears.

I think she got some soap in her eyes.
Now she's all clean. Take her out of the bath and wrap her in a towel.
Are you sure she is quite dry? (Fig. 8.4)

Similar directions can be given with regard to dressing the doll. It may be necessary first to provide a lesson to teach visual recognition of the names of various body parts, of the items used in bathing the doll, and of the various items of clothing. This should not be done by the use of stilted techniques, such as simply asking the child to point to the various objects named. When we place the name of the object in a sentence, we are using normal speech with a high degree of redundancy. We may, for example, first say the name of the object "shoes" and then say, "We must put her shoes on her feet. Where are her shoes?"

Another example of teaching auditory and visual communication through informal situations is to devote a lesson to making something. This is particularly useful where a number of children are involved. We may decide to make a paper hat, a mailman's bag, or even play-dough. First, we will talk about all the things that we are going to use. We might play

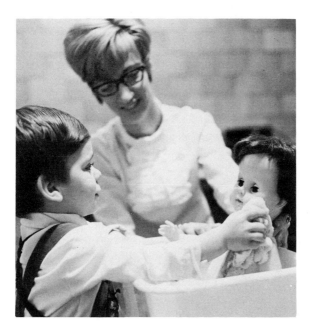

Fig. 8.4.   Informal lessons in visual communication may be structured around a play activity. (Courtesy of St. Mary's School for the Deaf, Buffalo, New York.)

"Kim's Game," with some of the items emphasizing visual cues. We will talk about the other things for which some of the other items might be used. Having insured that the children are able to speech read the important cue words, we may then begin the activity, providing visual cues at each stage of the process and always remembering to attract the children's attention before speaking. We shall also use the technique of verbalizing what the children are doing. This is meaningful communication to them and provides overlearning of the important words and phrases. We may ask a particular child what another child is doing.

> Today we are going to make play-dough.
> How many of you play with play-dough at home?
> Mary, what color play-dough do you have at home?
> Let's see what we need to make play-dough.
> What is this white stuff, John?
> Taste it. You still don't know?
> Let me tell you something about it.
> We get it from wheat; the baker uses it to make bread. We can also make paste with it if we mix it with water.
> Yes, that's right; it's flour.
> David, you'll know what this is if you taste it.
> That's right; it's salt.
> Mary, what do we use salt for?
> We also need water—one cupful.
> How much do we need, Mary? That's right. We are going to use one cup of water, one cup of flour, and this much salt—that's one-third of a cup.
> Three-thirds make a whole cup, but we only need one-third. David, can you measure one cup of flour?
> Mary, you measure one cup of water.
> John, show me one-third of a cup.
> Right. Now, will you mix them all together in a bowl and stir them with a spoon.
> Now it's mixed, we're going to knead it with our hands, just like when the baker makes bread.
> That word's the same as when you *need* something—like you need to go to bed when you are tired or you need to clean your teeth after your meals.
> This word looks and sounds the same. *Knead.*
> John, it's your turn to knead the dough now.
> Now we will make three piles of dough.
> That's one-third, that's one-third, and that's one-third.
> We will put the first one back in the bowl, and we're going to color it red with this special food color.
> Now the next one yellow, and the next one green.
> Now we've made play-dough.
> When we're finished playing with it, if we wrap it up tightly in a plastic bag, it won't get hard.

Such an activity as this provides abundant opportunities for the teacher to teach new vocabulary and language skills and to provide practice in the visual recognition of familiar and newly acquired words. The activity is naturally very stimulating, and the motivation to watch comes from a genuine involvement in what the children are doing. Learning of various types takes place, and speech communication, utilizing visual cues, becomes an integral part of learning through doing rather than an isolated exercise that, for young children, rapidly becomes boring. The scope of the informal lesson, using both visual and auditory presentations, is as large as the child's experiences. All the things that an enterprising mother or a nursery school or first-grade teacher will want to do for children with normal hearing are equally appropriate for the hard-of-hearing child.

Guessing games are much enjoyed by young children, and lessons can be built around such topics as animals.

I am very small.	Am I large or small?
I live in a hole in the wall.	Where do I live?
I like cheese for my supper.	What do I like for my supper?
I live in a hole in a tree.	Where do I live?
People say I'm very wise.	What do people say about me?
I can see in the dark.	What can I do in the dark?
I have a soft, woolly coat.	What kind of a coat do I have?
I follow my mistress wherever she goes.	Whom do I follow?
One day I followed her to school.	Where did I go one day?

Another type of lesson can be developed by giving to each of the children in the class three pictures or, if they are able to read, the written names of three things. The students are told that you will be saying some things about each of the pictures, but that what you say will always be wrong. They have to watch carefully to find out whether what you are saying is about one of the cards that they have and then to tell you why what you have said is wrong. For example, the statements might be:

Most people like salt in their coffee.
Owls have very small eyes.
We pick apples in the spring.
We write with a carrot.
An airplane sails on the ocean.

Practice of specific words can be provided by including those words in each of the sentences. Groupings, such as animals, occupations, days of the week, or various foods, that may have already been studied can be used.

Concentrated practice on the recognition of particular speech sounds can also be provided through an informal approach. In order to do this, the therapist will need to select a group of pictures, each of which contains a particular sound with which she wishes to provide the child practice in recognizing. She will also need a second list that will provide a contrast sound. The pairs are numbered and the matching pair of numbers placed in a paper bag. One at a time, the children are asked to come up and pick from the bag a number that will identify the pair of words between which they will discriminate. The child is told that you will say something about one of these two pictures and that what you say will contain the name of the item represented. First, the names of the items are spoken one after the other several times in order to permit the child to observe the contrast between the articulatory movements involved in saying the two names. Then he is given a sentence about the object. Initially, the required response may simply be correct identification. When the child is able to differentiate between the objects fairly easily, then the task can be made more difficult by asking him not only to identify the object, but also to respond to what you have said. When the children are able to do this, the activity can be modified by simply removing the contrast word and asking the child to identify a picture on the basis of the sentence. The pictures used are selected to give further recognition practice for the articulatory movements being worked on.

Every small child enjoys being told a story. It is easy for the therapist to capitalize on this motivation by using story telling to give speech-reading practice. No story should be told to young children without ample illustrative material, since this provides the situational constraints about which we talked earlier and enhances the child's interest in the task. Criteria for selecting appropriate books were mentioned in the chapter on auditory training. For younger children, the importance of selecting books that contain clear, simple illustrations is again stressed. As the complexity of the picture increases, the probability of making accurate predictions decreases, making it more difficult for the child to make use of situational constraints. We should also remember that very few of the stories written for children can simply be read to the hard-of-hearing child. It is necessary to go over the story carefully before the lesson and to rephrase it according to the language level of the children. Key words that may be unfamiliar to the children or that are difficult to speech read should be taught before the story is presented. In telling the story, the therapist should allow the children to look at each illustration first and then tell them to watch the story teller closely while she tells about the picture. Questions or comments that arise from the children as the story progresses should be encouraged, since this means that they are involving themselves in a communicative situation. They should also be encouraged to seek more information concerning things about which they may not be certain, to find out more about things that interest them, and to relate them to their own personal experiences. When the story has been told, it is often wise to provide a synopsis of it. Comprehension may be tested through a series of questions. For beginning speech readers these questions should follow the same sequence as the story. Since we know that breaking up the exact context within which the question is asked makes speech reading more difficult, the advance speech-reading student may be asked questions in a nondevelopmental pattern, jumping around in the story sequence.

A modification of story-telling activities can be achieved with sequenced pictures such as are available in the See-Quees series [13]. The complete story is first told with the pictures in order. The pieces are then removed and mixed up. The story is then retold, with each child taking a turn to select the next appropriate piece as the teacher describes it. The children should be told that what you are saying may not necessarily be about the item that should go next and that, for this reason, they will have to watch you carefully to make sure that you don't make a mistake. This provides the children with motivation for paying attention to what you are saying. As with the storybook, more advanced children can learn to identify parts of the story out of order. The sequence cards by Developmental Learning Materials serve the same purpose (Figs. 8.5 and 8.6).

Stories can also be used to train the child in the ability to make closure by presenting a series of pictures illustrating key items or people in the

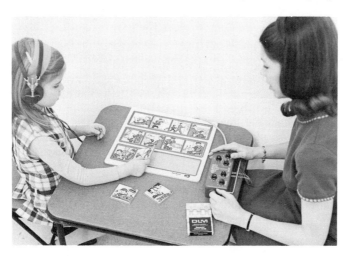

Fig. 8.5. The Judy See-Quees boards are being used with this child to combine visual communication training with language development. (Courtesy of Department of Speech Communication, State University of New York at Buffalo.)

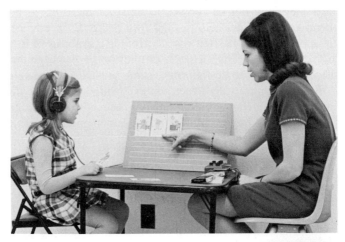

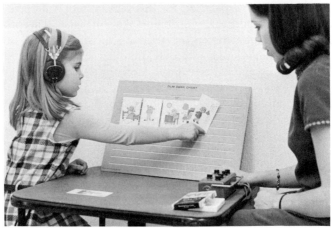

Fig. 8.6.   The Sequential Picture Cards, published by Developmental Learning Materials, are being used as stimulus materials for visual communication and language training. (Courtesy of Department of Speech Communication, State University of New York at Buffalo.)

stories and then giving sufficient cues for the child to be able to predict the completion of the sentence about them. For example, in a story about a farm, the pictures of the farmer, his wife, and the people who work on the farm and the pictures of the animals and farm buildings may provide the stimulus material. The story may then be built up in the following manner:

It was early morning. The farmer was awakened by the crowing of the _____. He had many things to do. He had to milk the _____, which would still be in the _____. Then he had to feed them some _____. While he was milking and feeding the cows, his wife would be giving corn to the _____. It is soon time for the breakfast. The farmer is hungry. For breakfast he eats a bowl of _____, two fried _____, and three pieces of _____, and he drinks several cups of hot black _____.

It will be clear to you now that there is, in fact, no such thing as an informal lesson plan. The informality refers to the method the therapist uses to achieve the goals of visual communication training. It is the difference between, for example, the freedom of the Montessori method of teaching young children and the more formal approach used in many public schools. Both methods are seeking to achieve the same end, though the way in which they go about it is different. Because in the informal approach the children are not conscious of the underlying principles that lie behind the type of activities in which they are being encouraged to take part, it is absolutely essential that the therapist should at all times be conscious of what it is she is seeking to achieve with a particular activity and the way in which the activity serves her purpose. In brief, before you decide to choose a particular activity, know exactly why you are doing so.

The Formal Lesson Plan

As one might expect, formal lipreading lessons are highly structured. They set out to achieve visual communication goals in a direct manner. The lesson is divided into separate units, each of which concentrates upon a particular aspect of visual communication. The following outline is based upon the approach suggested by Nitchie, but modified to include some of the principles advocated by the other major schools that we have discussed.

In Chap. 3 we discussed the problem that is presented to the lip-reader by the factor of homopheneity. You will recall that this refers to the close similarity in the visible articulatory movements (revealing movements) that cause some sounds, which differ in auditory characteristics, to appear the same visually. We pointed out that homopheneity may apply to groups of phonemes and to words, as well as to individual phonemes. Table 8.1 shows clusters of homophenous consonants, together with a description of the revealing movement. Alice Streng has suggested that homophenous words can be identified by using a chart in which an "initial consonant-vowel to word-ending comparison" may be made to establish which combinations are meaningful [23]. This is illustrated in Table 8.2. The formal lesson plan takes the factor of homopheneity into account in the manner in which sounds are grouped according to revealing characteristics.

STAGE ONE. INCREASING AWARENESS OF ARTICULATORY MOVE-MENTS. Our first stage is devoted to increasing the student's awareness of the revealing characteristics of specific movements. Though we are con-

TABLE 8.1. Revealing Movements Associated with Homophenous Phonemes

PHONEMES	REVEALING CHARACTERISTICS
p b m	Lips come together and are released through the following phoneme movement. In the final position before a pause, the lips are relaxed after the air pressure is released.
f v	Lower lip is brought into light contact with upper teeth.
θ ð	Slight protrusion of tongue; lip between teeth.
ʃ tʃ dʒ	Lip rounding and lip protrusion.
s z	Lips spread slightly; teeth visible. This revealing movement is noticeably influenced in character by the succeeding phoneme movement.
t d l n	Lips open in neutral position; elevation of tongue; lip to alveolar ridge may be visible.
k g ŋ	Lips open in neutral position; elevation of back of tongue to soft palate barely visible.
j	Lips open in neutral position; forward movement of tongue in assuming articulatory position may be slightly visible between the teeth.
h	No revealing movement.

cerned with movements rather than articulatory positions, groups of sounds do have peculiar revealing characteristics. Nitchie urges the teacher to describe the revealing features of the various sounds in order to define the student's knowledge more specifically. To illustrate this he suggests that we have all observed a cow's horns, but that few of us could say offhand whether the horns are above, below, in front of, or behind the ears. An artist, on the other hand, could tell you, because he is obliged to observe definitely. Nitchie says that the student should in the same manner be obliged to observe definitely the distinctive features of the articulatory movement. We should emphasize whatever is visible and ignore all aspects that are not.

Our explanation of the revealing characteristics of, for example, the movement that is visible in the production of /p, b, m/ would be

'For /p/ as in pay, apple, and cup
/b/ as in ball, table, and cab
/m/ as in my, summer, and home,

the lips are placed together and opened onto the movement that follows. When the movement occurs at the end of a word, before a pause, the lips may simply relax instead of opening onto the next sound. For example:

Can you read this *map*?
I just got *home*.
Do you like corn on the *cob*?'

TABLE 8.2. A Method for Determining Homophenous Words.* Illustration of the Technique Used in Combination With the Vowel æ

VOWEL æ

WORD ENDINGS

	p	b	m / t	d	n	nt	nd	l / f	v / θ	ð / s	z / ʃ	tʃ	dʒ / k	g	ŋ
p			pam pat	pad	pan	pant	panned		path	pass		patch	pack		pang
b			bat	bad	ban		band banned		bath	bass	bash	batch	badge back		bang
m	map		mat	mad	man		manned			mass	mash	match	Madge Mac		
t	tap	tab			tan		tanned						tack	tag	tang
d		dab		dad	Dan										
n		nab	gnat		Nan								knack	nag	
l	lap	lamb		lad			land	laugh		lass	lash	latch	lack	lag	
f			fat	fad	fan		fanned							fag	fang
v			vat		van										
θ															
ð			that		than							thatch			
s	sap		Sam sat	sad			sand		salve	sass			sack	sag	sang
z															
ʃ			sham			shout		shall					shack		
tʃ	chap		chat			chant									
dʒ		jab	jam								jazz		jack	jag	
k	cap	cab	cam cat	cad	can	cant	canned								
g	gap														
ŋ															

*From a suggestion made by Alice Streng at a lecture given at State University of New York at Buffalo.

STAGE TWO. RECOGNITION OF ARTICULATORY MOVEMENTS. Having defined and drawn the student's attention to the articulatory movements, the second stage provides the initial practice in the recognition of these movements. By the inclusion of rhythm practice, as suggested by the Jena method, this stage also attempts to incorporate into the total perception of the sound the motor-kinesthetic impressions associated with its production.

The movement for /p/ /b/ /m/ is one of the first to be studied. The contrast movements have been selected because they are distinctly different and have high visibility. For a more advanced lesson, the contrast movements should be selected from those previously studied. In this way, previously learned material can be reviewed, while insuring that only one new item is presented at a time.

she	fee	pea	shed	fed	bed
shy	fie	by	ship	fin	pin
show	foe	mow	shine	fine	mine

There are several things to note about the lists of words. For beginning lessons it is helpful to hold the vowel in each group constant. This pemits the student to concentrate his attention on comparing the consonants. Once he has become fairly confident in speech reading the movement words in each unit of three, then they should be presented so as to vary the accompanying vowel. For example, from the first unit one might present:

she	foe	buy
show	foe	pea
shy	fee	mow

Note that in each case the movement being studied occurs in the third word in the list. In more advanced lessons this insures that the student is always presented with familiar movements first, followed by the more difficult new movement. After practice, the order of the movement words can be rearranged to deprive him of this reassurance.

Movement words should also be given in which the movement being studied occurs at the end instead of the beginning of the word.

which	wife	whip
cash	cough	cab
leash	leaf	gleam

Note also that practice is given in recognizing the movement in combination with various vowels. This is out of respect for what we know about the effect that transitions have on speech sounds. We attempt to expose the student to the various modifications that transitions will have on the speech movement being studied.

Practice should initially be given by asking the student to watch the teacher carefully as she reads the lists of words previously written on the blackboard. She should first present them full-face and then at an angle of 45° to permit a semiprofile view. When the therapist is working with an individual student, it helps to sit before a large mirror and to have the student repeat the words after her. This provides simultaneous visual and motor-kinesthetic impressions, which it is hoped will strengthen the total perception of the movement. Mirror practice of words may be made part of the one assignment to augment the class work.

The teacher should avoid the tendency to move too quickly from the movement words to the third stage, which involves practice words. We have agreed that underlying the gestalt is the ability to recognize the individual movements that constitute a word or a phrase. Adequate practice should be devoted to this second stage, constantly remembering that our aim is to achieve accuracy at speed. As the student's familiarity with the movement words grows, the rate of presentation should increase until he is able to correctly recognize them with considerable rapidity. You have achieved success when he is able to sit back in his chair and, in a relaxed manner, identify the words as they are spoken to him, regardless of the pattern in which they are presented.

STAGE THREE. PRACTICE WORDS. This section further utilizes the aspects of visual training that will have been developed for a particular movement in stage two. This newly learned movement will also be presented in a variety of different vowel-consonant combinations. From this stage will be developed stage four, which consists of a series of sentences built around the practice words. For this reason, in choosing the words you should be careful to insure that they are within the student's vocabulary or that you have taught him their meanings, so that he will recognize them when you use them in the sentence practice. Following are our practice words for this lesson.

PRACTICE WORDS

pancake	milk	tame	cub
baseball	paint	lamp	wrap
peal	money	lamb	lip
male	peach	seam	rope
mask	brine	shape	dam

Once again, the words are first read one line at a time to the student while he watches carefully. He may then read the list himself for mirror practice, and finally read them together with the therapist to provide the motor-kinesthetic practice. Then, taking a line at a time, individual words are presented for speech-reading practice. Several combinations of the words in a given line may be presented. When this has been done with each of the lines, the student is told that the therapist will say one or two words from a line and he is to identify the group of four from which these come.

Finally, you can break up the predictability completely by simply combining, in any order, any of the words from the twenty present. The same task can be made somewhat easier by limiting the number of words from which the combinations will be drawn, for example, to the first and last column or the second and last column.

All of this involves training in visual retention and recall. Further emphasis of this aspect of communication training can be provided by progressively increasing the number of words in a presentation.

STAGE FOUR. SENTENCES UTILIZING PRACTICE WORDS. Stage four consists of a list of sentences utilizing the practice words. Initially, each practice word is identified for the student before he is given the sentence that will contain it. Later on, sentences can be presented without previously identifying the practice words. The difficulty of this task will be increased as the number of items from which his choice must be made is increased.

1. What do you need to make pancakes?
2. How much milk will we need for the pancakes?
3. What time do you get up?
4. What baby animal do we call a cub?
5. What is the name of a famous baseball team?
6. What color do most people paint a house?
7. What do we call the lamp that stands outside a house?
8. What do we wrap a baby in?
9. What is the easiest way to peel an orange?
10. What would you do if you won a lot of money?
11. What do we get from a lamb?
12. What does a man sometimes wear on his upper lip?
13. Tell me the name of a male movie star?
14. Which is the peach state?
15. What is the seam of a garment?
16. Where would you expect to find a tightrope?
17. At what kind of a ball would you wear a mask?
18. What would you need to make brine?
19. What shape is an orange?
20. Tell me the name of a famous dam in the United States?

You will note that each of the sentences has been presented in question form. The reason for this is to avoid developing the habit of simple repetition of what is said. The student is required to respond to the question he is asked, thus permitting the therapist to ascertain that he has understood the communication. Once the habit of responding appropriately has been developed, it is possible to present lesson activities that use the practice words in sentences in which one would normally have to rely upon repetition in order to ascertain that comprehension has occurred. However, in later stages of visual communication training, when the relationship has been established between the teacher and the student, there is no need to make this check constantly. One can rely upon the student to indicate to the teacher that he has or has not understood. This can in itself be an essential part of training since it shifts the responsibility for deciding that he has correctly identified the message to the student, which is what will occur in a normal communication situation. A modification of the technique is to provide the student with 20 cards, on each of which is written an answer appropriate to one of the questions; the student responds by selecting an appropriate answer. This is easier than responding to the question directly, since the answers limit the possible questions that the student needs to anticipate. The same method can be used, but instead of the student having the answers, the teacher can ask the question and then hold up the answer cards one at a time, asking the student to determine whether each one is appropriate or inappropriate. Finally, the teacher can present the answers, asking the student to identify the appropriate question. A more synthetic approach to the use of sentences in speech-reading training involves the use of the practice words as key words to a series of related sentences that, as far as possible, emphasize the movement being studied. For example:

> pancake
> Mother often makes pancakes for breakfast.
> She mixes milk, flour, and eggs to make the batter.
> She cooks the pancakes in butter.
> I prefer the buckwheat mix best.

> baseball
> Baseball is a very popular game in America.
> Every year the baseball teams compete in a World Series.
> My favorite team is the Boston Red Sox.

Other ways of providing sentence practice include activities that require the student to identify the content of the sentence as true or false, to provide the opposite of the statement given, or to complete a sentence. These may pertain to a particular topic of interest to the student, or they may be unrelated statements, which are harder to predict. For a businessman, a series of questions or statements might well be devised around a newspaper report concerning the stock market. The student is asked to respond to the questions or statements, or verify them where necessary, by consulting the report and by examining statements and questions pertaining to such things as the price of particular commodities, whether a commodity has risen or fallen in value, bull and bear markets, dividends, mutual funds, etc. Requiring the student to respond with a meaningful comment avoids the problem of using repetition as a form of response. This type of activity bridges the gap between the speech reading of sentences constructed to emphasize heavily a particular movement and the ability to follow the connected discourse.

The anecdote may be used as a method of training the student to follow progressively developing ideas. In selecting the anecdote, care should be taken to insure the story line develops as simply and quickly as possible, uncomplicated by an abundance of less relevant details. This may necessitate rewriting material to eliminate all but the salient points. An attempt should also be made to rewrite the material into the style of spoken English rather than that of the written form. Key words, including proper nouns, and new vocabulary should be gone over before the anecdote is presented. Comprehension can be tested by using a question-and-answer technique.

In a group activity, the teacher and one of the members of the group can set up a dialogue situation, reading the lines from a script. Such a story as the following might be used:

A minister's son is introducing the new deacon to his hard-of-hearing father.
Son: Father, I'd like you to meet our new deacon.
Father: New dealer?
Son: No, no, not new dealer, Father, new deacon. He is the son of a bishop.
Father: (nodding wisely) They all are.

The formal approach to lesson planning, in spite of its structure, should not detract the teacher from grasping every opportunity to meet the needs, as they arise, both of individual students and of the group. She should be ready to digress from the prepared material whenever the opportunity occurs to teach any aspect of communication skills.

The formal lipreading lesson is traditionally thought of as an approach applicable for use with older children and adults. However, it has been found that, providing the materials are prepared and selected with careful attention to interests and vocabulary, an enthusiastic response can be obtained by this approach to visual communication training with children as young as nine or ten years of age. The key to success with this type of lesson underlies all aspects of teaching—namely, the sincerity and, particularly, the enthusiasm of the teacher. If the activity can be made enjoyable, the students will participate and they will learn.

The Correlated Approach

The correlated approach to teaching visual communication skills evolves from the recognition that, although the hard-of-hearing child faces a communication problem that results initially from an impairment of auditory input, the problem is rapidly compounded by an ever-increasing language comprehension gap. Deficiencies in vocabulary and syntax result in deficiencies in language concepts upon which the major part of successful communication is dependent. When we provide training in auditory and visual communication skills, we must recognize that we are working only with the first stage of the process. The success of our attempts to improve communication will depend upon how well the student is able to establish a meaningful concept from the verbal directions that he will receive.

The correlation in this approach is between training in the techniques of visual communication skills and the broadening of language concepts. Where appropriate, communication training is also correlated with the provision of specialized knowledge in particular scholastic subjects. In the latter case, lessons may preview or review academic subject matter in which the need for help is anticipated. The teacher or therapist sets out to cover the major concepts that will be encountered in a particular classroom lesson. Using both visual and auditory stimulation, she will go over with the student any vocabulary that may be new to him, or that might be difficult to discriminate or speech read. Visual and auditory discrimination training is then carried out with these words, which are presented in isolation and in appropriate sentences and phrases. In this way, the child has an opportunity to learn to recognize the visual and auditory aspects of the spoken word and to become familiar with the meanings usually attributed to it. This is made possible not only because the child has far greater contact with the teacher than is possible in the normal classroom situation, but also because, in the therapy situation, the material is presented in a way more appropriate to the hearing-impaired child's needs. It may be presumed that the teacher will have made every effort to obtain the best available physical situation for learning to occur and that she will make maximum use of auditory and visual aids. Key words and contextual cues will be presented and frequent checks made to insure that comprehension has occurred. The students are encouraged to use the dictionary as a constant source of definition of new words and are given practice in identifying the correct and incorrect use of those words, as well as to identify them when they are seen and heard in speech. The teacher also goes over the pronunciation of new words and provides mirror practice, seeking to establish an auditory-visual motor-kinesthetic gestalt (Fig. 8.7).

Unlike the teacher of children with normal hearing, you must constantly be on the alert to build relationships between words and phrases that occur in the lesson and other concepts with which the child with normal hearing is presumed to be familiar. The regular classroom teacher is primarily concerned with the imparting of information. You must, in addition, be concerned with the establishment of language concepts, particularly with the subtle aspects of speech communication that are generally completely beyond the comprehension even of children with only moderate losses.

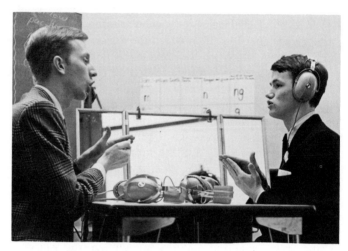

Fig. 8.7. The teacher seeks to reinforce word recognition by establishing an auditory-visual motor kinesthetic gestalt. (Courtesy St. Mary's School for Deaf, Buffalo, N.Y.)

Where the therapy session is designed to preview academic material to be presented in the regular class, an attempt should be made to provide the hearing-impaired child with information that his classroom peers may not have covered. This gives the child the experience of being able to contribute to the classroom lesson, and it reduces the sense of isolation that he may begin to feel as a result of his communication difficulty.

The following is an example of a lesson using the correlated approach. From this, it will be apparent that it is very difficult to indicate on paper how this type of lesson differs from a regular classroom lesson, since the difference is not so much in the content as it is in the techniques by which it is presented.

CORRELATED LIPREADING PLAN

Reading-age
    level: 6–9 years.
    Subject: People's homes in other lands.

Introduction: The material is designed to prepare the children for a social-studies lesson to be taught in the regular classroom. The topic includes a consideration of why people have come to build homes and why they differ in various parts of the world. Different kinds of shelters will be studied in relation to the parts of the world in which they are found, the regional climatic conditions, the pattern of life of the people, and the supply of available building materials.

Materials. A large map of the world, a globe if available, and a map of the United States will be needed. Pictures and photographs of various kinds of shelters will be used as visual aids, together with color slides or film strips, if available. Some of the raw materials out of which homes may be built, for example, brick, wood, clay, straw, a twig with leaves on, and perhaps even some ice cubes from the school kitchen will enrich the children's concepts.

Methods. The lesson begins with a general discussion of the types of houses in which the children live. They can discuss the materials out of which they are constructed and the purpose the house serves. The concept of protection against the elements, against animals, and against other people will be considered. The factor of climate will then be discussed in more detail.

The types of climate and the names of the climatic zones will be written on the blackboard, and the associated areas found on the map. The names of some of the countries to be found in each zone will also be written up, together with words describing the type of scenery one would find, such as sand, mountains, snow and ice, or swamps. Visual and auditory training is then given to insure that the children are able to recognize the word when it is spoken. The words are first read aloud after the children watch and listen to the therapist say them, and then they are identified in isolation and in appropriate sentences both with and without visual cues. The discussion may then center around what types of homes you might build in particular areas, what you would need protection against, and the materials available to you in meeting these needs. Pictures depicting actual homes from the areas being discussed can then be shown to the children, adding such words as follows:

eskimo	thatch	oasis
lapps	stilts	swamp
bushmen	bamboo	desert
troglodytes	abode	rain-forest
pygmies	sampan	mountain cave

The lesson may be concluded with a series of visual and auditory training activities, which also serve to check on the learning that has occurred. The teacher may make a series of statements about the lesson content, asking the children to judge them as true or false. If the statement is false, the child should then be asked to correct it.

The Eskimo's home is made of adobe.
Thatched roofs keep out the rain.

Houses built on stilts protect the inhabitants either from wild animals or water.
Nomadic tribesmen build houses on stilts.
Norway is in the subtropical zone.

Sentences may also be presented in simple question form requiring a response from the student. Another method might require the student to listen to a statement by the teacher and then to respond with another piece of information about the same topic.

It should be clear from the previous discussion that *the purpose of the correlated lesson is twofold: namely, to open up the avenues through which information can reach the children and at the same time to develop the language concepts essential to the utilization of that information.*

In concluding our discussion of visual communication training, it must be stressed that the three approaches that have been outlined constitute little more than illustrations of the different frameworks within which training in visual and, indeed, in auditory training skills can occur. The value inherent within each approach can only be assessed in terms of the effectiveness with which it achieves the ultimate goal of improving overall communication. Fortunately, you are not required to commit yourself to any one of them. You may decide to use each of the approaches as distinct parts of a series of lessons, or you may choose to combine certain aspects of each approach into a particular lesson plan. To these types of lessons should be added activities that involve such tasks as recognizing familiar or new proverbs, colloquialisms, synonyms and antonyms, and rhymes or riddles. You should make use of every available activity and technique that may serve to provide training in any aspect of communication. It must, however, constantly be borne in mind that whenever you are working with young people the reinforcement of language concepts constitutes as important a role as the provision of training in the use of the channels through which the directions to select these concepts will be received.

REFERENCES

1. Bruhn, Martha. *The Mueller-Waller Method of Lipreading for the Hard of Hearing.* (7th ed.) Washington, D. C.: The Volta Bureau, 1960.

2. Bunger, Anna M. *Speech Reading: Jean Method.* Danville, Ill.: The Interstate Press, 1944.

3. DeLand, Fred. *The Story of Lipreading, its Genesis and Development.* Revised and completed by Harriet Andrews Montague. Washington, D. C.: Alexander Graham Bell Association for the Deaf, 1968.

4. Developmental Learning Materials. Chicago: Scott, Foresman & Company, Educational Publishers.

5. Kinzie, Cora, and Rose Kinzie. *Lip Reading for Children (Grade I, II, III).* Seattle, Wash.: n.p., 1936.

6. Kinzie, Cora. *Lip Reading for the Deafened Adult.* Chicago: The John Winston Company, 1931.

7. Luzerne, Rae. "A Monument to Heinicke." *American Annals of the Deaf* 1(1848): 166–70.

8. Luzerne, Rae. "Thomas Braidwood." *American Annals of the Deaf* 3 (1851): 255–56.

9. Nitchie, Edward B. *Lipreading: Principles and Practice.* New York: Frederick A. Stokes Company, 1912.

10. O'Neill, J., and H. Oyer. *Visual Communication for the Hard of Hearing.* Englewood Cliffs, N.J.: Prentice-Hall, Inc., 1961.

11. Oyer, H. *Auditory Communication for the Hard of Hearing.* Englewood Cliffs, N.J.: Prentice-Hall, Inc., 1966.

12. "Peabody Language Development Kit." Circle Pines, Minn.: American Guidance Service.

13. "See-Quees." New York: The Judy Company, General Learning Corporation.

14. Stetson, R. H. *Motor Phonetics.* Amsterdam, North Holland: n.p., 1951.

15. Streng, Alice. Lecture given at State University of New York at Buffalo, 1963.

CHAPTER NINE

The Integration
of Vision and Audition

In our discussion of the act of total perception (Chap. 5) we referred to studies that investigated the effect of interchannel interaction of sensory data. While it has been generally accepted that information received through one sensory pathway can influence information received through another, it has been assumed by most writers that this arises by a process of association. Joseph Church does not agree with this opinion [4, p. 12]. He states, "This view overlooks the evolution of the senses, which indicates that specialized modalities have differentiated out of a sensorium commune or generalized (probably electrochemical) receptor surface."

J. Donald Harris supports Church's argument [11, p. 41]. He suggests that it makes sense neurologically to assume that the auditory and visual pathways are capable of directly influencing each other, since the two systems are directly interconnected at several points along the neural tract to the cortex. On the basis of the neural anatomy and the results of experiments on auditory-visual facilitation, he too refutes the widespread belief that the intersensory effects are to be explained on the basis of attention rather than on a more direct neurological basis. In his conclusion he states, "The weight of evidence is in favor of one organ enhancing the sensation from another organ, though there are negative findings" [11, p. 47].

George Ettlinger has also been interested in determining the nature of cross-modal interaction [7]. His experiments have been directed toward ascertaining whether the discrimination and perception of an object or event involves a neural system common to all modalities (supramodal), or whether recognition occurs independently in each modality (unimodal). He reviews experimental findings pertaining to the following:

1. The transfer of specific discrimination habits from one sense modality to another
2. The transfer of learned principles
3. The ability to match equivalent stimuli in different modalities

An example of an experiment to assess whether cross-modal transfer of discrimination habits can occur is provided by a study conducted by M. Cohl, S. L. Chorover, and Ettlinger [5]. They attempted to determine whether the learning of an auditory rhythm-discrimination task by adults facilitated performance of the same task by vision. No evidence was found to indicate that cross-modal transfer occurred in this particular experiment. In a similar study by M. Blank and W. H. Bridger, children were taught to discriminate between a single and double flash of light and then were asked to make the same discrimination between a single and double sound [1]. Significant transfer of the learned discrimination habit occurred in only one group of children, those for whom the learning procedure involved verbalization.

The second type of transfer, that of derived principles or hypotheses, involves the subject developing certain response techniques in one sensory channel and then utilizing them in another sensory channel. For example, a visual-motor task may be based upon the principle that the relationship between stimuli consists of each subsequent stimulus being a multiple of the previous one. When this principle has been learned, the subject can then make correct predictions. He is then presented with an equivalent task in a different sensory modality and a comparison is made of the time taken to learn the second task relative to the first. A shortened learning time indicates that the principle has been transferred.

The third type of behavior with which Ettlinger has been concerned involves the matching of equivalent stimuli between sensory modalities. In experiments investigating this ability, the subject is permitted to experience an object through one sense alone and then is asked to identify the object when it is presented for inspection through a second single channel. He may, for example, first taste it and then be required to select the substance from a group purely on the basis of its visual appearance.

In summarizing the experimental findings, Ettlinger concludes that "cross-modal transfer of a specific discrimination habit only occurs when language can be utilized" [24]. On the other hand, the research suggests that the cross-modal transfer of behavioral tendencies, or the ability to match across sensory modalities, may occur with or without verbalization. More recently, A. E. Brown and H. K. Hopkins, utilizing information-theory techniques, attempted to achieve a precise measurement of the interaction occurring between the auditory and visual sensory modalities [3]. They determined the optimal probability of detection of a 1000-Hz tone presented against a background of white noise as a function of the signal-to-noise ratio. The corresponding visual task required the subject to detect a 1000-Hz signal presented on an oscilloscope trace against a predetermined level of visible noise. You will note that this task involves the use of equivalent sensory stimuli. Thresholds were first established for the visual and auditory systems independently. The signal was then presented to both sensory systems simultaneously and a bimodal threshold obtained. A comparison of the two unimodal thresholds and the bimodal threshold indicated that the redundancy of information that results from combining two sensory channels in a bimodal presentation significantly improves signal-detection performance.

It seems that there is general acceptance that there exists interaction between data obtained through various modalities. The current discussion centers around the questions of the level at which this takes place and whether or not it is an association function depending upon language. We know that there exists neuro-anatomical evidence that the sensory areas of the brain are interconnected; we also know that there are subcortical interconnecting sensory neurons. Ettlinger suggests that the processing of sensory information may indeed occur at two levels. He proposes two mechanisms. The first, a unimodal system, involves a separate neural system for each sensory modality. Each modal system is responsible for the recognition of those sensory attributes relative to its particular function. All systems are related through a higher center, which receives the identifications (specific sensory perceptions) from each subsystem and uses them to evoke the total perception and its associated name or symbol value.

The second mechanism involves a cross-modal process that utilizes a single neural system concerned with those forms of behavior involving a general principle that holds true regardless of the particular type of sensory input.

What relevance do these suggestions have to our understanding of visual and auditory communication? If we follow Ettlinger's proposed model, we would envisage auditory and visual information being analyzed by the neural centers of each appropriate channel. The process of checking information received against the predictions made takes place first within each sensory channel. The individual auditory, visual, or tactile perceptions are then conveyed to a higher neural system, where each is evaluated in the light of the others. This concept is supported by the findings of George A. Miller and Patricia A. Nicely who, in an analysis of perceptual confusions among some English consonants, found that "the place of articulation which was hardest to hear correctly in our tests is the easiest to see on the talkers' lips. The other features are hard to see but easy to hear" [15]. Thus, we have another instance of the redundancy of intersensory information that the system of human communication has evolved. It is on the basis of this integrated data constituting total perception that the meaning, concept, or word value is assigned.

To incorporate the fact that there exist interconnecting neural fibers between the auditory and visual systems at several levels below the cortex, we might suggest that the intersensory comparisons are made at several stages below the level of perception. This would involve the process of cross-modal matching of equivalent stimuli, which is essential to the inter-channel trial-and-check stage that we discussed in Chap. 5. This would be equivalent to a situation in which two students are attempting to solve a common problem. Although they are using different approaches and the numerical results they obtain are different, they are able to compare their equivalent findings at several stages of the analysis in order to reassure themselves that they are on the right track.

We know that the early stages of learning to communicate involve the acquisition of certain fundamental principles by which sensory data is processed. We might interpret the cross-modal principle as suggesting that a basic processing rule learned with reference to a particular type of sensory information, whether it is visual or auditory, may be generalized to the processing of equivalent data in another channel. It has been shown that this type of behavior is not necessarily dependent upon verbalization and may, therefore, constitute the subconscious learning of communication principles that occurs in the early developmental stages of language learning. Nitchie, in his discussion of visual communication training, devotes a considerable amount of attention to what he refers to as the "mental factor" [17]. Among the labels he uses for the behavioral characteristics that he includes in this category are such words as synthetic power, intuitive power, and quickness and alertness of mind. Perhaps the possession of these attributes by an individual is a manifestation of a highly developed system of evaluating sensory information at pre-perceptual levels. We have already referred to the fact that human subjects are capable of improving their performance on repeated problems without being able to transfer anything specific about the stimuli involved in one problem to subsequent problems. We can attribute this to the establishment of a perceptual set. The improvement in the ability to learn a discrimination task may then be transferred across sensory modalities to a second channel. For this reason, we may be justified in suggesting that the analysis of vision and auditory information represents two aspects of the same behavior. Two levels of information processing appear to be involved: (1) the conscious or perceptual (cognitive awareness), in which the student and the instructor are dealing with verbalized principles, and (2) a pre-perceptual level (subconscious), where certain aspects of information processing are carried out automatically without reference to consciousness [2]. At present we know very little of the mechanisms involved at this level of analysis, though there is an increasing amount of evidence available to indicate that it takes place. It is this level that is involved in the implementation of discrimination habits. Some of these may have been consciously learned and then delegated to the habitual level; others are still beyond the awareness of the most distinguished psychologist or linguist. One cannot help being impressed by the realization that one's brain is so highly skilled in utilizing psycholinguistic principles, most of which we consciously know so little about, and many of which we remain unaware.

Our understanding of the processes involved in perception and learning will be greatly enhanced by research evidence to clarify the nature of some of the mechanisms involved in these two processes. Fortunately, however, we are not dependent on the resolution of these problems to justify an integrated approach to the teaching of auditory and visual communication. Such a philosophy may be supported on the basis of evidence that indicates that, when noise levels in any sensory channel are high, bimodal presentation of information is superior to unimodal.

Several studies have contributed to this evidence. John J. O'Neill reported the results of an experiment designed to assess the relative contribution that lipreading made in person-to-person communication [18]. He used 32 undergraduate students with normal hearing and no special experience in visual communication skills. The students were grouped into four listening panels, each of which observed the test items spoken by three speakers from a distance of eight feet. The materials used were comprised of seven vowels, each combined with the initial consonant "p," seven consonants each preceding the vowel "i," and twenty-four word lists of twenty-one items each. The total test items were presented at four signal-to-noise ratios, which served to progressively reduce the amount of information available in the auditory channel. The test items were presented through the visual channel alone, through the auditory channel alone, and through both channels simultaneously. The results indicated that speech reading facilitated communication under all conditions, but that the contribution it made progressively increased as the signal-to-noise ratio decreased, i.e., deteriorated. As might be expected, no relationship was found between the visibility of the various phonemes and the intensity at which they were produced. O'Neill provides a detailed breakdown of comparative recognition scores for each of the vowels and phonemes used under conditions of simultaneous presentation of visual and auditory stimuli and under conditions of auditory results superior to the unimodal.

In his conclusions, O'Neill states, "If the auditory channel of communication is employed alone, a high level of noise tends to make communication more difficult. When the visual channel supplements the auditory channel, there is an increase in the understandability of the vowels, consonants, words, and phrases that are transmitted."

W. H. Sumby and I. Pollack utilized the information found by O'Neill in a study that examined the contribution that the visual aspects of speech make to intelligibility [24]. They used bisyllabic spondees, monosyllabic words, and trisyllabic phrases for the speech sample. These items were presented to 129 subjects with normal hearing and no formal training in visual communication skills. They, too, presented the materials through the two unimodal channels of vision and hearing, and then through the bimodal channel of vision and hearing combined. The amount of information available in the auditory channel was varied by the manipulation of a speech-signal intensity against a constant noise level. The results of this experiment confirmed the findings of O'Neill, which indicated that as the signal-to-noise ratio is decreased the visual contribution to intelligibility increases.

Keith K. Neely attempted to further quantify the effects of visual cues on speech intelligibility as a function of distance and the angle from which the listener observes the speaker [16]. Using a trained speaker and 35 male listeners with normal hearing and vision, he compared the scores obtained by the subjects on a multiple-choice intelligibility test at 11 different seating positions. These positions represented distances of three, six, and nine feet and angles of 0, 45, and 90 degrees from the speaker. The results indicated a significant difference of 20 per cent between the intelligibility of speech received through hearing only and that received through hearing and vision simultaneously. Distance, within the limits tested, was not found to affect intelligibility, though the scores obtained by subjects directly facing the speaker were higher than those obtained for positions of 45- and 90-degree angles from the speaker.

In each of the three studies mentioned above, the variation in the amount of information available in the auditory channel was achieved through manipulation of the signal-to-noise ratio. S. J. Goodrich, in a study of the relative contribution made by the visual and auditory components of speech to speech intelligibility, manipulated the amount of information in the auditory channel by subjecting the speech material to four conditions of frequency distortion [10]. Using phonetically balanced word lists drawn from the CID Auditory Test W–22, she presented normal hearing students with the test items under the three conditions of vision, audition, and vision and audition together. Comparisons were made of the scores obtained under these three conditions for four conditions of frequency filtering. The filtered conditions were:

1. A wide bandwidth passing frequencies from 100 to 3000 Hz.
2. A low-pass filter passing only frequencies below 500 Hz.
3. A high-pass filter passing only frequencies above 200 Hz.
4. A 15,000-cycle bandwidth passing frequencies between 500 and 2000 Hz.

The results indicated that the mode of presentation (audition, vision, audition and vision combined), the filter frequency bandwidth, and the interaction of the mode of presentation and the frequency filter bandwidth all affected the subject's discrimination of the speech sample. It was found that, by audition only, speech discrimination was most seriously affected by the low-pass filter. Both the 1500-Hz band pass and the high-pass filter reduced auditory discrimination performance, but not to any serious extent. The effect of the bimodal presentation was to increase the discrimination performance for all frequency conditions. The increase was greatest for the low-pass condition, which produced the greatest reduction of information in the auditory channel. This is clearly illustrated by the mean and median percentage values for each of the three conditions. By vision alone, the mean percentage of words correctly identified by the 20 subjects was 12.6 per cent, the median 11.8 per cent; by hearing alone, the mean and median values were each 24 per cent; while for the bimodal presentation of vision and hearing, the mean value was 78 per cent with a median of 79 per cent.

The above experiments were all carried out using subjects with normal hearing. Similar studies have been reported using subjects with impaired hearing. C. V. Hudgins reported on the discrimination performance of a group of children, aged from ten years eight months to sixteen years two months, with average hearing losses in speech frequencies ranging from 82 to 108 decibels [12]. The speech sample was presented visually, auditorily, and through vision and audition combined. The results for each modality are shown in Table 9.1. It will be observed that only four of the fourteen subjects obtained any score at all through the auditory channel alone, and that only one of these received any significant degree of information. Yet a comparison of the visual and the combined visual-auditory presentation clearly indicates that the bimodal presentation provides considerably more information than the unimodal channel of vision, even though the scores obtained for hearing alone suggests that the auditory pathway contributes no information. Furthermore, a comparison of the additive scores for lip-reading and audition indicates that for all but three subjects the integrated score is greater than can be accounted for by a simple additive function.

J. C. Kelly reported the scores obtained by six hearing-impaired children on a discrimination task requiring the identification of spoken words

TABLE 9.1. The Average Score of a Group of Profoundly Deaf Pupils Obtained from Tests of Lipreading, Hearing, and Lipreading and Hearing (After C. V. Hudgins [11])

PUPILS	AVERAGE HEARING LOSS IN DECIBELS LEFT EAR	RIGHT EAR	AGE	LIPREADING	HEARING	BOTH
1	98	95	13–8	58	7	70
2	78	92	14–0	42	0	53
3	87	88	12–7	52	41	72
4	77	78	14–0	40	0	40
5	82	83	11–9	30	0	44
6	108	105	14–8	44	7	74
7	97	97	15–0	40	0	42
8	103	105	14–10	30	0	45
9	78	100	16–2	40	0	66
10	75	78	15–7	36	10	76
11	88	92	11–4	30	0	42
12	93	95	12–3	32	0	76
13	83	87	11–7	37	0	50
14	98	95	10–8	40	0	40

and spoken names of letters of the alphabet [13, p. 7]. The test items were presented through vision, audition, and vision and audition combined. A comparison of the results is presented in Table 9.2. Note first of all that the scores obtained for the recognition of the names of letters of the alphabet are considerably higher than those for word recognition. This we can understand in the light of our discussion of redundancy. The choices available to the subject are limited by the letters of the alphabet. Note also that under both conditions vision contributed less information than audition. This we would expect, since we have already said that the visible aspects of speech contain less information than the auditory. Once again it is clearly seen that bimodal presentation of speech material conveys more information than either the visual or auditory channel alone. This finding is further supported by Josephine Prall [21], who tested hearing-impaired children in a school for the deaf (Table 9.3). The results indicate that a subject's speech-discrimination performance is substantially enhanced when visual cues are presented together with the acoustic signal.

As part of a larger investigation, I studied the speech-discrimination performance of 50 primary-school-aged children with hearing losses ranging from 55 to 110 decibels [22]. The subjects were grouped into four hearing-loss categories: (A) 55 to 64 dB, (B) 65 to 74 dB, (C) 75 to 94 dB, and (D) 95 to 119 dB. Test materials consisted of a multiple-choice picture identification task. Four conditions of presentation were used: (1) unaided hearing without visual cues, (2) unaided hearing with visual cues, (3) aided hearing (personal hearing aid) without visual cues, and (4) aided hearing with visual cues.

A comparison was made of the group mean scores for each category under each condition. The results obtained are shown in Table 9.4. These indicate that the amount of information that the children were able to obtain from the auditory channel without amplification decreased as the hearing loss increased. For hearing losses in excess of 75 decibels, the auditory channel alone was insufficient to permit the recognition of the names of familiar objects on the basis of the auditory cues alone, even when the choice of alternatives was limited to six items. The benefit derived from amplification was also shown to be in an inverse relationship to the severity of the hearing impairment. In other words, even with amplification, the amount of information that the auditory channel is capable of contributing to speech discrimination becomes progressively less as the amount of residual hearing decreases.

TABLE 9.2. Visual, Auditory, and Audio-Visual Communication of Hard-of-Hearing Subjects (After J. C. Kelly [13])

SUBJECT	WORDS	LETTERS
Visual Only		
A	30	65
B	21	63
C	33	60
D	52	75
E	10	45
F	50	78
Mean Per Cent	32.67%	64.33%
Auditory Only		
A	88	98
B	81	86
C	56	73
D	38	77
E	25	30
F	19	57
Mean Per Cent	51.17%	70.17%
Audio-Visual		
A	93	100
B	93	96
C	82	100
D	75	96
E	69	63
F	88	94
Mean Per Cent	83.33%	91.50%

TABLE 9.3. Average Scores for PBK Lists: Lipreading Alone, Hearing Aid Alone, and Lipreading and Hearing with Aid Combined (After Josephine Prall [20])

PUPILS	BETTER EAR AVERAGE IN DECIBELS	GRADE	LIPREADING ALONE	HEARING AID ALONE	LIPREADING AND HEARING AID COMBINED
P.A.	70	5	28	0	33
M.B.	63	6	27	10	41
L.C.	57	5	30	27	47
J.C.	68	8	24	3	44
C.H.	52*	2	30	26	43
J.H.	45	5	29	22	47
C.L.	63	7	27	16	45
M.T.	57	8	27	27	45

*Better ear average here represents loss in left ear only. Average loss in right ear for the three frequencies is 70 decibels. Pupil uses aid in right ear.

TABLE 9.4. Mean Percentage Discrimination Scores for Hearing Loss Against Conditions of Presentation for Fifty Primary School Children (After Derek A. Sanders [22])

HEARING LOSS IN DECIBELS	UNAIDED, WITH NO SPEECH READING (PER CENT)	AIDED WITH SPEECH READING (PER CENT)	AIDED, BUT WITH NO SPEECH READING (PER CENT)	AIDED WITH SPEECH READING (PER CENT)
A 55–64	41	60	79	93
B 65–74	21	74	55	90
C 75–94	0	74	36	88
D 96–110	0	78	6	79

In all categories of hearing loss the number of items correctly discriminated without amplification increased when visual cues were made available. The least increase occurred in the category of children with the greatest amount of residual hearing. The possible explanation for this may be that the children in this group had sufficient residual hearing to obviate the need for heavy dependence upon the visual cues of speech and were, therefore, less skilled in speech reading. This assumption is supported by the score of 79 per cent that the children in this category obtained for amplified speech without visual cues.

Under the most favorable communication condition (amplified speech with visual cues), the children in hearing-loss categories A, B, and C obtained significantly better discrimination scores than under any other condition. The children in category D, however, were clearly so dependent upon the visual channel as the major source of information and derived so much from visual cues (78 per cent by vision alone) that the amplified speech signal contributed no significant additional information.

The study of the value of bimodal presentation of information to deaf subjects has not been confined to a combination of the visual and auditory channels. J.M. Pickett has reported on experiments involving the encoding of speech information into vibro-tactile information to provide an information source complemental to the visual and the auditory channel [19]. He designed an instrument known as a "vocoder" to transpose the frequency vibrations of the spoken message signal into an equivalent vibratory signal. This signal is received by the student through the finger tips. Using the vocoder with deaf children, he compared the discrimination of speech sounds through the tactile sense with discrimination of the same sounds through vision. He then compared scores obtained under the bimodal condition of touch and vision with those obtained through vision alone. It was demonstrated that sufficient information can be presented by vibro-tactile means to permit speech discrimination. Furthermore, it was shown that better discrimination can be obtained for some speech sounds using vibro-tactile information than can be obtained through visual information. For example, using vibratory information one can distinguish between /m/ and /b/, a discrimination not possible on the basis of differential visual cues. A comparison of the bimodal performance, using vision and touch, and the unimodal scores, obtained through vision alone, indicated that a greater amount of information was received through the bimodal presentation.

The available research data strongly indicates that multisensory presentation of related information results in the integration of that information into a perceptual gestalt at some level of processing. It is not clear whether this process involves a common sensory pool from which a total perception is finally structured, or whether each sensory system is responsible for the perception of those stimuli appropriate to its own sensitivity. In both cases, the information is presumed to be transmitted further to the associative areas in order that meaning may be attributed according to a personal value system. The work of Ettlinger seems to suggest that both theories may hold true, each being applicable to different types of perceptual experiences.

Regardless of which theory ultimately proves valid, the results of the studies concerning the interaction of sensory systems in the process of speech communication clearly emphasize the superiority of bimodal over unimodal systems. Pickett has expressed very succinctly the contribution that a bimodal system makes to communication.

In general, when information is added to a sensory communication link of limited capacity, such as lipreading, the added information can improve communication in two ways. First, if the added information conveys dimensions of the source code that are poorly transmitted by the existing sensory channels, then the total channel capacity is increased (for that particular source). Second, even if added information is partially or totally redundant and there is little or no increase in total capacity, the added redundancy will improve the resistance of the link to interference or distraction in one of the existing sensory systems.

We must insure that our aural rehabilitation techniques are designed to improve communication in both of these two ways. We should not assume that the ability to communicate through a single channel with a reasonable degree of adequacy obviates the need for attention being paid to developing the awareness of available information in the second channel. In Chap. 5 we developed a philosophy of speech perception that emphasizes the importance of the integration of information. Following this line of thought it does not seem justifiable to accept the idea of a bimodal system as constituting two unimodal systems. The concept of a simple adding of information obtained from two channels is found untenable. We can agree that the addition of the second channel increases the amount of available information, but we propose that it does more than this. It is suggested that *effective bimodal function involves a modification of the perceived data in both channels.* You will recall that in the studies by J. W. Gebhardt and G. H. Mowbrey [9] and by T. Shipply [23] the perception of a visual stimulus was modified by a change that was made in the auditory input. In other words, we may in fact perceive the auditory stimulus differently when it is presented together with the visual information, and vice versa. Thus, the purpose of visual communication training is not simply to provide supplemental information to that obtained through the auditory channel, but to increase the probability of making correct predictions concerning the received auditory signal. As a result, the subject may actually derive more information from audition when it is presented together with vision than he would be able to derive from audition alone.

If we can accept such an explanation of the nature of bisensory function, it is easy to incorporate the concept of interchannel trial-and-check, which we discussed in relation to the act of perception. We can also include the idea of an internal and external scanning process that seeks to establish congruency (between channels) and seeks to exclude that which is noncongruent. The use of a bimodal system is therefore seen as affecting not only the amount and nature of the information received, but also the perceptual mobilization or set that the person will assume.

Finally, we need to translate this philosophy into the actual techniques of visual and auditory training. Our goal is twofold: firstly, to insure that maximum information is derived from each sensory input channel; and secondly, to insure that intersensory interaction may take place during the learning experience.

Fortunately, we are able to conclude that we need reject neither the system of training that advocates a unisensory approach nor that which suggests a bimodal or multisensory approach to training. In discussing a unisensory approach to aural rehabilitation, Doreen Pollack states, "If an impaired modality is to function maximumly it must be trained intensively and systematically. Other cues must be de-emphasized in training" [20]. If we are to insure that the student becomes fully aware of a particular aspect of a stimulus complex, i.e., the auditory or the visual components, then we will focus upon this aspect by means of a unisensory presentation. In doing so, we magnify these characteristics and permit a more discriminatory observation, which yields more information. The student may consciously or unconsciously become aware of cues previously embedded within the total gestalt. As Pickett has pointed out, these cues may, under good listening conditions, constitute part of the redundancy and, therefore, not be essential to comprehension. However, when communication conditions deteriorate, comprehension may depend upon their availability. Through unisensory training, we seek to increase the total amount of redundancy available within that channel, for various types of material, under varying conditions of communication. Our training techniques should, therefore, allow for specific consideration of the particular characteristics of the unisensory (visual or auditory) message signal. We must present sound auditorily without visual cues and encourage the student to close his eyes and to concentrate upon what he hears. We must draw his attention to such valuable paralinguistic cues as rhythm, pitch, stress, and loudness, which also serve to add constraints, reduce choice, and thus improve predictability. Techniques employing the judging of paired stimuli as same or different can be helpful in improving auditory perception of these aspects of a spoken message. Training in the recognition of individual phonemes by their acoustic characteristics alone can greatly enhance the amount of information a student can derive from hearing.

We should also pay attention to visual communication cues, depriving the listener temporarily of the redundancy provided by auditory cues, and thus, necessitating more careful processing of visual information. We will make use of contrast words to heighten the perception of the differences, however slight they may be, between the articulatory movements of different sound groups. We should use practice words and sentences to provide repeated exposure to the newly learned articulatory movements, as well as using exercises and games selected to improve visual memory span and to develop the student's ability to make closure.

At this point our philosophy diverges markedly from that of Pollack, who seems to suggest that vision plays no part in the acquisition of speech and language in the child with normal hearing. The rejection by Pollack of the multisensory approach to aural rehabilitation is incompatible with the concept of communication as involving the utilizing of information, regardless of the sensory channel through which it becomes available. The greater the number of constraints that operate when we make our predication, the more accurate we are likely to be in our interpretation of the message signal. Pollack suggests that there is sufficient information available in the auditory channel of the hearing-impaired child for him to be taught to be independent of vision. To support this contention, she refers to Joseph Carl R. Licklider's work, which shows that speech remains intelligible even after severe peak clippings. She concludes, therefore, that "the limited hearing child can be taught to interpret correctly the signals coming over a communication channel of minimal capacity, if those signals are heard consistently." Such reasoning is in error on two points. The effect of peak clipping and the effect imposed upon the speech signal by most hearing losses are not comparable. Rather than clipping off peaks, hearing impairment causes the peaks only to cross threshold. Peak clipping is an amplitude distortion function. Most hearing losses, on the other hand, add to the intensity distortion—the far more limiting factor of frequency distortion. The second error is the assumption that constant exposure to a distorted sound pattern will ultimately result in its recognition. We will certainly agree that practice in listening or watching, which involves focusing the student's attention on particular characteristics of the message signal, may make available to him a greater amount of information, sometimes even enough to permit recognition to occur. However, the amount can never exceed that which is within the channel. The effect of hearing loss is to reduce the total amount of available information, frequently to the point at which it constitutes too little for recognition to be possible. When this occurs, the student will either fail to comprehend the message signal or will seek additional information from the complementary channel. Pollack rejects this concept, claiming that it involves a cross-modality transfer, which tends to confuse the subject. We have attempted to show that, rather than confusing, cross-modal transfer enhances total perception, a belief that is supported by the results of a number of studies, including those of Pickett. In designing his study of the use of tactual communication as a complementary channel to vision, he recognized that "there is the remote possibility that the use of tactual information may interfere with the use of lipreading." When analyzing the results he concluded, "In tests with combined lipreading and tactual reception, the tactual information on consonants and the number of syllables was found to improve transmission without detracting from lipreading the visible features of other sounds." In the perception of some sounds it was found that discrimination improved dramatically with the addition of tactual information to vision.

More recently, John Gaeth published data concerning the audio-visual approach to deaf education, which merits careful consideration because of the implications that it might have for our understanding of the processes with which we are dealing. Gaeth's work was carefully conducted under controlled conditions. He attempted to produce evidence concerning the relative effectiveness of unimodal and bimodal presentation of communication and material to be learned. In a paper presented to the National Symposium on Deafness in Childhood held at Vanderbilt University in 1966, Gaeth reviewed a series of experiments that he conducted between 1957 and 1966 [8]. He defined the aim of these experiments as: "to investigate bimodal versus unimodal methods of presentation of material to be learned." The results seemed to provide evidence contrary to our basic assumption that bimodal presentation provides a greater degree of information than unimodal.

In his studies, Gaeth used the method of paired-associate models, requiring the individual to respond with the second of a pair of stimuli when presented with the first. Six to ten paired items were used. These consisted of simple words, nonsense trigrams, nonsense drawings, and novel noises. The presentation was made auditorily, visually, or audio-visually, with the criterion for learning being either the number of trials taken to reach a certain level of performance, or the number of correct responses obtained for a specified number of trials. In addition to controlling the method of presentation, the method of learning and practicing was also controlled, providing a total of nine different conditions represented by nine groups of children.

Gaeth provides the learning curves for 90 fourth-grade children divided into three equal groups. The three groups learned by the three methods of presentation. The results showed that no difference occurred in the learning curves, regardless of the methods of presentation; that is to say, the combined auditory-visual presentation was not superior to that achieved by either of the unimodal presentations.

When the material was presented to a group of hard-of-hearing children with losses of between 16 and 30 decibels ASA, no significant difference was found between the rate of learning attained through the audio-visual and that attained through the visual presentation. However, a significant deficiency in learning was demonstrated when the material was presented through the auditory channel alone. (These same findings were obtained for two other groups of children with hearing losses ranging from 31 to 45 decibels and from 45 to 60 decibels in the better ear.)

With a group of children whose hearing losses fell within the range of 61 to 75 decibels, the resultant learning curves indicated that the combined presentation actually produced a poorer learning rate than the visual presentation alone. In reacting to these findings, Gaeth comments:

A reasonable inference seems to be that for the groups with the milder hearing loss the auditory material was meaningful or at least intelligible to the children and thus did not interfere with the performance, though it did not help it either. In the case of the children with the hearing losses between 61–75 dB, the material was not intelligible and either confused the tasks somewhat or distracted the children from functioning as efficiently as they did visually.

He goes on to state:

The first major experiment showed repeatedly that the combined method of presentation was not superior to the visual method with hard-of-hearing children, nor superior to either the visual or the auditory with children with normal hearing. Secondarily, it highlighted the fact that hard-of-hearing children, in regular schools, were not performing auditorily as well as might have been expected from their audiograms or from their speech discrimination scores.

Using large numbers of children with normal hearing, Gaeth also conducted experiments of a similar nature with the same basic results, using as the items to be learned three syllable nouns, nonsense syllables, and a set of nonverbal, nonmeaningful visual symbols.

From the results that he obtained in his experiment he concluded:

1. The combined auditory-visual presentation of simple words, pronounceable nonsense syllables, or nonmeaningful symbols and noises does not result in improvement of performance over single modality presentations.
2. When there is a difference in performance between the auditory and visual method of presentation, the combined presentation is never better than the better of the two unimodal presentations, although it may occasionally be slightly poorer but usually not significantly so.
3. When different materials are presented via the auditory and visual channels (e.g., the visual symbols with the pronounced syllables), the performance with the combined presentation tends to be between the two individual performances when they are significantly different, or to approximate the better condition when the two unimodal conditions do not deviate markedly.

Such results as these cannot be passed over lightly, for they seem to stand in contradiction to the whole basis of our approach to auditory-visual training. Certain factors need to be considered when examining these results. (1) The bulk of the data presented was obtained from children with normal hearing, although a small sample testing of hearing-impaired children indicates the same learning behavior. (2) The performance on the tasks presented did not involve the attributing of meaning to the stimulus complexes but specifically measured learning on the identification of a missing paired associate.

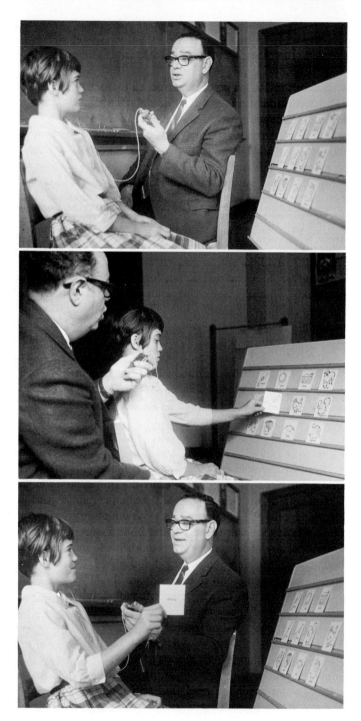

Fig. 9.1. Information is provided first through each sensory modality separately, then simultaneously. (Courtesy of St. Mary's School for the Deaf, Buffalo, New York.)

340

Gaeth suggests that, when faced with a new learning situation, the child initially uses only one modality, that with the highest degree of redundancy, and that a multisensory presentation constitutes two learning tasks that must be separated for unisensory learning to occur.

It would seem important to differentiate between those tasks involving the memorization of test items or their relationships and tasks requiring the development of new concepts or involving the identification of previously acquired concepts on the basis of the information potential contained within the stimulus complex. Furthermore, in the process of speech communication, the degree of redundancy within each channel shifts markedly from moment to moment and seldom permits the multiple exposure to the stimulus that was an important component of the learning task in the studies by Gaeth.

In his paper, Gaeth briefly directs his comments to the benefit that individuals have been shown to derive from bimodal presentation by suggesting that the improvement in such situations results, not from the "integration of simultaneous bimodal presentation, but from the integration of rapidly alternating unimodal stimulation." He also, in another part of the paper, suggests that perhaps the bimodal presentations may be critical in situations in which the young hard-of-hearing or normal child encounters new words or new concepts.

The challenging ideas that Gaeth's data provide still await careful examination and further testing by those concerned with the education of the hearing-impaired child. They constitute the kind of challenge that should keep us aware of how little we still understand about either the communication or learning processes of the hearing-impaired subject. They should stimulate us to conduct more of such experimental studies, broadening the avenues of investigation to include the study of the relative ease with which meaning can be attributed through a unisensory versus a multisensory approach. We must be particularly concerned with situations that will have direct bearing on the normal communication environment of the child. In the meantime, we appear to continue to be justified in proposing that unisensory training in visual and auditory perception of speech does serve to improve the total perception that occurs when a multisensory presentation is given. We can state, in the light of Gaeth's work, that the material should be presented for discrimination, first, through the channel in which an attempt is being made to improve perception and, then, through the alternate modality. This represents the initial unisensory presentation referred to by Gaeth. Finally, bimodal presentation—e.g., visual cues, auditory cues, visual and auditory cues combined—should be made in order that the maximum potential information is made available (Fig. 9.1).

To this bimodal approach we should add the use of mirror practice to visual communication training in order that the child not only can see the way in which he produces certain sounds, but also can become aware of the motor-kinesthetic sensations occurring as he produces them. We justify the approach of speech by reference to the theory of the motor-kinesthetic perception of speech proposed by Alvin M. Liberman [14]. Similarly, when we are presenting a sound auditorily we should not only ask the child to listen and identify the sound, but also to repeat it several times after the auditory model is presented by the teacher. Feedback of his own speech production should be provided and then, through the use of a tape recorder, contrasted with the model presented by the teacher in order that he can more correctly approximate her normal speech production.

The lesson plans that we develop for the child with impaired hearing will not on paper reflect the integrative nature of the sensory training that we seek to give. It is the method of presentation rather than the content that provides the unisensory and then multisensory experience. If you accept the training model we have developed, you will subscribe to the theory that the student should be given the opportunity to utilize both vision and audition in speech comprehension. You will agree that he needs to be able to integrate the information within these channels to the limits of his own particular communication system. The division of visual and auditory training into separate lesson periods, each with its own lesson plans and procedures, cannot be justified according to our philosophy. The integration must beome an integral part of special periods devoted to the enhancement of speech comprehension. Activities designed to improve the ability to utilize visual cues simply emphasize the visual first; they then present the auditory cues associated with the visual cues and, finally, blend them in the audio-visual presentation. Auditory training simply reverses the order of precedence of vision and audition.

For this reason, this chapter does not contain sample lessons; those provided in the previous two chapters will incorporate the integration of vision and audition within the method of presentation.

We can conclude this discussion of the integrated approach to aural rehabilitation by making a contrast between the efforts we must make in order to increase the total amount of information available to the hearing-impaired person and the ease with which you and I understand speech. The immense gap that exists between the conditions under which the hard-of-hearing person must operate and those with which the person with normal hearing experiences is made clear by the description of normal speech perception provided by Peter B. Denes and Elliot N. Pinson:

> When we listen under favorable conditions, the clues available are far in excess of what is actually needed for satisfactory recognition. Indeed, general context is often so compelling that we know positively what is going to be said even before we hear the words. This is why under normal conditions

we understand speech with ease and certainty, despite the ambiguities of the acoustic cues. It is also the reason that intelligibility is maintained to such an astonishing extent, despite the variability of speakers, in the presence of noise and distortion [6, p. 146].

Unfortunately, this is not so for the person with a hearing problem.

REFERENCES

1. Blank, M., and W. H. Bridger. "Cross-Modal Transfer in Nursery-School Children. *Journal of Comparative Physiological Psychology* 58(1964): 277–82.

2. Bocca, E., and C. Calearo. "Central Hearing Processes," in *Modern Developments in Audiology*. Ed. J. Jerger. New York: Academic Press, 1963.

3. Brown, A. E., and H. K. Hopkins. "Interaction of the Auditory and Visual Sensory Modalities." *Journal of the Acoustical Society of America* 41(1968): 1–6.

4. Church, Joseph. *Language and the Discovery of Reality*. New York: Random House, Inc., 1963.

5. Cole, M., S. L. Chorover, and G. Ettlinger. "Cross-Modal Transfer in Man." *Nature* 191(1961): 1225–26.

6. Denes, Peter B., and Elliot N. Pinson. *The Speech Chain*. Murray Hill, N.J.: Bell Telephone Labs, 1963.

7. Ettlinger, George. "Analysis of Cross-Modal Effects and their Relationship to Language." *Brain Mechanism Underlying Speech and Language*. Edited by Frederick L. Darley. New York: Grune & Stratton, Inc., 1967.

8. Gaeth, John. "Deafness in Children." *National Symposium on Deafness in Childhood*. McConnell Freeman and Paul H. Ward, editors. Nashville, Tenn.: Vanderbilt University Press, 1967.

9. Gebhardt, J. W., and G. H. Mowbrey. "On Discriminating the Rate of Visual Flicker and Auditory Flutter." *American Journal of Psychology* 72(1959): 521–29.

10. Goodrich, S. J. "The Relative Contributions of the Visual and Auditory Components of Speech to Speech Intelligibility under Varying Conditions of Auditory Distortion." To appear in a forthcoming issue of the *Journal of Speech and Hearing Research*. M.A. Thesis, State University of New York at Buffalo, 1967.

11. Harris, J. Donald. *Some Relations Between Vision and Audition*. Springfield, Ill.: Charles C Thomas, Publishers, 1950.

12. Hudgins, C. V. "Problems of Speech Comprehension in Deaf Children." *The Nervous Child*. 9(1951): no. 1.

13. Kelly, J. C. *Audio-Visual Reading: A Manual for Training the Hard of Hearing in Voice Communication.* Urbana: University of Illinois Speech and Hearing Clinic, 1967.

14. Liberman, A., et al. "Perception of the Speech Code." *Phychological Review* 74(1968): 431–61.

15. Miller, George A., and Patricia E. Nicely. "An Analysis of Perceptual Confusions among Some English Consonants." *Journal of the Acoustical Society of America* 27(1955): 338–52.

16. Neely, Keith K. "Effect of Visual Factors on the Intelligibility of Speech." *Journal of the Acoustical Society of America* 28(1956): 1275–77.

17. Nitchie, Edward B. *Principles and Methods of Lipreading.* New York: The Nitchie School of Lipreading, n.d.

18. O'Neill, John J. "Contributions of the Visual Components of Oral Symbols to Speech Comprehension." *Journal of Speech and Hearing Disorders* 19(1954): 429–39.

19. Pickett, J. M. "Tactual Communication of Speech Sounds to the Deaf: Comparison with Lipreading." *Journal of Speech and Hearing Disorders* 28(1963): 315–30.

20. Pollack, Doreen. "Acoupedics: A Uni-sensory Approach to Auditory Training." *Volta Review* 66(1964): 400–409.

21. Prall, Josephine. "Lipreading and Hearing Aids Combine for Better Comprehension." *Volta Review* 59(1957): 64–65.

22. Sanders, Derek A. "A Follow-up Study of Fifty Deaf Children Who Received Pre-School Training." Unpublished Ph.D. thesis, Royal Victoria University of Manchester, Manchester, England, 1961.

23. Shipply, T. "Auditory Flutter-Driving of Visual Flicker." *Science* 145(1954): 1328–30.

24. Sumby, W. H., and I. Pollack. "Visual Contributions to Speech Intelligibility in Noise." *Journal of the Acoustical Society of America* 26(1954): 212–15.

CHAPTER TEN

Case Management

In each of the previous chapters we have been concerned with a specific aspect of the process of aural rehabilitation. We have examined the structure and function of the human communication system and have looked in some detail at the nature of the information embodied within the visual and acoustical aspects of the verbal and nonverbal message signal. We have discussed the way in which we learn and maintain the process of attributing meaning to the communication code and have studied the effect that an impairment of auditory function is likely to have upon this process. In the chapters on hearing aids, visual and auditory communication training, and the interaction of these two sensory modalities, our discussion centered around the nature and rationale for the specific techniques that we use in attempting to improve the communication function of the hard-of-hearing person. We must now once again attempt to step back and obtain a similar overview of the problem to that which was presented at the beginning of this book. It is hoped, however, that the difference will be that we are now better equipped to perceive the details of the total pattern.

THE CASE HISTORY

When we see a hearing-impaired child or adult for the first time, we find ourselves ignorant of the nature of the communication problem. Our first task is to gain information. For this, we turn initially to the case history, which may have already been taken by the otologist or audiologist who carried out the diagnostic evaluation. It represents a record of the chronological development of the communication problem as recalled and perceived by the person who is doing the reporting. Its value lies in the implications that reside in the information it provides. It places constraints upon the predictions we make concerning the areas in which the person will need help and the relative urgency for action in each of the particular areas.

Specific attention should be paid to the age of the subject at the time of the deafness. The relevance of this must be understood in the terms of auditory-perceptual development, which we discussed in Chap. 5. The child who was born profoundly deaf will have developed a communication system that ignores auditory phenomena. He will not be capable of utilizing amplified sound until he is given intensive training designed to develop auditory behavior. When the onset of deafness has occurred after birth, the amount of auditory cues that have been unconsciously internalized and structured will depend upon the period of learning that occurred before the deafness was acquired. The longer the period of normal hearing, the greater the auditory-perceptual resources we have to tap.

The etiology and type of deafness should also be noted. In as much as 50 per cent of all cases of deafness the causation of the auditory disorder is unknown. Among those for whom there is an established etiology, we should be particularly alert to children whose problems have been attributed to maternal rubella (German measles during pregnancy), particularly when it occurred during the first three months of pregnancy; incompatibility of the maternal and fetal blood groups (Rh factor); prematurity; anoxia; and encephalitis. These etiologies are known to be associated frequently with specific and generalized defects of pre- and postnatal development. With this group of children in particular, you should remember that a clear-cut diagnosis of sensori-neural deafness as the single cause of the child's communication problems is difficult to make. This is particularly true during the early years of the child's life. No qualified otologist would wish a diagnosis of sensory-neural deafness to inhibit a teacher or therapist from observation of behavior that tends to suggest that the problem is more complicated than it originally appeared to be. A great deal of information concerning the nature of the child's problem can be learned by attempting to teach him to overcome it. Every classification of the child's difficulty must be tentative, made within the limits of information available at the time. It should most certainly be open to reappraisal in the light of further information obtained by the teacher or therapist through observation and testing.

We have already talked about the information that can be derived from the otological and audiological data concerning the type, the extent, and the configuration of the hearing loss. This information, interpreted in the light of the other findings, will make it possible for you to make predictions concerning how well the child should respond to amplification and the extent to which you might expect him to come to depend upon the auditory signal as a primary source of information. You will expect to be able to verify this through various tests of progress conducted after a period of training. Indications that the child or adult is not performing according to your expectations should cause you to re-evaluate the nature of the difficulty and to inquire whether, in fact, you are dealing with the type of problem you thought you were, and whether the therapy and methods you are using are appropriate to the person's needs. In the case of a child, the level of speech and language development should be commensurate with the age of onset, the pattern and severity of loss, and the age at which the diagnosis was made. If, after working with the child, it becomes apparent that there is a discrepancy between the child's performance and that which you would predict from the available data, you should not hesitate to seek further diagnostic evaluation.

The therapist or teacher is fortunate if she receives a complete case work-up on a hard-of-hearing person, including his academic or occupational performance and his social adjustment. It is not unreasonable to expect that you will have to collect this sort of information yourself. It is vital to the successful outcome of a program designed to help school-age children that the therapist should not play an isolated role. She should not be simply someone who works on auditory and visual communication training once or twice a week without contact with the classroom teacher who is responsible for the child's academic achievement. An effective program must involve the joint efforts of all who are concerned with preparing the child to be a self-supporting and competent member of society. We shall discuss this later when we consider the role of the school in the rehabilitation program. It is, however, important to your work in aural rehabilitation that you familiarize yourself not only with how a child functions in communication situations that you establish in the clinic, but also with the type of behavior that he manifests both in the classroom and at home. The difficulty of the communication situations he will encounter in these environments is considerably different. Furthermore, a knowledge of what he is doing in these two situations will help you to evaluate certain patterns of behavior that he may manifest with you and may also enlighten you to some of the patterns of behavior that he may not exhibit to you, but which may be characteristic of his relationship with other people.

If you are to make use of the information that parents and teachers provide, it will be necessary for you to be able to evaluate it. You must know the background of attitudes and feelings against which to interpret the comments made about the child. You should attempt, therefore, to find out how the adults responsible for him perceive the problem and the child's difficulties, what they think he ought to be achieving, the interpretations they place upon his behavior, and how they attempt to handle it. It is one thing to learn about a child's behavior, but another to be able to interpret it in the light of the knowledge of the climate in which it occurs. So often the frustrations that a child experiences, either in class or at home, are to a great extent the results of a failure on the part of the adults to understand the real nature of the problem he faces. This type of ignorance is generally in no way the fault of the people concerned; they simply do not have the background knowledge necessary in order to place a different interpretation upon this behavior. A great deal of inappropriate handling of hard-of-hearing and other handicapped children is done with the best of intentions; the people involved are simply acting within the limits of their understanding of the difficulties. It falls to those of us who have greater insight into the nature and implications of hearing impairment to do the best we can to inform and, therefore, to better prepare those people in the child's life who have infinitely greater influence upon his perceptions of the world and, ultimately, upon the way he sees himself, than we are ever likely to have.

In addition to the case history and audiological data, the teacher or therapist should also seek whatever additional information she feels important to a fair understanding of both the child's problem and his potential for overcoming it. You are entitled to copies of information relating to the child's intellectual ability, his performance in classroom subjects—particularly in reading—and his social and emotional maturity. If these are not available, then you should discuss with the school principal or counselor the possibility of obtaining such evaluations. If the child is to be seen again at a speech and hearing clinic, a request could be made to them to see if they would agree to undertake or arrange for such testing.

With all the data available, it is a worthwhile investment of time and energy to attempt to summarize it, together with its implications, in the form of a written report. The amount of time that this involves for a busy teacher or school therapist is not underestimated. However, the report is primarily intended for your own use. It serves as a means of clarifying the picture by relating and correlating the various types of available information, thus permitting you to plan for the subject's needs more appropriately. Reading through the various sources of information does not provide the same degree of clarity as summarizing it in writing. Apparently the verbalization of ideas serves to clarify them. One might, perhaps, claim that we have little more than a gist of an idea until the details are "spelled out." Such a description of a child and his problem, written in a logical and organized manner, will serve as an excellent basis for communicating with other specialists who may be requested to see the child. It is also useful in talking with the classroom teacher and school principal, and with a certain amount of judicious editing, it can be used as a basis for counseling the parents.

COUNSELING

The role of counseling in aural rehabilitation is one to which, we said earlier, we would give more consideration. The therapist or teacher sometimes feels apprehensive about accepting responsibility for this aspect of rehabilitation. The opinion is often voiced that the responsibility for such guidance rests with the more highly qualified staff of a speech and hearing center. For the majority of cases, I reject such a viewpoint. It overlooks the fact that an effective program must be comprehensive and that, in all probability, a conscientious and concerned therapist will create a suitable climate of mutual trust between herself and the children or adults with whom she is working. As your students and parents develop confidence in you, first as a practitioner and then as a person, they are far more likely to seek and accept advice and guidance from you than they are from a relative stranger in a speech and hearing clinic. Furthermore, unless a student is enrolled in a continuous program in the clinic, the guidance he receives is likely to be periodic and may not be readily available at the time when it may be most effective.

The major purpose of this counseling is to reduce anxiety and so to improve a person's overall adjustment. The two types of guidance, informational guidance and personal-adjustment guidance, are closely related. Much of the anxiety that a hearing-impaired person or the parents of a hearing-impaired child experience arises from ignorance of the nature of the problem with which they are confronted. Problems always seem much worse when they are ill-defined and amorphous. The provision of significant information permits the therapist and the individuals concerned to clarify the issues and to break down the rather overwhelming concept of hearing impairment into a series of manageable components or problems. This is important since it enhances the possibility of the student or his parents experiencing the satisfaction of seeing early progress in at least some areas of the total picture. While it takes time to bring about change in the person's actual performance in social situations, it is generally possible to modify the perspective from which he views the problem and, therefore, to develop a more positive perception of it.

We quite reasonably expect that the person who suffers from a handicap imposed by an impairment of hearing will be in need of some degree of adjustment counseling. E. S. Levine has listed five personality factors that may be encountered to a greater-than-normal extent in a hearing-impaired person [4]. These are deficiencies of concept development, emotional immaturity, rigidity and egocentricity, poor social adaptability, and limited interests and motivations. H. R. Myklebust is of the opinion that the anxiety and depression experienced by hearing-impaired people arises as much from the difficulty of maintaining social contacts as it does from the imposed auditory isolation [5]. He also points out that the greatest adjustment problems arise when the deafness is acquired after the normal personality has stabilized. This is understandable, since each of us comes to think of ourself in a certain way. Such a self-concept has to take into account our various minor deviations from that which we consider to be desirable. You will note we sometimes go to considerable length to conceal these deviations from others. The onset of deafness in later childhood, adolescence, or adult life presents considerable personal-adjustment problems since it constitutes a major threat to the self-image. It involves the exceptance of limitations frequently considered as weaknesses. In reaction to such self-evaluation, the hard-of-hearing person with acquired deafness is liable to deny the problem, becoming extremely resistant to suggestions that he seek help. He may assume an aggressive attitude or may progressively withdraw from situations in which he experiences difficulty. The congenitally deaf child, on the other hand, knows only one world and one self. He shows a certain unawareness of his problem and is less threatened by the concept of himself as an imperfect person. The social problems that he will encounter are relatively well defined by society, facilitating the modification of behavior in such a way as to circumvent them.

The group that appears to have the greatest amount of difficulty are those individuals whose hearing losses are mild to moderate, less than 50 decibels [1]. This group live in a border area between the deaf and the hearing. Identification with either group is difficult. The penalties that the hearing society places upon the person's behavior are not clearly defined nor easily predictable; thus, the person tends to experience a much greater degree of uncertainty and frustration than the severely handicapped child or adult whose role has been clearly defined.

In addition to counseling the person with a hearing impairment, we should anticipate the anxieties that will be experienced by the parents of a deaf or hard-of-hearing child or by the married partner or fiancé of an adult. It is important that the counseling that you are prepared to give should also be extended to people close to the hearing-impaired person, since they constitute an influential factor in determining whether or not one will be successful in enabling the hearing-impaired person to make the necessary adjustment. It is frequently quite helpful to invite these persons to the early counseling sessions concerned with the definition of the problem. Not only are they likely to benefit from such information, but they are also likely to contribute to your understanding of the total emotional climate in which the hard-of-hearing person must function. Later on in the counseling sessions, when the discussion turns to the more personal aspects and implications of the hearing problem, you may find it advisable to have separate meetings with the relatives in order not to limit, by their presence, the student's expressions of his true feelings. It is, however, frequently helpful to bring the people concerned together in order that they can communicate with each other about their anxieties, with you, as the therapist, playing the role of an objective arbitrator. This type of guidance situation is particularly valuable when working with adolescent hard-of-hearing students and with married partners.

Such discussion of the more personal anxieties that result from the handicap must occur as a natural result of mutual confidence and respect between the teacher or therapist and the student. It is difficult to find guidelines concerning the limits of competence that a therapist or teacher should observe in counseling situations. This is, to a great extent, due to the fact that even stringent limits might still be too liberal in some situations. On the other hand, to remove this responsibility totally from the therapist would be to deny any help for all but a few fortunate individuals. You must rely on common sense to indicate when the topic is becoming too involved and is showing indications of falling outside your own feeling of competence. You should not hesitate to state that you do not feel qualified to voice an opinion on a particular matter and should be prepared to seek outside counsel if and when appropriate.

SPECIAL CONSIDERATION FOR THE PRESCHOOL CHILD

The program of communication training for the preschool child is invariably one of habilitation rather than rehabilitation. That is to say, when a child is born with an impairment of hearing, every aspect of his communicative development will be affected from birth onward. Our task is one of education in its broadest sense. In setting up a program designed to achieve this, we must be extremely conscious of the many factors that contribute to the development of normal communicative behavior in the hearing child. It is important to remember that the whole structure of human communication is based upon an organized perception of the external world and our relationship to it. We spoke in Chap. 5 of the way in which this perception develops as a holistic schema, and we mentioned the ways in which an impairment of hearing is likely to impede such development.

The earlier we are able to identify the presence of defective hearing, the better chance we have of structuring the child's environment in such a way as to minimize the handicap represented by his hearing impairment. Early diagnosis makes possible the provision of amplification for the child at the critical time at which the child with normal hearing is setting up an inventory of the auditory impressions received of the noisy world in which he is born. The subtle learning processes involving reception, discrimination, and classification of auditory input are well established in the hearing child by the time his attention begins to be drawn to the noises that human beings make when they communicate. The acquisition of spoken language comprehension and then of speech is not so much a distinct developmental step as it is a point on a long continuum of auditory-perceptual development that begins at birth.

An effective program of communication training for the young deaf child must be conceived with the awareness of this fact. It starts as soon as the problem is identified by familiarizing the parents with the complexities of the problems that they and their child will face. It must provide hope and encouragement of an honest and realistic nature. The program must be structured to make it apparent after a short time that the goals you and they have set for yourselves and for the child are indeed attainable. Each stage of the training program must be shown to be dependent upon what has been achieved before and to be intimately related to the steps ahead. The parents should be led to realize that the problem of their deaf child is no longer theirs alone, but is shared by the therapist, teacher, and to a lesser degree by a number of other specialists. This also means that, although they will always be the most important members of the team, the responsibility for success and failure no longer rests entirely upon their shoulders.

It would be unrealistic to attempt to describe a comprehensive program of parent guidance and child training for the young deaf child. Those who are particularly interested in this aspect of communication training are referred to Irene Rosetta Ewing [2], Grace M. Harris [3], and Edith Whetnall and D. B. Fry [9]. The point, however, should be made that the success of an early guidance program depends almost exclusively upon the extent to which the parents can be persuaded that the child's speech and language development is dependent upon the establishment of a language-rich home environment. The training program should, therefore, be directed at the parents rather than the child. The major aim is to pattern their communicative behavior with the child in such a way as to insure that he is constantly exposed to verbal language. This must occur in a form that embodies a high level of redundancy and must be presented in a manner that provides both auditory and visual stimulation in a meaningful context. The parents must train themselves to verbalize continuously what they are doing when they are with the child. What begins as a conscious effort should ultimately become an unconscious pattern of communicative behavior.

Parents of young hearing-impaired children need particularly careful guidance and training in the role that the hearing aid will play in the child's education. They should be quite clear about what might reasonably be expected from the provision of amplification, and they should be perfectly familiar with the aid and its controls. Training sessions should teach them how to help the child derive the maximum benefit from the aid and how to use it when they are working with the development of specific language concepts, during story telling, or during language-play activities. The parents should feel completely at ease in dealing with the aid and must be convinced of the need for the child to wear it at all times, since their attitude toward the aid will greatly influence the child's acceptance of it.

In Chaps. 7 and 8 we discussed some of the techniques that we use in providing auditory and visual communication training for the very young deaf child. The aim of the parent training program is to demonstrate these techniques and then to train the parents to use them. This training is generally given to the mother. The emphasis should be upon demonstrating the ways in which she can utilize, for language training, everyday activities around the house, particularly those that involve meeting the child's own needs. The preschool training program must depend heavily upon the parents providing most of the child's early education. It is doomed to failure if it does no more than concentrate on structured activities. The average mother has little time to devote to working in structured situations with one of what may be several young children. If, on the other hand, the program can be designed to demonstrate to the parents that they can utilize as language-stimulation activities the very tasks that keep them occupied during the day, it is likely to produce a learning situation that begins with the mother's first contact with the child in the morning and does not cease until the child is put to bed at night.

One of the major goals of preschool training is to prepare the child for placement in a full-time educational program. The questions of school enrollment should be discussed well in advance with the parents. The available educational facilities should be considered in relation to the child's demonstrated and assessed potential. His emotional and social development and the wishes of the parents must also be taken into account. Wherever possible, arrangements should be made for the parents to visit those educational facilities that might reasonably be considered to be appropriate to the child's needs. When the parents' wishes conflict with what seems to be an advisable recommendation, it will be necessary to provide very careful and considerate counseling in order to help them see the gap between what they wish for the child and what he is realistically capable of handling. It should always be borne in mind that, however unreasonable the parents may seem, their burden is no small one, and they invariably believe that they have the child's best interests at heart.

THE SCHOOL-AGE CHILD

The guidance and supervision that begins with the preschool child is equally important when school placement is made. This is particularly true when the child enters into a school system for hearing children. The informational aspects of counseling must reach into the school environment. Without this, the aural rehabilitation program for the child in the regular school system will probably consist of little more than one or two half-hour periods each week, which is unlikely to have any significant affect on his overall behavior pattern.

It is recognized that one cannot ask the teacher in a regular school classroom to devote an undue amount of time to the needs of the hard-of-hearing child. It has, however, been my experience that most teachers, when placed in this situation, do in fact go out of their way to provide the best possible help they can without neglecting the other children in the class. The classroom teacher is, perhaps, the most influential person in determining how much the child's potential will be achieved in a regular school situation. Her positive approach to the child and his difficulties is likely to give rise to a similar response pattern in the other children. Her role should involve both evaluation and education. All the advice and recommendations made in the clinical situation are essentially generalizations made on the basis of experience with a large number of other children with similar types of problems. However, even children with apparently identical-type losses frequently function quite differently in the classroom. So much depends on parental attitudes and support, the utilization of resources in the school, the understanding and self-confidence exhibited by the teacher, and a number of other variables. The teacher is not concerned with predictions made on the basis of knowledge of children with similar difficulties, but with the actual day-to-day successes and failures she observes in a particular hard-of-hearing child in a particular situation. She can observe his behavior and make notes of particular difficulties that he exhibits in communication, social relationships, and academic work. As the school year draws to a close, she will then be in a position to compose a short meaningful report concerning the general pattern of behavior shown by the child. She will also be able specifically to mention progress made in particular areas, together with her personal feelings concerning how the child's needs for the coming year might best be met.

Special educational needs of the hard-of-hearing child in a school classroom for hearing children are often initially a source of concern to the teacher, who is uncertain of what might be required of her. It can be stated quite definitely that the teaching techniques that benefit the hearing-impaired child are essentially those that are recognized as constituting good classroom procedure for the hearing child. Every effort should be made to insure that the child is seated in a position that permits a clear view of the teacher's face, but that at the same time permits him to direct his attention to other children in the classroom when necessary. This generally involves a seating placement at the front of the class, toward one side. The most successful position is often found to be one on the window side of the room. Placement here means that, for the most part, the teacher will be talking with the light falling on her face, facilitating the use of visual cues as an aid to communication. The effect of eliminating the visual cues upon the communication ability of most hard-of-hearing children should be pointed out to the teacher. Some simple but helpful techniques include standing fairly still when giving instructions, avoiding speaking with her back to the class when writing on the blackboard, maintaining good eye contact when reading orally, rephrasing important ideas, and presenting new vocabulary orally as well as in writing. These techniques will benefit not only the hard-of-hearing child but some of the other slower learners in the class. It often reduces the load on the teacher if she pairs the hard-of-hearing child with one of the more reliable hearing students. This provides him with someone to whom he can turn for confirmation of directions or assignments that he may have missed or of which he may be unsure. Making available to the child, the parents, and even the speech therapist an outline of future lesson topics will make it possible for extra preparation to be given at home and for academic work to be woven into auditory and visual communication training sessions.

Since most of the hard-of-hearing children will be wearing hearing aids in school, some comment on its value to the teacher is pertinent. Unfortunately, as we have already pointed out, the role of the hearing aid in rehabilitation is often misunderstood by the lay person. It is falsely assumed that once the hearing aid has been fitted, the child no longer hears distorted speech. This conclusion is based on the incorrect belief that the hearing aid is a device that corrects, or at least compensates for, the deficiencies in hearing. Thus, it is difficult for the teacher or parent to understand why the child does not show a marked improvement in his ability to communicate once he has been fitted with a hearing aid. It should be explained that, generally speaking, the role of the hearing aid is simply to make sound louder. Since most children wearing hearing aids suffer from sensori-neural-type deafness, the problem is not only one of loudness but also one of distortion. It should be explained that the hearing aid is not able, to any marked degree, to compensate for this distortion. As a result, the amplified speech may be comfortably loud, but may also appear to be blurred. Furthermore, because of the small size of the hearing aid, the quality with which it reproduces speech falls far short of that which a person with normal hearing will find acceptable. Thus, the hearing aid itself adds a certain amount of additional distortion. Nevertheless, the child will benefit from the fact that speech that was previously not loud enough to be useful has now been brought within the range of hearing. It should, however, be explained that, unless the child is taught to differentiate between and recognize the sounds now audible to him, he will find speech little more intelligible than it was before.

Close contact should be maintained between the classroom teacher and the speech therapist to eliminate many of the misunderstandings that might occur concerning the child's auditory performance in the classroom, and to permit a carry-over into the classroom situation of the abilities that are developed in the therapy sessions. The therapist is also able to familiarize the teacher with day-to-day operation of the hearing aid and to explain to her how she may deal with such minor servicing of the aid as changing the battery or cord or seeing that the earmold is kept free of wax.

The role of the school principal should not be overlooked, since he is the person with authority in the school. He is in a position to serve as the coordinator of the total educational and rehabilitation program setup for the child. Since the responsibility for the actual classroom placement or the recommendation for the transfer of the child to a special-education program ultimately rests with him, he should receive the reports from the various individuals who have had contact with the child. It will be in his office that a master file containing all these reports will be kept. If this file is to have any value, it must be readily accessible to any staff member who may wish to consult it.

In acting as a consultant to a number of principals faced with the responsibility for making placement decisions, I have found that the initiation of an annual meeting of all staff members concerned with each handicapped child proves to be the most successful method of reaching a sound decision. This meeting should occur toward the latter part of the school year in order that decisions reached concerning the child can be implemented in time for the beginning of the new school year. This involves the annual referral of the child and his parents back to the speech and hearing clinic for re-evaluation of the child's needs. The staff meeting will not occur until the new report from the speech and hearing clinic has been received. At the same time, each staff member who has contact with the child will be requested to draw up a summary of his observations and to report on any specific findings. This report goes directly to the school principal. He insures that a copy of each report is provided for the meeting to each appropriate staff member; thus, each of these staff members are familiar with the total picture of the child's progress. If possible, the meeting, called by the school principal, should include the educational psychologist, the speech and hearing therapist, the school nurse who probably did the audiometric evaluation, the reading consultant who may be involved, and the classroom teacher. It is also important to have present the classroom teacher in whose class the child may be placed for the coming year. In this way, she will be familiar with the complete background of the child with whom she will be asked to work. At some time during the staff meeting it is necessary to have the parents meet with the group to discuss their own feelings about the child's progress both at home and at school and to express their opinions concerning the future educational placement of the child. Such a meeting brings to light much information that would not otherwise be available. It also indicates the degree of cooperation that the principal may expect from the parents in implementing the final decision.

Once the opinions of the various people working with the child are known, it is necessary for them to reach a concensus concerning how the child's educational needs might best be met for the coming year. It will be the responsibility of the school principal to personally produce a final report or to delegate this responsibility to one of the other members of his staff. He must accept the ultimate responsibility for conveying this information to the parents of the child and for insuring that copies of the final report and the recommendations made are sent to the appropriate educational authorities, the speech and hearing clinic, and the pediatrician or family doctor.

All this may sound rather idealistic, yet if we are to adequately meet the needs of the hard-of-hearing child, we must turn such idealism into practice. The cost of habilitating the hearing-impaired child is high both in time and in terms of specialized resources; however, the cost of failure to pay the price is ultimately a far greater expense to society. The provisions that have been outlined above are not, in fact, just theoretical proposals, but constitute the description of the organization that was established for handling the needs of the hearing-impaired child in a normal school system in Michigan. Such a coordinated approach to the problems of rehabilitating the hearing-impaired school child is the only way of making the maximum possible use of the various services available.

It is a far more difficult task to convince the adult that the time and, possibly, the expense that he will need to invest in an aural rehabilitation program will significantly improve his ability to function in society. If you are to achieve this, it is necessary to insure that the rehabilitation sessions take place within a framework that is meaningful to the student. It is essential that the materials used and the situations simulated should be relevant to what the individual considers to be his major needs. You should, at all costs, avoid prepackaged lesson plans, the primary purpose of which is to make life easier for the therapist but which, as a result, deprive the lesson activity of any kind of individuality. They leave the student to conclude that what he is being asked to do has little relevance to his particular needs.

The provision of a high-quality, meaningful aural rehabilitation program is a very time consuming and demanding task. For the business or professional man, you must be prepared to design special lessons that are built around situations, terminology, and phraseology that he will encounter in his work. Similarly the garage mechanic, waitress, or department-store assistant will also need appropriate lesson materials. The special consideration that must be given to the differences in professional or occupational communication needs must also be given to the different social needs of people. It is just as important that training materials for the teenager should reflect the specific vocabulary, phrases, and interest topics of the current teenage or early twenties culture as it is that those used with the professional man respect his particular needs. Concern for the individual's needs is likely to make him feel that there is a close relationship between what he does in training sessions and what he encounters in everyday situations. This is not to exclude the use of any other kinds of training materials. Any lesson activity that combines a useful purpose, clear both to the therapist and the student, with an enjoyable activity is certainly well justified.

The program must also be flexible enough to encourage the students to suggest ways in which he might obtain more help. It may be necessary to discuss the communication problems that arise for a teenager when on a date, the problems of whether or not to discuss the hearing problem with a new boyfriend or girlfriend, and if so, when and how it should be done. A teenager might find more motivation from training conducted in the realistic conditions of a coffee bar, or he may request that he be allowed to bring his girlfriend to several of the lessons. You must decide what is reasonable and worthwhile, but you must avoid doing so on the basis of preconceived ideas concerning what a lesson should involve. Throw away the straitjacket of the formal lesson structure and seek more meaningful approaches to rehabilitation. The therapist or teacher who is prepared to take the risks involved in being creative is likely to achieve far greater success than is possible within the confines of highly structured classroom activities.

Counseling the adult hearing-impaired person should also include familiarizing him with some of the special devices available to assist him in functioning more adequately in our sophisticated auditory society.

One of the inventions that has had the greatest impact upon human communication has been the telephone. You will remember that it was Alexander Graham Bell's search for a means of amplifying speech for the deaf that ultimately led to his invention of the telephone. The Bell Telephone System has shown great concern for the communication needs of the handicapped person, particularly those with hearing impairment. The company established a special Committee for the Handicapped to stimulate and guide the development of special tele-communication devices for people with all types of physical handicaps that interfere with communication.

The tele-communication devices that have been developed for persons with impaired hearing are illustrated in Figs. 10.1 through 10.6. These major developments were summarized in the summer 1965 issue of *Bell Telephone Magazine:*

> Because partially deaf people vary in their hearing needs almost as widely as people who need prescriptions for eye glasses, there has to be a good deal of flexibility in the telephone equipment designed to aid them. And so

there is. One relatively familiar item of telephone equipment is the special hard-of-hearing telephone set with a small volume control knob in the receiver which amplifies the sound reception comfortably to the proper level within hearing range [Fig. 10.1]. There is a similar telephone that amplifies the voice of a person with weak speech who is talking on it. Another telephone, which looks like the other two, has a "push to listen" button beside the volume control knob and works effectively in noisy locations for both hard-of-hearing and normal hearing persons [Fig. 10.2]. The "push to listen" button amplifies the voice at the other end of the line and cuts out most of the noise from the background.

For certain types of serious ear damage, such as the loss of capacity to hear by air conduction, we also offer a "bone-conduction" receiver, from which sound vibrations are conducted through the skull, then analyzed by the inner ear and heard in the brain as in normal hearing [Fig. 10.3]. Another solution for those with serious hearing problems is the "watch-case receiver" which enables a third person to "plug in" on a conversation and

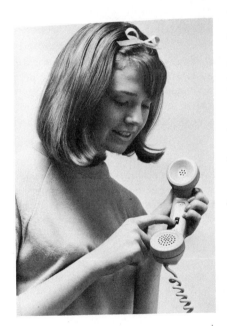

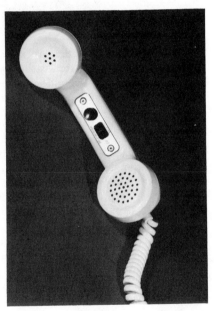

Fig. 10.1. Hard-of-hearing handset equipped with a volume control on the underside of the handset. (Courtesy of AT&T.)

Fig. 10.2. The handset provides amplification for both receiving and transmitting in noisy locations. It has a built-in transistorized amplifier with volume control and push-to-listen switch. (Courtesy of AT&T.)

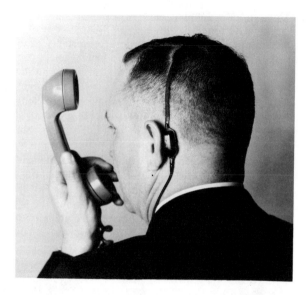

Fig. 10.3. "Bone conduction" receiver—principally designed for those who have lost capacity for hearing by way of air conduction. This device permits sound vibrations to be conducted through the skull, analyzed by the inner ear, and heard as in normal hearing. (Courtesy of AT&T.)

repeat what is being said on the other end of the line to a deaf person so that he can lip-read what is being said and yet carry on his side of the conversation on his own. It might be additionally noted here that the Teletrainer—a device originally designed for teaching telephone usage—is being used experimentally to enable deaf children to learn to make brief but necessary calls.

By the way, you might think that, of all people, switchboard operators would be expected to have adequate, if not better than average, hearing capabilities. The truth is we've supplied thousands, in all kinds of businesses, with small transistorized amplifier devices that plug into their switchboards. When an operator plugs her headset into one of these amplifiers, she can adjust the volume to her most comfortable level by turning a volume-control knob.

When the Telephone Rings

Of course, conversing on the telephone is just one of the communications problems faced by the person with impaired hearing. First, he has to be made aware of the fact that somebody is trying to reach him—in other words, that the phone is ringing. There are various methods of tackling this, depending upon the degree of his deafness. We can, for example, provide a louder signal [Fig. 10.4]. We can also provide a signal in a different frequency range, where his hearing might be less impaired. Indeed, the standard telephone can be equipped with bells with any one of six different frequency ranges at no extra cost. In the area of sound, we offer such extra-strength signals as horns and large gongs (recommended only if you have distant or very understanding neighbors). We can also provide buzzers, which are particularly good when attached to some kind of sounding board, and the Bell Chime* signal device, which usually is adequate for those with only moderate hearing impairment.

If the hearing problem is particularly acute, we can supply what we call an "Auxiliary Signal Control" device. This is an electrically controlled switch that causes an appliance to go on when the telephone rings and off when the phone stops ringing. It will control any appliance, such as lamp to catch his eye or an electric fan to feel on the back of his neck [Fig. 10.5]. We have also provided, in some cases, "beehive" lamps (called that because of their shape) that can be used in place of, or in addition to, bell signals [Fig. 10.6]. They light when the telephone rings and, naturally, can be seen to best advantage in subdued illumination [10].

*Trademark of the Bell System.

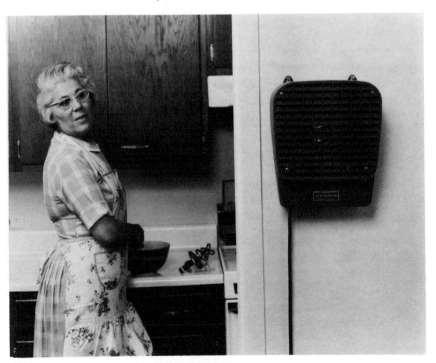

Fig. 10.4.   Ringing signal for people with impaired hearing. (Courtesy of AT&T.)

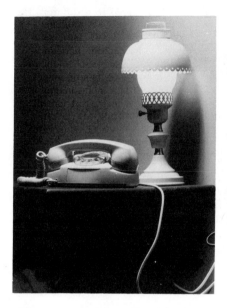

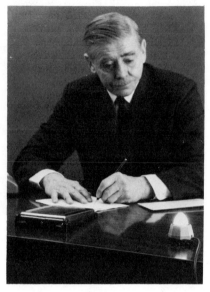

Fig. 10.5. Auxiliary signal control. This is an electrically controlled switch that goes on when the telephone rings and off when the phone stops ringing. It will control any appliance the user wants to connect with it, such a lamp or an electric fan. (Courtesy of AT&T.)

Fig. 10.6. "Bee hive" lamp, named after the shape. Used in place of or in addition to bell signals. It lights when the telephone rings, and can be seen to best advantage in dim light. (Courtesy of AT&T.)

Other useful commercially available accessories include a unit known as the "Servo-Switch," which, when wired to a lamp near to a telephone, will cause the lamp to flash on and off as the phone rings [8]. Another device constitutes a hearing-aid accessory that permits the hearing-impaired person to amplify the radio or television audio signal to meet his personal loudness needs without disturbing others in the room. Designed to fit standard or custom earmolds, it may also be used with dynamagnetic receivers.

Knowledge of the availability of such communication aids as those described helps the therapist to provide more adequately for the total rehabilitation of the hearing-impaired person.

CONCLUSIONS

In July of 1968, an Institute on Aural Rehabilitation was held at the University of Denver [7]. The delegates who attended this meeting represented the major contributors to research and therapy in aural rehabilitation. They reached the rather sad conclusion that we have, for the most part, not been successful in convincing the adult of the value that rests in auditory and visual communication training. This was not easy for a group of committed workers to admit. It was even more disappointing for those of us in attendance to realize that not only have we failed to convince the public of the value of this service, but in spite of our personal commitment, we have also failed to provide any clear-cut evidence that their confidence is justified.

This may seem to be a rather despondent note on which to draw our discussion of aural rehabilitation to a close. I believe, however, that the future of our efforts in this total field of rehabilitation is dependent upon our having the courage to be honest about what we have achieved so far and what we are practicing at this time. Without a deep commitment by the therapist and teacher to the concept of rehabilitation, all the research in the world will not help the hearing-impaired person.

Those of us in the profession who are responsible for training student therapists, teachers of the deaf, and audiologists, and those of you who will have this responsibility in the future must be prepared to dispense with the traditional wisdoms that make us feel secure, to reject familiarity of theories or techniques as an adequate justification for acceptability, and to subject the whole process of aural rehabilitation to careful scrutiny. Perhaps the most basic need is that we should each begin to question seriously the nature of the communication process with which we are working. We cannot hope to develop an adequate technique in auditory and visual communication training until the process of human communication is more accurately defined. You will recall that throughout this text it has been repeatedly necessary to admit that, because of the lack of research evidence, our justification for certain procedures must rest entirely upon empiricism or a pragmatic approach to the problem. This situation will not change until the process of aural rehabilitation is given the same attention by the audiologist, hearing therapist, and teacher of the deaf as has been given to the clinical diagnostic aspect of audiology. The difficulties involved in isolating, defining, and quantifying the many aspects of speech communication are indeed monumental, but no more so than the problems faced by any specialist studying human behavior. The discipline of psychology has not been daunted by such a task. Why, then, should we fail to accept the challenge to describe those aspects of human communication related to the training or retraining of the hearing-impaired person.

The problem in the past has, perhaps, rested primarily in the fact that those of us who have shown concern for aural rehabilitation have been handicapped by the type of training that we, ourselves, received. The understanding of communication requires specialized knowledge in a variety of areas that, in many cases, were in their infancy when we were trained, or that were not considered relevant by our mentors. Unlike the students of today, we were not encouraged to study acoustics, psychoacoustics, linguistics, psycholinguistics, neurophysiology, or cybernetics. Furthermore, we did not have available the vast potential afforded by the field of computer science. Perhaps the hope for the future rests in the training programs of today, which are, without a doubt, beginning to qualify a group of people, such as yourselves, who may be, for the first time, capable of approaching the problems of aural rehabilitation from the viewpoint of a behavioral scientist rather than that of an educator.

In this text we have aimed to broaden the traditional approach to the study of rehabilitating the hearing-impaired person. An attempt has been made, albeit at a very elementary level, to introduce you to some of the fundamental contributions that fields other than our own have made to the understanding of human communication. As was mentioned in the preface, the major aim has been to convince you of the importance of looking beyond our profession for information that will better enable you to comprehend the nature of the task before you. We have done no more than scratch the surface of the contributions that these related areas can make to our own profession.

It is not important whether you accept or reject the concepts that have been put forth in the preceding chapters. Like any philosophy or theory, the ideas we have discussed should be received with skepticism. However, the true skeptic neither accepts nor rejects ideas without scrutiny. Thus, the challenge is not to agree with them, but to think about them. It is hoped that some of the things we have talked about will spark in some of you an interest that will cause you to dig more deeply into the subject. The only idea that I would urge you to accept is the belief that a sound understanding of the nature of the task you are undertaking constitutes the essential basis of a meaningful program of aural rehabilitation. Beyond this, it falls to you, the teacher or therapist, to translate the principles and techniques that you find meaningful into the practicality of everyday therapy situations.

The effectiveness of any philosophy or technique rests not with its proponent, but with its practitioners. As a teacher or therapist, you should know and understand the rationale for what you do. Your confidence in its effectiveness should arise from familiarity with the evidence available to support your approach, from a confidence in the internal logic of the theoretical model, and in the evidence of concurrence between your theory and your empirical observations. At the same time, however, it is crucial to remember that your commitment to a philosophy should be tentative. We are dealing with theoretical models, oversimplifications, perhaps even misrepresentations of the dynamic processes of human communication. We must take care to avoid becoming the disciples of a particular school (even though it be our own), lest we too find ourselves no more than exponents of traditional wisdom. For the sake of those individuals who seek our assistance, we are morally bound to remain open minded in our search for some better way.

REFERENCES

1. Elser, R. "The Social Position of Hearing Handicapped Children." *Exceptional Child* 25(1959): 305–9.

2. Ewing, Irene Rosetta. *New Opportunities for Deaf Children*. Springfield, Ill.: Charles C Thomas, Publisher, 1958.

3. Harris, Grace M. *Language for the Pre-School Deaf Child*. 2nd ed. New York: Grune & Stratton, Inc., 1963.

4. Levine, E. S. "Studies in the Psychological Evaluation of the Deaf." Edited by F. M. Lassman. Reprinted from the *Volta Review Research* (1963).

5. Myklebust, H. R. *Your Deaf Child*. Springfield, Ill.: Thomas Bannerstone House, 1950.

6. _____. *The Psychology of Deafness*. 2nd ed. New York: Grune & Stratton, Inc., 1966.

7. *Proceedings of the Institute on Aural Rehabilitation*. Denver, Colo.: University of Denver, 1968. Supported by the Social and Rehabilitation Service Administration (Grant #212-T-68), and sponsored by the University of Denver Program in Communication Disorders.

8. Servo-Switch. Boston, Mass.: Radio Shack, n.d.

9. Whetnall, Edith, and D. B. Fry. *The Deaf Child*. London: William Heinemann, Ltd., 1964.

10. Whitney, L. Holland. "Services for Special Needs." *Bell Telephone Magazine* (Summer 1965). Reprint.

Index